# Leading and Managing in Contemporary Health and Social Care

# Leading and Managing in Contemporary Health and Social Care

*Edited by*

**ELIZABETH ANNE ROSSER, DPhil, MN, Dip N Ed, Dip RM, RN, RNT, PFHEA**

*Professor Emeritus*
*Faculty of Health and Social Sciences*
*Bournemouth University*
*Bournemouth*
*Dorset, United Kingdom*

**CATE WOOD, PhD, BSc (Hons), BA, PGCHE, DN, RGN**

*Researcher*
*Faculty of Health and Life Sciences*
*Oxford Brookes University, Oxford*
*Clinical Facilitator*
*RCGP, London*
*Honorary Clinical Fellow*
*Plymouth University*
*Plymouth, United Kingdom*

ELSEVIER

---

**Notice**

Practitioners and researchers must always rely on their own experience and knowledge in evaluating and using any information, methods, compounds, or experiments described herein. Because of rapid advances in the medical sciences, in particular, independent verification of diagnoses and drug dosages should be made. To the fullest extent of the law, no responsibility is assumed by Elsevier, authors, editors, or contributors for any injury and/ or damage to persons or property as a matter of products liability, negligence or otherwise, or from any use or operation of any methods, products, instructions, or ideas contained in the material herein.

---

ISBN 9780702083112

*Executive Content Strategist:* Robert Edwards
*Content Development Specialist:* Denise Roslonski
*Project Manager:* Poulouse Joseph
*Designer:* Renee Duenow
*Illustration Manager:* Teresa McBryan

Printed in the United Kingdom

Last digit is the print number:   9   8   7   6   5   4   3   2   1

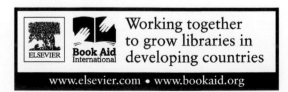

# CONTRIBUTORS

**SARAH E. ABEL, DNP, RN, CEN, FAEN**
Director of Educational Resources, Global Initiatives,
    and Marketplace
Sigma Theta Tau International Honor Society of
    Nursing
Indianapolis, Indiana
United States

**SIVA ANANDACIVA, MSC PSYCHOLOGICAL
RESEARCH METHODS, BSC(Hons) PSYCHOLOGY**
Chief Analyst
Policy, Events and Partnerships
The King's Fund
London, United Kingdom

**SUZIE BAILEY, MSc LEADERSHIP (QUALITY
IMPROVEMENT), MSc MANAGEMENT (HEALTH),
BSc(Hons) SOCIOLOGY**
Director of Leadership and Organisational
    Development
Executive Team
The King's Fund
London, United Kingdom

**CAROL J. CLARK, MCSP, MSc, MMACP, PhD,
SFHEA**
Professor and Head of Department
Rehabilitation and Sport Sciences
Bournemouth University, Bournemouth
Dorset, United Kingdom

**LOIS FARQUHARSON, PhD, MSc, BA**
Executive Dean
The Business School
Bournemouth University, Bournemouth
Dorset, United Kingdom

**LEE-ANN FENGE, DProf, MSc, BA(Hons)**
Professor of Social Care
Social Sciences and Social Work
Bournemouth University, Bournemouth
Dorset, United Kingdom

**CAROL L. HUSTON, MSN, MPA, DPA, FAAN**
Professor Emerita
School of Nursing
California State University
Chico
United States

**ELIZABETH MADIGAN, PhD, RN, FAAN**
CEO
Executive Services
Sigma Theta Tau International Honor Society of
    Nursing
Indianapolis, Indiana
United States

**CLARE FELICITY JANE PRICE-DOWD, DR OF
HEALTH & SOCIAL CARE PRACTICE, MA, MA,
BSc(Hons), RGN, RHV**
Head of Leadership and Lifelong
    Learning–Midlands
People Directorate
NHS England & Improvement
United Kingdom

**ELIZABETH ANNE ROSSER, DPhil, MN, Dip N
Ed, Dip RM, RN, RNT, PFHEA**
Professor Emeritus
Faculty of Health and Social Sciences
Bournemouth University, Bournemouth
Dorset, United Kingdom

**SARAH SCOBIE, BA, PHD, MSC**
Deputy Director of Research
Nuffield Trust
London, United Kingdom

**TONY SMITH, PHD, MSC, PGCERT, PGCE, BA**
Senior Lecturer, Leadership and Organisation
    Development
Centre for Leadership in Health and Social Care
Sheffield Hallam University
Sheffield, United Kingdom

**DEBBIE SORKIN, MA, MBA**
National Director of Systems Leadership
The Leadership Centre
London, United Kingdom

**LIZ WESTCOTT, DCM, MSC, DM, RGN, DR**
School of Nursing and Midwifery
Oxford Brookes University
Oxford, United Kingdom

**NIGEL L. WILLIAMS, PHD, PMP**
Reader in Project Management
Co-Founder of Responsible Project Management
Operations and Systems Management Subject Group
Faculty of Business and Law
University of Portsmouth
Portsmouth, United Kingdom

**CATE WOOD, PHD, BSC(Hons), BA, PGCHE, DN, RGN**
Researcher
Faculty of Health and Life Sciences
Oxford Brookes University, Oxford
Clinical Facilitator
RCGP, London
Honorary Clinical Fellow
Plymouth University
Plymouth, United Kingdom

# PREFACE

■ ■ ■ ■ ■ ■ ■ ■ ■ ■ ■ ■ ■ ■ ■ ■ ■ ■ ■ ■ ■ ■ ■ ■ ■ ■ ■ ■ ■ ■ ■ ■ ■ ■

Advances in the delivery of global health and social care have increased the demands made on leaders and managers in today's contemporary societies. Global health and social care systems are witnessing many long-term trends and demands associated with a recognized need for change to allow services not only to keep pace but be fit for purpose. To meet these critical demands, overarching organizational systems are being encouraged to move toward a context that promotes interaction between multiple professional groups. For the next generation of leaders and managers to function successfully in this evolving environment, it is necessary for them to have the requisite skills and knowledge, irrespective of whether they are working at a policy or organizational level, as educators, or as service providers. Therefore, this first edition comprising 15 chapters provides a comprehensive and authoritative text to support this context.

We are delighted to welcome colleagues from home and abroad who, with their different outlooks, provide a richness of perspectives. The authors' backgrounds mirror a wide-ranging readership and span theoretical and practical viewpoints from national and international perspectives. We anticipate that this book will assist in empowering new and established leaders and managers to successfully lead and manage, and facilitate their understanding of the emerging policies, processes, and available resources that can assist them in their endeavors. We have chosen topics from a wide-ranging health and social care standpoint, given the international move toward integration. We note that, especially across UK universities, education relating to leadership and management is targeted at an interprofessional audience rather than any one specific professional group,

allowing students to understand differing perspectives through an interprofessional lens.

The reader may also like to consider that several months after writing the first chapter, the global COVID-19 pandemic erupted. This has had a significant impact on many issues, not the least of which has been the exceptional pressure placed on global health and social care services, and, of course, the requirement that leaders and managers within these services step up and deal with issues never previously experienced. As vaccinations are rolled out across the world, it is hoped that we will learn from experience and discover how best to address such a global emergency by taking note of examples of good practice.

We hope that this book will assist those who wish to broaden their knowledge of leading and managing in contemporary health and social care environments. The chapters seek to assist leaders and managers and those learning their craft achieve this goal and deliver efficient, effective, and financially viable services to diverse populations; many capable, enthusiastic, and committed people have been involved in the preparation of this textbook, and credit must be given to them.

## Organization of the Book

The text is organized into 15 discrete chapters, which can be read sequentially or as standalone areas of interest:

Chapter 1: With her interest in workforce development and global health care, Professor Emeritus Elizabeth Rosser sets the scene both globally and more specifically in the UK with regard to the common goals and challenges of health and social care services and their workforce. Elizabeth analyzes the impact of integrated services and digital transformation in the UK on day-to-day services and on the workforce. Shortages in global workforces and the impact of mass migration are explored before providing a brief overview of selected leadership theories.

Chapter 2: Debbie Sorkin, National Director of Systems Leadership at the Leadership Centre considers the notion of leadership for the 21st century and presents a window to the broader societal context for recent innovations in leadership. She focuses particularly on innovation related to staff and professionals, providing vivid examples of leadership innovation both at home and abroad. Finally, she recognizes the success of emerging patient leadership in embracing the goal of person-centered care.

Chapter 3: Dr Carol Huston is Professor Emerita, School of Nursing at California State University. She is an international nursing leader, motivational speaker, and acclaimed nursing educator. Carol, who has authored many leadership texts, examines the crafting of organizational culture and behavior. She explores the vital role of positive work cultures in ensuring organizational success. She examines the role of leaders in creating and sustaining a positive work culture and the strategies they can use to achieve this.

Chapter 4: Suzie Bailey, Director of Leadership and Organisational Development at the Kings Fund, is an able author of strategic and executive leadership. She views this through the lens of politics and power and recognizes how these aspects help shape the leadership and structure of local systems. She particularly examines the role of the board of directors and the range of issues they are required to make decisions about and the changing role of leaders toward greater system leadership.

Chapter 5: Dr Lee Ann Fenge, Professor of Social Work at Bournemouth University, discusses the notion of strong leadership and its link to quality of care, safety, and safeguarding. After acknowledging the challenges facing leaders in health and social care, she discusses the importance of strategic partnerships for strengthening leadership and the human factor in learning from past mistakes. She gets to the crux of how strong leadership is critical for ensuring client safety and safeguarding and emphasizes the importance of clear communication and accountable processes that work effortlessly across boundaries.

Chapter 6: Dr Tony Smith, Senior Lecturer in Leadership and Organisation Development at Sheffield Hallam University, is an authority in the field of leadership and interprofessional and team working. Tony considers the challenges facing health and social care teams and the importance of creating a successful group dynamic. He recognizes the key elements of effective leadership and the importance of interdisciplinary teams within health and social care services.

Chapter 7: Dr Carol Clark is Professor and Head of Department for Rehabilitation and Sport Sciences at Bournemouth University. As leader of a large team of academics, she supports others in managing risk. She reflects on factors that have contributed to her own resilience and that of others and identifies how to build and maintain this strength as a leader. She explores factors that are used to recognize and successfully manage risk and how the reader might build their own and others' resilience throughout their careers.

Chapter 8: Dr Clare Price-Dowd is Head of Leadership and Lifelong Learning for the Midlands region at NHS England and Improvement and has worked in the NHS her entire career. Clare is passionate about the importance of effective communication, and her chapter systematically explores the importance of this in the leadership and management of health and social care services. She critically analyzes the changing face of communication with the increasing use of technology and offers a range of communication tools to maximize the impact of individual practice.

Chapter 9: Dr Sarah Scobie is Deputy Director of Research at the Nuffield Trust and is particularly interested in making use of integrated data to understand and improve population health. Her chapter considers how to make data matter for strategic leadership. She explores the scope of using data to improve health and care management and how they can enhance decision-making at different levels of an organization. She discusses the impact of digital technology on the availability and use of data and the emerging challenges and opportunities. She ends the chapter by emphasizing the importance of leadership for analytics and the role of all leaders in making effective use of data.

Chapter 10: Siva Anandaciva is chief analyst in the policy team at the Kings Fund and leads projects related to NHS funding, finances, productivity, and performance. Siva considers the trends in health and social care expenditure and the current and future financial issues challenging the health and social care systems.

He examines the approaches of different countries to the funding of health and social care systems and their impact on equitable access to health care. He ends the chapter by discussing the measures that leaders and managers can use to reduce the growing costs of care.

Chapter 11: Dr Lois Farquharson is Executive Dean of Bournemouth University Business School. Lois employs the positive philosophy and practice of continuous improvement, working in collaboration with various organizational stakeholders to develop teams and individuals in the context of the organizational vision, mission, and goals. Lois is therefore well positioned to explore leading and managing change with the reader, by analyzing contemporary approaches in the context of health and social care. She identifies some of the main challenges services face when implementing change programs.

Chapter 12: Dr Nigel Williams is Reader in Project Management at Portsmouth University, with a special interest in Responsible Project Management. Nigel identifies different perspectives and discusses the process of project management from the optimizing, adaptive, and responsible perspectives. Before joining academia, Nigel worked for 15 years as a manager and business consultant for enterprises in the Caribbean region. His research examines stakeholder interactions using social network analysis, the project capacity of organizations in post-conflict countries, and the evolution of project capabilities in organizations.

Chapter 13: Dr Liz Westcott is an Executive Coach and Coaching supervisor and a Nursing and Midwifery Council assessor. She is President of the Phi Mu Chapter of the international nursing organization, Sigma Theta Tau International Honor Society of Nursing. Liz worked with Professor Emeritus Elizabeth Rosser to discuss coaching and mentoring for successful leadership. They analyze the effectiveness of coaches, mentors, and practice supervisors for

today's leaders and managers in health and social care and the impact of creating a successful coaching and mentoring culture. They end the chapter by analyzing the value of generating an effective learning organization and the role of coaching, mentoring, and reflection in its success.

Chapter 14: Dr Liz Madigan, Chief Executive Officer of Sigma Theta Tau International, and Dr Sarah Abel, Director of Educational Resources, Global and Marketplace, also at Sigma, the largest global nursing organization by individual membership, share authorship of this chapter. With their global reach, they are ideal for exploring the global challenges facing health and social care leaders. They recognize the unprecedented rise in global migration and the importance of creating cultural sensitivity and, as leaders and managers, acting as role models for the organization. They analyze the need to provide resources to help develop cultural competence in the workforce and adhere to ethical recruitment. They conclude the chapter by emphasizing the importance of effective communication in enhancing successful delegation and how global organizations can improve the delivery of health and social care across the world.

Chapter 15: Dr Cate Wood has clinical, leadership, managerial, and academic expertise in striving to develop behaviors and strategies fundamental for the delivery of high quality, safe, and compassionate health and social care. In the final chapter, she brings the book to a close by exploring future implications for leaders in health and social care. She analyzes why health and social care organizations need to invest in new types of leadership and management development and the cultural values, characteristics, and skills required of them. She emphasizes the importance of interprofessional education to assist in preparing the next generation of leaders for successful integration of health and social care services globally.

# CONTENTS

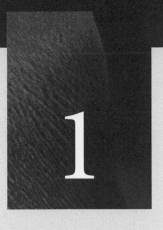

# 1

# SETTING THE GLOBAL AND REGIONAL CONTEXT IN CONTEMPORARY HEALTH AND SOCIAL CARE

ELIZABETH ANNE ROSSER

## OBJECTIVES

*After reading this chapter, you should be able to:*

- Identify the major challenges facing global health and social care leaders and the lessons that can be learned from each other.
- Analyze how integrated care services in the United Kingdom impact the workforce and the delivery of day-to-day services.
- Critically discuss how digital transformation affects current and future health and social care leaders.
- Critically analyze how global workforce shortages compounded by mass migration impact the global health and social care workforce.
- Briefly discuss six theories/approaches to leadership and identify how they apply to specific situations in your practice.

## INTRODUCTION

Successful leadership and management in contemporary health and social care depend on having a sound understanding of the current landscape in which these services are delivered, as well as a vision for the future. This chapter sets the scene with a brief overview of the challenges countries worldwide face in their quest for quality, fundable services. It offers a snapshot of the continued journey of radical change in the United Kingdom (UK) National Health Service (NHS) and social care with a focus on England. Finally, against an overview of select leadership theories, the reader is invited to think about their own relationship with "self" as a leader or manager and consider their position with regard to the changing association between those who deliver services and those who receive them.

## COMMON GLOBAL HEALTH AND SOCIAL CARE CHALLENGES

Globally, health and social care systems in resource-rich countries share the common challenges of aging populations, the need to incorporate advances in technology, and the ongoing rise in the cost of services. Indeed, these have as great an impact on health as they do on social care. Resource-poor countries face the double burden of communicable diseases such as malaria, HIV/AIDS, diarrhea, and infectious diseases, as well as the problems presented by an increase in non-communicable diseases such as obesity, diabetes, and cancer. Resource-rich countries also have the ongoing challenges of lifestyle-related conditions such as cardiovascular disease, age-related conditions such as dementia, and other long-term conditions. However, accidents such as those posed by road traffic exist on a worldwide scale. In addition, migration and world travel influence the nexus between communicable and non-communicable diseases in both resource-rich and resource-poor countries, with impacts upon us all. Strategic leaders and managers worldwide must support the global efforts to combat diseases with scientific research that will result in vaccines, pharmaceuticals, effective systems of disease prevention, and lifestyle changes.

Robertson et al. (2014) provide a good overview of the entitlements, funding arrangements, delivery approaches, and key issues for the health and social care services of nine resource-rich countries—Australia, France, Germany, Ireland, Japan, the Netherlands, the Republic of Korea, Sweden, and the United States. What is clear from this 2014 study is that all countries referred to had either recently reformed their health or social care systems or were in the process of doing so at that time. Ensuring consistent funding and resource allocation—especially during the global financial crisis of 2007, when many governments cut or froze spending on welfare—has been especially challenging (Robertson et al., 2014). As in all businesses, health and social care services need to keep abreast of both the ongoing needs of the population and current developments in medical, scientific, and social research. Leaders and managers are advised to adopt a positive philosophy of accepting "change as the only constant" to survive and thrive.

Thanks to the strategic leadership of many countries, the willingness of leading scientists and medical personnel to work together, and advances in digital technologies, much has been achieved in the last decade. Nevertheless, a great deal remains to be done. As we move into the 2020s and scientists continue their search for new solutions, the western world faces new challenges of maintaining funding and strategic visioning both globally and regionally, embracing the new digital transformation of services, and developing the next generation workforce. In particular, service leaders and managers must overcome these challenges against a backdrop of global shortages of professionals.

Deloitte's analyses (Allen, 2019) identify a number of countries that have met with success in recent years, including the United Kingdom, the Netherlands, China, Germany, and the United States. However, they also recognize these countries' continued struggle to achieve financial sustainability in their complex and dynamic environments, and they anticipate the trend will continue beyond 2020. Factors contributing to the struggles of these countries include the considerable increase in their ageing populations, an increasing number of whom have long-term conditions; costly investments in infrastructure and technology; rising workforce costs against a backdrop of staff shortages and increasing demand for improved service infrastructure, such as the provision of general practitioners, community care, and rising mental health problems (Allen, 2019). In response, Chokshi

(2019) recognizes that the commonalities in the problems experienced by countries globally suggest that there are generalizable solutions. He proposes four principles to underpin a strategy toward population health and recommends that all four principles be actioned for success:

1. Identifying the scope of the population for which they are responsible
2. Developing a sound foundation of effective, high-quality, community-based care
3. Delivering care close to the patients, integrating their physical, emotional and social care with the additional use of digital technology
4. Using data to guide care delivery and push forward improvement.

He cites examples where global convergence, using these principles, offers countries the opportunity to learn from each other, with innovative local adaptations being employed to apply successful solutions in one country for success in others. Each of these principles is alluded to in the subsequent paragraphs.

## Population Health Management

Moving forward in this new decade, many public health and social care systems, such as those in the United Kingdom and across the world, are working with partners in private care systems to introduce population health management (PHM) in order to enhance the physical and mental health of patient populations over both their individual life spans and across generations (Taylor et al., 2019). Indeed, Orlowski (2019) emphasizes PHM's global reach because of its ability to assist world leaders in better managing their resources and delivering value. He argues that PHM is different from public health as it focuses on key outcomes for identified groups that share specific common characteristics, and not merely a disease diagnosis. PHM emphasizes resource management for wider or social determinants of health so as to enhance individual well-being and move away from the traditional focus on illness. Through big data, PHM brings together an understanding of the scope and needs of specific groups (Fig. 1-1) (Chokshi's principles 1 and 4) and engagement with consumers in care delivery to capture the four goals of health care:

1. Improvement in the health of the population.
2. Improving their experience of care delivery.
3. Health and wellbeing of the workforce.
4. Reduce the overall cost of care.

(Bodenheimer & Sinsky, 2014).

With PHM's emphasis on value, Orlowski (2019) underscores the importance of using the most efficient intervention when resourcing care and identifying who would benefit most across the care pathway, while allowing comparison of entire pathways.

Leaders and managers of health and social care services need to proactively drive the development of new PHM solutions and innovative business models to enhance service delivery and improve outcomes. Allen (2019) identifies a number of initiatives by Japan, the United States, India, and Brazil, in which the countries are working to consolidate their assets to improve efficiency. However, more fundamentally, leaders and managers must acknowledge the need to become more proactive and focus on well-being, changing from a purely systems-driven approach to one that includes a change in attitude toward greater consumer engagement and empowerment. Once passive recipients of care, consumers are now insisting on transparency, convenience, access, and individualized service, which they already receive in other aspects of their lives (Allen, 2019).

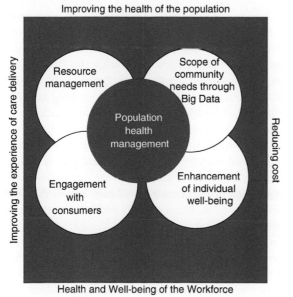

Fig. 1-1 ■ Population health management

## Digital Transformation

Fueled by unparalleled developments in digital solutions in both health and social care, digital transformation (Chokshi's principle 3) is set to underpin new models of care; drive cheaper, more precise, and less invasive treatments; and shape new ways of working for health and social care professionals. There are clear examples of how digital transformation has aided in early detection, intervention, and care for those in Japan who have dementia. The use of a mobile application in India has aided communication and supervision for community health workers and improved maternal and infant health outcomes in their rural communities; similar technological developments have also occurred in Chile, Thailand, and Germany (Allen, 2019). Nevertheless, Jones et al. (2019) recognize that significant barriers to its widespread adoption remain. They suggest that culture and mindset, organizational structure, and governance are the three barriers to adopting digitalization that are most mentioned by leaders in the pharmaceutical and medical technology industry. They review 30 countries that best supported the introduction of digital solutions in health care, and as success factors, identified such issues as involving government in the introduction of such solutions, focusing on the tangible benefit to consumers, and encouraging stakeholders to invest in the right skill mix. In spite of considerable advances in the global adoption of digitalization, there remains a good deal to be done.

While Jones et al. (2019) acknowledge that health care organizations globally are redirecting their budgets to digitalize entire systems, gaps remain in terms of quality, access, and financial support. Collaborative work across stakeholders appears to be the key to success. Within the UK NHS, as Maguire et al. (2018) confirm, introducing the radical change to digital at a time when services are already under considerable pressure prevents the workforce from readily adopting such change. Additionally, the cost to purchase new hardware and software can be prohibitive when budgets are already stretched. Last, some organizations face challenges in engaging service users in such cultural change, while others have struggled with their partner organizations. Still others have been seriously challenged by the process of introducing large-scale change. Whatever the challenges, it seems crucial for strategic leaders and managers of health and social care services to keep pace with developments, purchase sustainable systems with an eye to the future, and develop their workforce and service users to adopt cultural change.

## SUMMARY POINTS

- Resource-rich and resource-poor countries share common health and social care problems.
- Common problems can be addressed with generalizable solutions.
- With a focus on well-being, consumers of health and social care need to be empowered to improve population health outcomes.
- Leaders and managers need to accept change as the only constant and continue to adapt.
- Keeping pace with developments in digital transformation is crucial for successful health and social care outcomes.

## HEALTH AND SOCIAL CARE IN THE UNITED KINGDOM

At a regional level, the United Kingdom has been witnessing unprecedented change. However, it is important to recognize that, since the devolvement of the four countries comprising the United Kingdom, each individual country has interpreted and managed its health and social care systems differently to meet the needs of its population. For the purposes of this chapter, the focus will mainly be on the health and social care services in England, with reference to Scotland, Wales, and Northern Ireland where appropriate. Nevertheless, irrespective of where leaders and managers are situated, there is a great deal to be learned from each other as all countries within the United Kingdom and across the world strive to achieve the best quality health and social care at the best value to meet the needs of the population that they serve.

The two systems comprising the delivery of health care and social care services, particularly in England, have traditionally been funded and managed differently. In spite of the close interface and impact they have on each other (for example, is "caring" for an elderly person in their own home, attending to their hygiene and personal needs, a health care or social care issue?), the two systems have been led and managed completely separately. In many areas of England, the systems have not connected either digitally or through face-to-face communications, and different terminology is used by each discipline to refer to similar issues. Nevertheless, for over three decades, there have been a number of strategic attempts to integrate the two through ambitious innovations and policy changes (e.g., Ham & Murray, 2015; HM Government, 2019). Indeed, the Health and Social Care Act of 2012 (HM Government, 2012) placed integration at the center of policy reform with the idea that care should revolve around the person using the services and not the systems providing them. However, as Smith et al. (2018) recognize, integrating services is not straightforward and essentially contradicts many of the assumptions of professionalism, with health care leaders sharing responsibility for the delivery and outcomes of care spanning different services. Even in the context of the separate health and social care systems, there have been considerable efforts to develop interprofessional teams with a focus on collaborative working, unlike traditional "multi-professional" teams. In their review of the literature, Smith et al. (2018) find these traditional teams have no focus on collective working; instead, their attention on the patient is individual, without recourse to the wider "team," and each professional group functions independent of the other. Interprofessional working, however, embraces the fundamental premise of teamwork, where outputs are assessed and based on the team's collective effort. Nevertheless, despite considerable advances in integration since 2015, such as through the Better Care Fund (HM Government, 2019), Smith et al. (2018) acknowledge that interprofessional working remains an ideal that health and social care organizations are working to achieve.

As organizations work toward the outcome of interprofessional working, leaders and managers at all levels of the health and social care systems will have to think differently and understand each other's different worlds as well as those of their patient/client. Whole system change has had to become a reality; the professional workforce has needed to become more flexible, multi-skilled, and more aware of how they fit within the grand scheme, and be accepting of new roles, new technologies, and new ways of working. Indeed, the Five Year Forward View (NHS England, 2014a) was published over 7 years ago to set out an ambitious vision to continue the ongoing program of radical change and identify why improvements were needed to achieve the goals of "better health, better care and better value." Taking the United States as an example, more focus has been put on care in the community and away from acute secondary care facilities (Chokshi's principle 2). Then, as the Five Year Forward View took shape, in 2015, there was a concerted effort in England to bring the health and social care systems together to form Sustainability and Transformation Partnerships (STPs); by June 2016, the geographical footprint of each of the 44 entities was decided, spanning the whole country. STPs set out to take collective responsibility for improving the health and social care of their local population by managing resources and delivering the NHS standards (NHS, 2017). It will take time for this partnership to be embedded and become a success at all levels. Since then, some areas have formed an even closer collaboration, a more advanced version of an STP, called an Integrated Care System (ICS). Although there have been attempts in the past to integrate services, this was a real strategic change to share funding, bring together people and systems, and encourage more connected services. Where they exist, ICSs allow the collective leaders to better understand their local population's available data and tailor care to individual needs. The plan has been that all the health and social care commissioners and providers will work with consumers and the public by gaining new powers and freedoms, and take on new responsibilities to improve the health and well-being of their local population (NHS, 2017). Indeed, by April 2021 there are now 42 ICSs covering every area in England and are expected to be fully operational by April 2022 (British Medical Journal, 2021).

In summary, in spite of a long history of health and social care services working in silos with separate and independent systems, over the past 30 years, there have been a number of strategic attempts in England to bring them closer together (HM Government, 2019). The publication of the Health and Social Care Act of 2012, mainly targeted at England and Wales, saw a concerted focus on their integration and a number of policy documents were published in an attempt to bring them together through STPs and ICSs (DHSC 2021; NHS, 2017, 2019; NHS England, 2014a). Nevertheless, such radical change will require different ways of working, cultural change, and a workforce flexible enough to adapt.

## Workforce

Consideration needs to be given to the changing face of the health and social care workforce to meet the evolving global population needs. With 234 million workers across the world, the health and social sector comprises one of the largest and fastest growing employers in the world; moreover, 7 out of 10 workers are women (half in the form of unpaid care work [Boniol et al., 2019]). Nevertheless, it is estimated that there will be a global shortfall of almost 18 million health workers by 2030, mostly in low- and middle-income countries (Boniol et al., 2019). It is necessary therefore that considerable investment be made, not only to help achieve universal health coverage, the sustainable development goals, and global health security, but also to assist in each country's economic growth and maximize women's economic empowerment (Boniol et al., 2019). The main barriers to achieving the World Health Organization's health goals seem to revolve around the number, distribution, and skills of the workforce (WHO, 2018).

Additionally, fueled by the collective global shortfall, globalization has encouraged widespread migration of the health and social care workforce, with various studies pointing to a pattern of movement from low- and middle-income countries to high-income countries in North America and Western Europe. Indeed, some high-income countries depend on low- and middle-income countries' highly skilled professional health workforce to meet their own shortfall (Aluttis et al., 2014). For example, WHO (2006) notes that Africa, with 10% of the world's population, bears 25% of the global disease burden, but has only 3% of the global health workforce. Health workforce migration only exacerbates the situation and impacts not only the "brain drain" on the services themselves, but, with estimates of losses from African countries to high-income countries of up to 70%, also the funds invested by low- and middle-income countries in developing a highly skilled professional workforce (Aluttis et al., 2014).

Within the United Kingdom, the situation mirrors the global shortages, with an estimated workforce shortage of 100,000 workers in health care and 122,000 in social care, with a quarter of the staff being on zero-hours contracts. Projections in the NHS estimate even greater shortages of up to 200,000 by 2023–24 and at least 250,000 by 2030. It appears that nursing remains the main shortage area (over 40,000), and it is anticipated that this could double by 2023–24 and reach 100,000 by 2028–29 (Gershlick & Charlesworth, 2019). However, the picture is complex, and the issue has been magnified by Britain's decision to exit from the European Union, which presents considerable uncertainty for Europeans wishing to live and work in the United Kingdom. There has been an 85% decline in the number of nurses coming to the United Kingdom from the European Union, with similar numbers estimated in adult social care. International recruitment is key to sustaining viable health and social care systems, and it is anticipated that a restrictive immigration policy will make this even harder (Gershlick & Charlesworth, 2019).

In an attempt to redress the global distribution of health workers, WHO (2018) has put a spotlight firmly on primary care (Chokshi's principle 2). They recommend developing "fit for purpose" community health workers (CHWs) across the range of qualified professionals through traditional practitioners, with a wide variety of sustainable skills and a more evenly distributed workforce. This, they believe, will result in fewer deaths and lower the burden of disease. The focus globally, therefore, is on developing primary care facilities, recognizing that CHWs are effective in delivering a wide range of services from preventative to curative care, and they contribute to reducing inequities in the population's access to care (WHO, 2018).

Within the United Kingdom, the NHS fully recognizes the need to strengthen primary care and indeed the need to reinforce the "triple integration" of primary and specialist care (Fig. 1-2), physical and mental health, and health and social care, as described in the NHS (2019) Long-Term Plan. The Long-Term Plan acknowledges the need to not only increase staff numbers but also retain those already in the system (NHS, 2019). Beech et al. (2019) reinforce that essential changes to staff terms and conditions are required. For example, with the integration of health and social care, both services often recruit from the same pool. They recommend that terms and conditions across the two services need to be equitable, for example, matching pay increases in the NHS would cost social care £1.7 bn by 2023–24 (Gershlick & Charlesworth, 2019). Additionally, the Long-Term Plan recommends making the NHS a better place to work, ensuring pay and rewards to attract staff to the new ICSs, addressing international recruitment, and

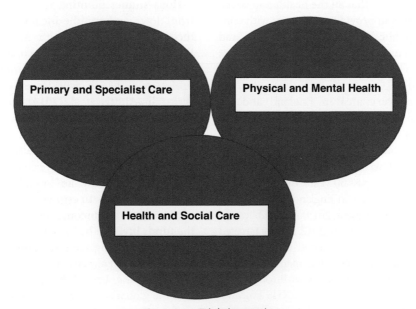

**Fig. 1-2** ■ Triple integration

improving efficiency through workforce redesign by having the right skills and technological support for change.

Workforce redesign (Fig. 1-3) will undoubtedly mean that new roles and new ways of working will emerge, and as a result, whole systems will need to change to allow these new roles to be established. Providing support for people to live independently will mean more care delivered at home, more use of new technologies, greater information sharing, and as a result, education to develop the workforce to work more autonomously. More importantly, workforce redesign will need clear leadership, in order to help staff integrate and adjust to new systems and educate them to adapt to new ways of working and new responsibilities. Continuity of leadership will be key as leaders develop a shared vision across the previously divided services, engage their workforce, develop relationships with their new partners, and drive enhancements in quality. However, real success happens at a much more fundamental level. Inevitably, there will be territorial issues that need to be addressed and so, taking time to develop the shared goals and values is important for success (Centre for Workforce Intelligence, 2013).

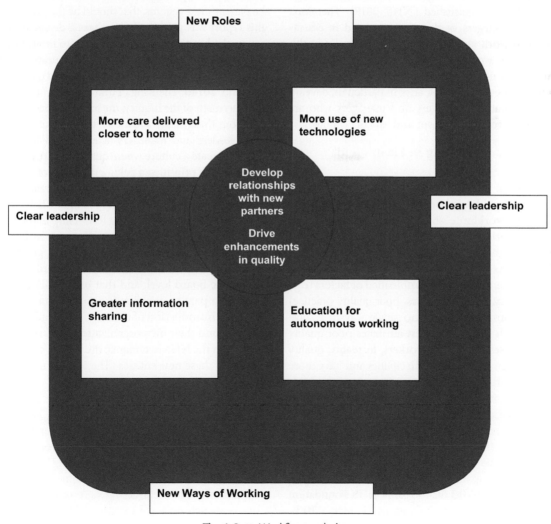

Fig. 1-3 ■ Workforce redesign

Therefore, in addition to safeguarding the equality of conditions, leaders and managers need to work hard to ensure that their workforce has the right people in the right place with the right skills to deliver the right care at the right time (Centre for Workforce Intelligence, 2013). A key issue will be ensuring that leaders and managers themselves have the right skills to deliver on the new agenda.

In summary, against the backdrop of global shortages in the health and social care workforce, the UK NHS and social care are also struggling to cope. Nevertheless, plans to continue to invest in the recruitment and retention of staff, address the terms and conditions across the services, and continue the program of workforce redesign have already been published (NHS, 2019). Therefore, leaders and managers of these services and in education need to work together to prepare both the health and social care workforce for ongoing radical change. Educators also need to think differently, prepare their vision for the new worldview, and, in particular, develop the next generation of leaders and managers who are strong in their resolve to accept and lead the change.

## "Wicked" Issues Arising in Health and Social Care Delivery

In addition to the ongoing radical change bringing together health and social care systems and the considerable workforce shortages, health and social care have experienced considerable and complex challenges, otherwise known as "wicked" issues (Ferlie et al., 2011). As Rosser et al. (2017) acknowledge, these "wicked" problems refer to a combination of factors (e.g., low competency, fewer resources, poor quality practice) that are so complex, there is no single way to resolve them. Although the media often attributes poor quality of care to nurses and social workers, in reality, quality issues have been found across disciplines and have more recently been attributed to strategic organizational leaders. Evidence from a number of inquiries indicate that the combination of these challenges can result in gross "systems" failure, leading to unacceptable and occasionally inhumane care (Francis, 2013; Keogh, 2013; McNicoll, 2017). Within the United Kingdom, the investigation that is often held up as an appalling example is the one associated with the Mid Staffordshire NHS Foundation Trust and its 290 recommendations (Francis, 2013), although there have been many incidents elsewhere in

health and social care, particularly in child protection cases (e.g., McNicoll, 2017). However, as an example, at a time when the Mid Staffordshire NHS Foundation Trust was seeking Foundation Trust status and national targets and financial balance took priority over delivering acceptable standards of care, Francis (2013) found that many patients had experienced inexcusable suffering. He concluded that the leaders of the organization, the Trust Board, failed to listen to its patients and staff or correct deficiencies that were reported to them. Additionally, and "above all, it failed to tackle an insidious negative culture involving a tolerance of poor standards and a disengagement from managerial and leadership responsibilities" (Francis, 2013, p. 1). Further, he concluded that it should be patients, not systems, that should be the priority. After this report was published, there was a deluge of activity across the health sector in an attempt to move practitioners away from merely focusing on measurable targets to focus more particularly on compassion and quality (NHS England, 2014b; The King's Fund, 2013). Importantly, in the aftermath of the inquiry, the focus has been on learning from these many situations, with a spotlight on the NHS leaders and managers at a national level urging them to create a culture where quality of care and patient safety are the priorities: a culture that promotes openness and honesty and allows staff at all levels to raise concerns without fear of reprisal (The King's Fund, 2013).

The development of strong leadership in individuals and teams has refocused the NHS on considering the importance of leadership style and recognizing that leadership exists at all levels of an organization, not just at the board level, and that each individual plays their own part in contributing to the quality of care. With the introduction of the new ICSs, leaders need to look beyond their own organization and engage externally with the NHS to enhance the improvements envisioned in these new entities (The King's Fund, 2013).

### SUMMARY POINTS

- The United Kingdom has spent the last 30 years seeking ways to bring the completely separate systems of health and social care services closer together.
- Taking the United States as an example, the United Kingdom began redirecting its resources away from an emphasis on acute care toward developing primary care services.

- Radical change in the vision for an integrated health and social care workforce will mean leaders and managers need to be strong and have clear vision and the right skills and energy for change.
- Considerable global workforce shortages indicate a need to reinvest, avoid the "brain drain" from low- and medium-income countries to high-income countries, and refocus on the community.
- "Wicked" issues require strong leadership and refocusing from measurable targets toward compassionate practice.

## THE NATURE OF LEADERSHIP AND MANAGEMENT

The purpose of this section is to introduce a small selection of contemporary theories and their application to leaders and managers in the health and social care services. With the many comprehensive texts dedicated to leadership (e.g., Dugan, 2017) and management theories (e.g., Kessler, 2013) there is no attempt to offer a comprehensive account but to give the reader an opportunity to understand the evolving approaches for leaders and managers of these services.

The goal of health and social care services is to attain high quality and high productivity, as well as safe and effective integrated care that achieves consumer satisfaction. Strong workforce leadership and management are seen as essential if lessons from the "wicked" issues already discussed are to be realized. Leadership has been variously defined as the relationship between those who lead and those who decide to follow, focusing on the behaviors of directing and coordinating a group of individuals toward a common goal (Sfantou et al., 2017). I would also argue that to achieve strong, confident leadership, it is important to consider the leader's relationship with self (Holroyd & Brown, 2011). Management, by contrast, is about monitoring and adjusting to today's work while regularly looking backward to ensure that set goals and objectives are being met (Kerr, 2015).

### Leadership Theories

Dugan (2017, p. 34) refers to "formal and informal theories." Formal theory often refers to ideas "derived over time through hypotheses that are empirically studied to generate relationships among concepts attempting to describe and explain a greater whole." Informal

theories, he suggests, refer to those who state, "I have a theory about that," implying an unconfirmed opinion or idea that lacks empirical authentication. Nevertheless, he recommends that, when consciously constructed, informal theories can be influential tools to help us create meaning. Formal theories (Fig. 1-4) are a way of explaining constructs and strategies to leadership and management students, and Kessler (2013) assures us that none are so pure as to enable us to pick them off the shelf and apply them without exception or complement. They merely help explain, predict, and influence leadership and management dynamics.

Health and social care services are complex entities, and their leaders will require flexibility in their approaches, as most theories were developed for business and will require adaptation for use in health and social care settings (Al-Sawai, 2013). I will introduce you to six approaches that I have selected and apply them to the world of health and social care for you to consider your own approach and how these may be relevant to you. With current theories favoring collaboration and teamwork within and across organizations, they are as follows:

- Transformational
- Transactional
- Authentic
- Shared
- Collective and collaborative
- Compassionate

### Transformational Leadership

Favored by many in the health and social care services, transformational leadership develops mutual relationships between leaders and followers, transforming followers to leaders and leaders to moral agents (Burns, 1978). The role of a leader is to inspire followers and instill in them a belief that they have the ability to do exceptional things. Leaders inspire confidence and respect in followers, motivate them to believe in a shared vision, strengthen morale, and enhance job satisfaction (Sfantou et al., 2017). Within the NHS, there has been a great deal of evidence of staff feeling overwhelmed and stressed; coupled with staff shortages, this has paved the way for transformational leaders to demonstrate an unwavering focus on their inspiring vision and strategy, spreading optimism and

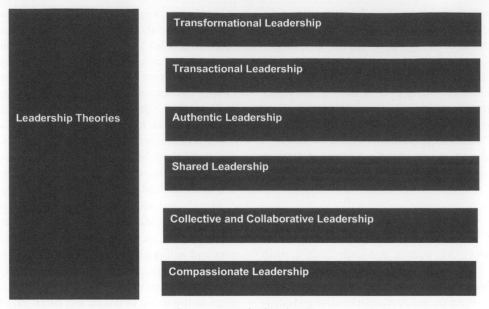

**Fig. 1-4** ■ Leadership theories

a sense of achievement to others (West et al., 2017). Within the workplace, individuals need to feel good about themselves and that they are doing a good job. Transformational leaders provide a supportive and informal culture for the workforce to not only survive but thrive.

### Transactional Leadership

Often suggested as a negative approach when considered alongside transformational leadership, transactional leadership still has its place in contemporary health and social care. Transactional leadership aims to maintain the status quo by following due process and is advocated when consistency and reliability are important. Leaders pay attention to followers' work to reward or find faults and deviations, and, using precise procedures, this leadership style is effective in an emergency situation or when quality assurance is important (Sullivan & Garland, 2010).

### Authentic Leadership

Leadership is genuine and transparent; a leader's legitimacy is built on honest relationships with followers whose input is valued. In a number of the "wicked" issues mentioned earlier, leaders in the past have influenced others in less than honest ways and created a culture that has fostered a change in their underlying beliefs and values, encouraging them to engage in "crimes of obedience" (Al-Sawai, 2013, p. 286). However, in authentic leadership, the relationship between leader and follower is built on an ethical foundation. For the most part, authentic leaders are positive individuals who promote openness, and their leadership has an explicit moral dimension (Dugan, 2017). In a negative climate in which leaders are ambitious and selfish, authentic leadership is favored, viewing leadership as trusting, balanced, and transparent with an interest in the common good.

### Shared Leadership

Increasingly, health professionals, like their social work peers, are working autonomously, and a number of studies have demonstrated that they do not respond well to authoritarian leadership. As illustrated in the section on ICSs, leaders have a role to play in developing collaborative relationships through support and task delegation, which fosters a model of shared leadership as it encourages shared governance, continuous learning in the workplace, and effective working relationships (Al-Sawai, 2013). Shared leadership builds on the empowerment principles of participative and transformational leadership and assumes that a highly professional workforce comprises many leaders (Sullivan & Garland, 2010). It empowers staff within the decision-making processes, encourages them to develop within a team, and is effective in enhancing the work environment and job satisfaction.

### Collective and Collaborative Leadership

Like shared leadership, collective and collaborative leadership encourages all staff to take leadership roles as well as responsibility for the organization's success, not just their own roles. It encourages colleagues to work together toward the mutual benefit of the organization and promotes open communication and sharing of knowledge and experiences across organizations and their different stakeholders. Given the radical changes taking place within the NHS and the integration of health and social care in the United Kingdom, the high levels of dialog, debate, and discussion implicit in collaborative leadership will achieve collective understanding of the problems and potential solutions. With the publication of a number of high-profile scandals in both health and social care (Keogh, 2013), there is a need to rebuild public confidence, increase patient/client safety, and reestablish quality care. Collective leadership, as West et al. (2014, p. 7) suggest, "represents a strategy for integrating leadership collectively across organizations," ensuring its distribution to every member of the workforce. Collaborative leadership capitalizes on expertise, motivation, and capabilities within the organization, encouraging colleagues to work together toward effective practices and processes and promoting understanding of different cultures and interdependence among multiple stakeholders. Indeed, the Kings Fund (2011) suggests that the notion of leaders as "superheroes" is long gone, as the complexity of today's health and social care and their integration call for a more collective and collaborative model of leadership to meet the new agenda.

### Compassionate Leadership

In recent years, following the scandals in the UK NHS, there has been much written about compassionate leadership, not as a theory but as a way of being and acting (e.g., Francis, 2013; Keogh, 2013). There has been a demand for compassion within health care

elsewhere as well, for example, as the first principle of the American Medical Association Code of Ethics and in New Zealand as a patient right (Sinclair et al., 2016). Compassion offers a philosophy or approach to underpin leadership theories. NHS England (2014b) recognizes the role of managers/leaders in connecting individuals and teams to their own humanity and core purpose, recognizing there is no finite "recipe" for success but an ability to respond in a humanized way to each individual patient/client. Defining compassion, de Zulueta (2016, p. 2) states it is "the altruistic concern for another person's suffering and the desire or motivate(ion) to alleviate it" and it "happens within and between people, is complex and dynamic and resists quantitative measurement but is easy to recognize." Developing a culture within organizations where compassionate care can flourish requires leadership that encourages learning and openness, so mistakes and hazards can be shared and discussed, and new learning can develop. As de Zulueta (2016) acknowledges, a disciplinary culture where fear and blame prevail will encourage individuals to hide their mistakes for fear of retribution. Berwick (2013, p. 4) states in his report on improving patient safety, "Fear is toxic to both safety and improvement… Abandon blame as a tool and trust the goodwill and intentions of the staff." However, compassionate leadership starts with each individual and their relationship with self; it happens from the inside out (NHS England, 2014b). As de Zulueta (2016) suggests, adopting elements of collective, shared, authentic, and transformational leadership combined with compassion is important for avoiding the often punitive culture existing in the health care context.

Management theories primarily focus on motivation and how we communicate, influence, lead, and, often, resolve conflicts with others. As with leadership theories, management theories merely help explain, predict, and influence management dynamics and are addressed comprehensively in Kessler (2013).

Concluding this section, a 21st century leader and manager needs to be able to address the needs of the changing population and the subsequent changes to health and social care services. Ultimately, leadership and management are about the relationship you have with yourself and the way we interact with and understand each other. Essentially, each and every one of us needs to believe in "self," create a questioning environment, listen to others, and instill a culture of development and learning from others (Holroyd & Brown, 2011).

## SUMMARY POINTS

- Formal theory helps explain, predict, and influence action.
- No leadership or management theory is "pure" or provides definitive answers.
- There is considerable scope for creating a different type of leader for 21st century health and social care.
- Successful leadership and management depend on the relationship that the leader and manager have with "self."

## CONCLUSION

This chapter has served to set the scene for the forthcoming chapters. It acknowledges the changing dynamic of health and social care across the globe, recognizing that although each country organizes its systems and services and sources its funding differently, there are common challenges facing all countries, with potentially generalizable solutions. In addition to leading and managing the different systems, each country has a political dimension that envelops its vision, which can negatively impact its ambitions. Whether rich or poorly resourced, global leaders need to turn their attention to developing a digital infrastructure that will enhance services; this will require investment, expertise, and ultimately, funding and education to support it.

From the UK perspective, the integration of health and social care is developing briskly. In response, leaders and managers should be strong in their resolve to sustain the trajectory of radical change and possess the skills and energy to achieve this. Against a backdrop of considerable global shortages in the nursing workforce, leaders need to think creatively to maintain service delivery and standards of care. Nevertheless, to avoid the pitfalls of the current "wicked" issues, leaders and managers need to move toward person-centered leadership, encouraging professionals to listen to their consumers. They must be mindful of government targets, yet focused on compassionate practice, with services revolving around the consumer and away from a focus on the services themselves.

A brief overview of leadership theories has set the scene for discussion on the different type of leader required by health and social care. For success, individuals need to focus on their relationship with "self" and use a combination of formal theories along with their own experience to shape their own direction.

## REFERENCES

Allen, S. (2019). 2020 global health care outlook: Laying a foundation for the future. *Deloitte Insights*. https://www2.deloitte.com/content/dam/Deloitte/cz/Documents/life-sciences-health-care/2020-global-health-care-outlook.pdf

Al-Sawai, A. (2013). Leadership of healthcare professionals: Where do we stand? *Oman Medical Journal*, *28*(4), 285–287. https://www.ncbi.nlm.nih.gov/pmc/articles/PMC3725246/ https://doi.org/10.5001/omj.2013.79.

Aluttis, C., Bishaw, T., & Frank, M. W. (2014). The workforce for health in a globalized context—Global shortages and international migration. *Global Health Action*, *7*(23611). https://www.ncbi.nlm.nih.gov/pmc/articles/PMC3926986/ https://doi.org/10.3402/gha.v7.23611.

Beech, J., Bottery, S., Charlesworth, A., Evans, H., Gershlick, B., Hemmings, N., … Palmer, B. (2019). *Closing the gap: Key areas for action on the health and care workforce*. The Health Foundation, Nuffield Trust, The King's Fund. https://www.kingsfund.org.uk/sites/default/files/2019-03/closing-the-gap-health-care-work-force-full-report.pdf

Berwick, D. (2013). *A promise to learn – A commitment to act: Improving the safety of patients in England*. National Advisory Group on the Safety of Patients in England. https://assets.publishing.service.gov.uk/government/uploads/system/uploads/attachment_data/file/226703/Berwick_Report.pdf

Bodenheimer, T., & Sinsky, C. (2014). From triple to quadruple aim: Care of the patient requires care of the provider. *Annals of Family Medicine*, *12*(6), 573–576. https://www.ncbi.nlm.nih.gov/pmc/articles/PMC4226781/

Boniol, M., McIsaac, M., Xu, L., Wuliji, T., Diallo, K., & Campbell, J. (2019). Gender equity in the health workforce: Analysis of 104 countries. *Health Workforce Working Paper 1*. World Health Organization. https://apps.who.int/iris/bitstream/handle/10665/311314/WHO-HIS-HWF-Gender-WP1-2019.1-eng.pdf?ua=1

British Medical Association. (2021). Integrated Care Systems (ICSs). https://www.bma.org.uk/advice-and-support/nhs-delivery-and-workforce/integration/integrated-care-systems-icss

Centre for Workforce Intelligence. (2013). Think integration, think workforce: Three steps to workforce integration. https://assets.publishing.service.gov.uk/government/uploads/system/uploads/attachment_data/file/507666/CfWI_Think_Integration.pdf

Chokshi, D. A. (2019, October 22). Four principles for improving health care around the world. *Harvard Business Review*. https://hbr.org/2019/10/4-principles-for-improving-health-care-around-the-world

Department of Health and Social Care (DHSC). (2021). Integration and innovation: working together to improve health and social care for all (HTML version). Updated 11 February 2021. https://www.gov.uk/government/publications/

working-together-to-improve-health-and-social-care-for-all/integration-and-innovation-working-together-to-improve-health-and-social-care-for-all-html-version

de Zulueta, P. C. (2016). Developing compassionate leadership in health care: An integrative review. *Journal of Healthcare Leadership*, 8(8), 1–10. https://www.ncbi.nlm.nih.gov/pmc/articles/PMC5741000/pdf/jhl-8-001.pdf

Dugan, J. P. (2017). *Leadership theory: Cultivating critical perspectives*. John Wiley & Sons.

Ferlie, E., Fitzgerald, L., McGivern, G., Dopson, S., & Bennett, C. (2011). Public policy networks and 'wicked problems': A nascent solution? *Public Administration*, 89(2), 307–324.

Francis, R. (2013). Report of the mid Staffordshire NHS Foundation trust public inquiry. https://assets.publishing.service.gov.uk/government/uploads/system/uploads/attachment_data/file/279124/0947.pdf

Gershlick, B., & Charlesworth, A. (2019). *Health and social care workforce: Priorities for the next government*. Health Foundation. https://www.health.org.uk/sites/default/files/2019-11/GE04Health%20and%20social%20care%20workforce.pdf

Ham, C., & Murray, R. (2015). Implementing the NHS five year forward view: Aligning policies with the plan. https://www.kingsfund.org.uk/sites/default/files/field/field_publication_file/implementing-the-nhs-five-year-forward-view-kingsfund-feb15.pdf

HM Government. (2012). Health and social care act. www.legislation.gov.uk/ukpga/2012/7/contents/enacted/data.htm

HM Government. (2019). 2019-20 Better care fund. Policy Framework Department of Health and Social Care and the Ministry of Housing, Communities and Local Government. https://assets.publishing.service.gov.uk/government/uploads/system/uploads/attachment_data/file/821676/Better_Care_Fund_2019-20_Policy_Framework.pdf

Holroyd, J., & Brown, K. (2011). *Leadership and management development for social work and social care: Creating leadership pathways of progression*. Learn to Care in collaboration with Bournemouth University. ISBN-13: 978-0-9560414-5-6.

Jones, G. L., Peter, Z., Rutter, K.-A., & Somauroo, A. (2019). *Promoting an overdue digital transformation in healthcare*. McKinsey & Company. https://www.mckinsey.com/industries/healthcare-systems-and-services/our-insights/promoting-an-overdue-digital-transformation-in-healthcare

Keogh. B. (2013). *Review into the quality of care and treatment provided by 14 hospital trusts in England: Overview report*. NHS. https://www.nhs.uk/nhsengland/bruce-keogh-review/documents/outcomes/keogh-review-final-report.pdf

Kerr, J. (2015). The leadership checklist: 10 principles that make leading easier. https://www.inc.com/james-kerr/the-leadership-checklist-10-principles-that-make-leading-easier.html

Kessler, E. H. (Ed.), (2013). *Encyclopedia of management theory*. Sage Publications.

MacGregor Burns. J. (1978). *Leadership*. Evans, Harper & Row.

Maguire, D., Evans, H., Honeyman, M., & Omojomolo, D. (2018). Digital change in health and social care. The Professional Association for Social Work and Social Workers. https://www.basw.co.uk/resources/digital-change-health-and-social-care

McNicoll, A. (2017). Ten years on from Baby P: Social work's story. Community Care. https://www.communitycare.co.uk/2017/08/03/ten-years-baby-p-social-works-story/

National Health Service England (NHS England). (2014a). Five year forward view. https://www.kingsfund.org.uk/projects/nhs-five-year-forward-view

National Health Service England (NHS England). (2014b). Building and strengthening leadership: Leading with compassion. https://www.england.nhs.uk/wp-content/uploads/2014/12/london-nursing-accessible.pdf

National Health Service (NHS). (2019). The NHS long-term plan. https://www.longtermplan.nhs.uk/wp-content/uploads/2019/08/nhs-long-term-plan-version-1.2.pdf

Orlowski, A. (2019). *Vive la révolution in population health management*. Nuffield Trust. https://www.nuffieldtrust.org.uk/news-item/vive-la-revolution-in-population-health-management

Robertson, R., Gregory, S., & Jabbal, J. (2014). *The social care and health systems of nine countries*. Commission on the Future of Health and Social Care in England. https://www.kingsfund.org.uk/sites/default/files/media/commission-background-paper-social-care-health-system-other-countries.pdf

Rosser, E. A., Scammell, J., Bevan, A., & Hundley, V. A. (2017). Strong leadership: The case for global connections. *Journal of Clinical Nursing*, 26(7–8), 946–955.

Sfantou, D. F., Laliotis, A., Patelarou, A. E., Sifaki-Pistolla, D., Matalliotakis, M., & Patelarou, E. (2017). Importance of leadership style towards quality of care measures in healthcare settings: A systematic review. *Healthcare*, 5(4), 73. https://www.ncbi.nlm.nih.gov/pmc/articles/PMC5746707/

Sinclair, S., Norris, J. M., McConnell, S. J., Chochinov, H. M., Hack, T. F., Hagen, N. A., … Bouchal, S. R. (2016). Compassion: A scoping review of the healthcare literature. *BMC Palliative Care*, 15(6), 6. https://www.ncbi.nlm.nih.gov/pmc/articles/PMC4717626/

Smith, T., Fowler-Davis, S., Nancarrow, S., Ariss, S. M. B., & Enderby, P. (2018). Leadership in interprofessional health and social care teams: A literature review. *Leadership in Health Services*, 31(4), 452–467. https://www.emerald.com/insight/content/doi/10.1108/LHS-06-2016-0026/full/pdf?title=leadership-in-interprofessional-health-and-social-care-teams-a-literature-review

Sullivan, E. J., & Garland, G. (2010). *Practical leadership and management in nursing*. Pearson Education Limited.

Taylor, K., Pettinicchio, C., & Arvanitidou, M. (2019). The transition to integrated care: Population health management in England. Deloitte. https://www2.deloitte.com/content/dam/Deloitte/uk/Documents/public-sector/deloitte-uk-public-sector-population-health-management.pdf

The King's Fund. (2011). The future of leadership and management in the NHS. No more heroes. Report from the King's Fund Commission on Leadership and management in the NHS. https://www.kingsfund.org.uk/sites/default/files/future-of-leadership-and-management-nhs-may-2011-kings-fund.pdf

The King's Fund. (2013). *Patient-centred leadership: Rediscovering our purpose*. The King's Fund. https://www.kingsfund.org.uk/sites/default/files/field/field_publication_file/patient-centred-leadership-rediscovering-our-purpose-may13.pdf

West, M., Eckert, R., Collins, B., & Chowla, R. (2017). *Caring to change: How compassionate leadership can stimulate innovation in health care*. The King's Fund. https://www.kingsfund.org.uk/sites/default/files/field/field_publication_file/Caring_to_change_Kings_Fund_May_2017.pdf

West, M., Eckert, R., Steward, K., & Pasmore, B. (2014). *Developing collective leadership for health care*. The King's Fund. https://www.kingsfund.org.uk/sites/default/files/field/field_publication_file/developing-collective-leadership-kingsfund-may14.pdf

World Health Organization (WHO). (2006). *The world health report 2006 – Working together for health*. Author.

World Health Organization (WHO). (2018). WHO guideline on health policy and system support to optimize community health worker programmes. https://apps.who.int/iris/bitstream/handle/10665/275501/WHO-HIS-HWF-CHW-2018.1-eng.pdf?ua=1

## REFLECTIVE QUESTIONS

- Based on your own experience, what can you learn from other countries to help you in your current decision-making?
- From your own experience, think of one leader and one manager who stand out as exceptional. What characteristics do they have that make them a good leader and manager?

- If you accept that we are all leaders, in practical terms, how might you create a climate of openness and honesty and allow your colleagues to raise concerns without fear of reprisal?
- From the theories that have been presented and from your own experience, what qualities do you think you possess and what might need further development to further your success?

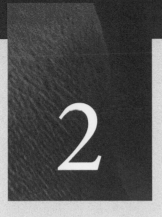

# 2

# LEADERSHIP FOR 21ST CENTURY HEALTH AND SOCIAL CARE: LEADING INNOVATION

DEBBIE SORKIN

## OBJECTIVES

*After reading this chapter, you should be able to:*

- Describe the broader societal context for recent innovations in leadership.
- Explain models of leadership across health and social care and from a national and international perspective, with their emphasis on actions and behaviors.
- Set out what leadership means in relation to complex issues.
- Illustrate what these innovations in leadership have looked like in practice.
- Identify the role and value of compassionate leadership, both in itself and as a driver of innovation.
- Provide examples of leadership innovation in and with communities.
- Summarize the direction of leadership in health and social care systems.

## INTRODUCTION

Chapter 1 discussed how major challenges facing global health and social care systems have driven change, including in approaches to leadership. This chapter takes a closer look at what this means for innovation in leadership, in both theory and practice, drawing on examples from the United Kingdom and around the world. Much of this innovation has been in response to two key drivers. On the one hand, we have seen welcome increases in life expectancy over the past half century. On the other hand, we continue to live with persistent health inequalities. Both of these have had a profound impact on health services. In 1948, the year

the UK National Health Service (NHS) was founded, life expectancy in England and Wales was 66 years for men and 70 years for women. By 2018, these figures had increased (for the United Kingdom as a whole) to 79.3 and 82.9 years for men and women, respectively. This reflects trends worldwide: the average life expectancy globally in 2017 exceeded 70 years, up from around 48 years in 1950, which is as far back as global records reliably go (ONS, 2015). Principal causes of death have also changed, away from infectious diseases and toward cancer, Alzheimer's, and the co-morbidities—kidney disease, diabetes, stroke—that ride on the coattails of old age and lifestyle factors (ONS, 2020). Both of these factors have financial consequences; we commonly spend more on health and proportionately more on caring for older people. In the UK context, the Institute for Fiscal Studies (IFS) estimates that 30p out of every £ spent on public services now goes toward health. The average 65-year-old costs the NHS 2.5 times more than the average 30-year-old, while an 85-year-old costs 7.5 times as much (Stoye, 2017).

Therefore, part of the new role of leadership in the 21st century is to think constantly about how to match the capacity of health and social care systems with this growing demand. Moreover, that capacity is not equally distributed, and not everyone gets the same access to a healthy old age. Within the United Kingdom, there are stark differences in health outcomes: The Health Foundation has calculated that there is a gap of almost 19 years in healthy life expectancy (that is, the number of years without significant illnesses or co-morbidities) between the most and least deprived areas of England. Marmot (2010) shows the importance of the social determinants of health—housing, education, employment, social relationships, and family ties—in addressing these outcomes. He calls for concerted action at the national, regional, and local levels. Progress has been slow; after 10 years, Marmot et al. (2020) note that improvements began to stall from 2011 onwards, with life expectancy actually falling in the most deprived communities.

To meet the changing health and social care landscapes, there are calls for a whole-system approach and new approaches to leadership, including creating conditions for individuals to take control of their own lives. In this chapter, consideration is given to some of the innovations in leadership and their outcomes.

## INNOVATIONS IN LEADERSHIP APPROACHES

One of the key innovations in health care leadership over the past 20 years has been to move away from the idea of a single leader at the head of an organization and place the focus more on modeling leadership through behaviors and actions. For example, NHS Scotland (2009, p. 2) notes that how people act and behave at all levels could "help make or break delivery of the change agenda in health." In an English context, the same ideas were reflected by Berwick (2013), who emphasizes how change and improvement come about through people at all levels modeling appropriate behaviors. This way of thinking envisages leadership less as a single role and more as a set of actions that drive continuous improvement in service quality. This has also been reflected in innovative thinking about leadership in social care. The National Skills Academy for Social Care (Department of Health and Skills for Care, 2014) published the first Leadership Qualities Framework for England's sector. The framework was predicated on leadership being about behaviors and grounded in everyday practice. It directly linked leadership, safety, and continuous improvement and spelled out what good leadership looked like in action, for people working at all levels in the sector.

The idea of linking leadership with behaviors has since been embedded in leadership frameworks in a number of health care systems worldwide. In England, the National Leadership Academy (2013, p. 5) emphasizes "behaving in a way that reflects the principles and values of the NHS." In Canada, the LEADS (LEADS Collaborative, 2015) health leadership capabilities framework sets out key skills and behaviors required to lead in all parts and at all levels of the health system. In addition, in New Zealand it is noted that "Organisations express leadership and capability not only through their systems and structures, but more importantly through their culture, values and behaviours" (New Zealand Health Quality and Safety Commission (2016, p. 9).

The emphasis continues; in England, the NHS Improvement and Leadership Development Board (2016) and NHS England (2020) both place good leadership practice as demonstrated through behaviors at the heart of high-quality clinical care and continuous improvement. How this leadership practice has been shaping up inside and outside the United Kingdom is the subject of the rest of this chapter.

### SUMMARY POINTS

- A key innovation in health care leadership in the 21st century has been a move away from the idea of a single leader and a move toward the idea of leadership based on behaviors and actions.
- As a corollary, leadership is described as something that can be practiced at any level in an organization.
- Leadership can be seen in an English context in social care as well as in health care.
- The approach is now embedded in leadership frameworks for health and social care systems within the United Kingdom as well as other countries and regions.

## THE RISE OF SYSTEM LEADERSHIP

Chapter 1 refers to "wicked" issues, and Chapter 5 mentions "wicked" problems arising in health and social care delivery. Another innovation for 21st century health care leadership, building on the idea of grounding leadership in behaviors but this time in response to wicked issues/problems, has been the application of system or adaptive leadership approaches.

There has been a growing understanding that many of the deep-seated or multi-faceted issues facing health and social care—changing demographics, more people living longer with chronic conditions, and increasing health and social inequalities—cannot be solved by traditional "command and control" leadership or by diktat from the center. Rather, what is needed is what Heifetz (1994) defines as adaptive leadership. This way of working, grounded in discussion, openness, and asking questions rather than jumping to solutions, was designed to help people approach challenges that were new or outside the familiar or that kept recurring and required long-term change where the solutions were unknown and therefore outside existing expertise. Senge et al. (2015) are among a number of management thinkers who take these ideas and apply them to systemic issues that require a cross-sector approach. Managing the care of older people, for example, needs professionals from the health and social care systems to work together and practice collaborative leadership. The authors note that leadership in these situations is about learning as much as doing. System leadership is less about forcing change to happen and more about creating the conditions that could produce and sustain change. Other writers, such as Snowden (2020), show how these approaches can help people lead in situations that are complex and inherently unpredictable. The understanding that many of the problems facing health and social care fit this description has led to system approaches gaining ground. In an English context, 2012 saw the coming together of the System Leadership Steering Group, comprising representatives from across the NHS, local government, public health, social care, and other sectors, who pooled funding to commission research into system leadership and provide on-the-ground support in places grappling with complex issues across health and social care.

Ghate et al. (2013) examine national and international experiences of system working across the United Kingdom, the United States, Canada, Australia, and Denmark, and the key leadership behaviors across different countries that has led to real change. The researchers identify six key ways of behaving (Box 2-1).

Ghate et al. (2013) go on to show how the current UK context of public service, the practice of system leadership, and the attributes of system leaders could fit together in a nested, integrative model (Fig. 2-1).

The model has three rings. The outer ring describes the environments in which people are working, while the middle ring describes the qualities or actions needed in those who lead complex change, that is, forms of system leadership. The inner ring describes the personal styles and behaviors that people leading in systems need. The model contributes to the evidence base by illustrating the complexity and intricate interconnections involved in systems leadership.

Many others have contributed to the evidence. In a UK context, the Centre for Health and Care Leadership (Weir, 2019) collates the views of health and social care leaders that apply system leadership principles in their work, noting how this involves shifts in mindsets, behaviors, and leadership practice. The King's Fund has contributed a steady stream of research covering England, Scotland, and countries outside the United Kingdom. In particular, Timmins (2015) corroborates many of the behaviors needed for effective leadership in systems, in order to keep the focus on patient outcomes. System thinking has increasingly come to the fore in innovative health service practice, both inside and outside the United Kingdom. NHS Scotland (2009, p. 12) talks about "engaging leadership," including building shared purpose across a range of stakeholders. The approach is mirrored in the health and social care service in Northern Ireland (Department of Health Northern Ireland, 2014), which defines

---

**BOX 2-1**

**Ways of feeling**: basing action around personal core values and commitment

**Ways of perceiving**: standing back, "getting off the dancefloor and onto the balcony," allowing for the unseen and unpredicted, seeking and listening to diverse views

**Ways of thinking**: synthesizing complexity and sense-making for other people

**Ways of doing**: enabling and supporting others, giving people the space and permission to think creatively, repurposing and reframing existing resources

**Ways of relating**: mutuality, empathy, authenticity, self-awareness

**Ways of being**: courage to take risks, resilience, patience, humility, persistence

Ghate, D. et al. (2013). Systems leadership: Exceptional leadership for exceptional times. Synthesis Paper, The Virtual Staff College. https://thestaffcollege.uk/wp-content/uploads/VSC_Synthesis_exec_complete.pdf

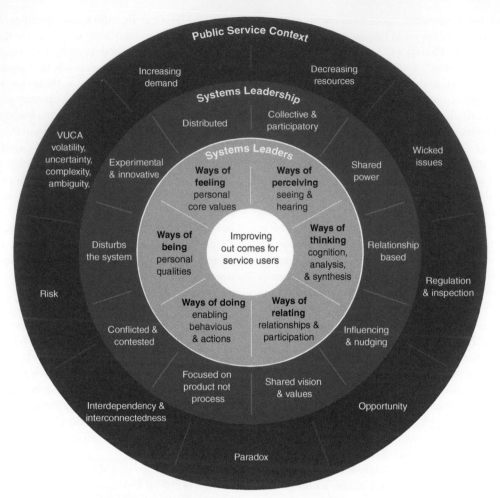

**Fig. 2-1** ■ Model for system leadership. (Reproduced with permission from the Staff College). Ghate, D. et al. (2013). Systems leadership: Exceptional leadership for exceptional times. The Virtual Staff College. https://thestaffcollege.uk/wp-content/uploads/VSC_Synthesis_exec_complete.pdf

collective leadership as including interdependent and collaborative system leadership.

In Australia, Health Workforce Australia (2013) refers to the "S" in *LEADS* as "shaping and aligning complex systems." Similarly, in New Zealand, the Health, Quality and Safety Commission New Zealand (HQSCNZ, 2016, p. 6) notes, "We need to appreciate the health system as a dynamic, adaptive collection of inter-related and interdependent components with a common purpose or aim." The Canadian Health Leadership Framework (LEADS Collaborative, 2015) demonstrates systems thinking as one of the six key attributes for successful leaders. In an English context, Sir Simon Stevens (NHS England, 2014, p. 16) nails his colors to the mast by stating, "Increasingly we need to manage systems—networks of care—not just organizations." The theme has carried through in the Long-Term Plan (NHS England, 2019a), which is predicated on systems working to build the health and well-being of local populations.

To conclude, there is a growing body of evidence arising from theory being put into practice to benefi-cial effect. This is not to say that leadership, or system leadership, is in and of itself a magic bullet. Stubborn factors—culture, history, or politics—can always get in the way. However, there has been progress, and some examples of that progress are set out in the next section.

## SUMMARY POINTS

- Many of the deep-seated, "wicked" issues/problems facing health and social care cannot be solved by traditional "command and control" forms of leadership or by diktat.
- Building on the idea of grounding leadership in behaviors and actions, a further innovation in 21st century leadership has been the drive to adopt system or adaptive leadership.
- System leadership includes working across professional boundaries, asking questions rather than jumping to solutions, and looking to achieve shared purpose across a range of disciplines and sectors.
- Leadership is about learning as much as doing: creating the conditions for change.
- National and international research has analyzed what comprises good system leadership behaviors, alongside an evidence base built on the experience of putting them into practice.
- A commitment to system leadership is now a common feature in health and social care leadership.

## INNOVATION IN LEADERSHIP PRACTICE

A troubling issue in health and social care has been the need to support people who are living longer, but not always in good health. Innovation in 21st century health and social care has meant applying new leadership approaches based on behaviors and system thinking to address this issue in practice. This has often been linked to integrating health and social care services around an individual, as set out in Chapter 1 and then explored as a general theme throughout this book. Chapter 1 emphasizes the importance of supporting this integration seamlessly and, where appropriate, in the community rather than in an acute hospital setting. In England, many reports have pointed out the lack of integration and adverse consequences for patients. For example, the Barker Review (2014, p. 1) describes the post-war health and social care settlement as no longer fit for purpose, calling for "far better integration of health and social care…so that services are built

around people's needs." The baton was picked up in the NHS Five Year Forward View (NHS England, 2014), which was founded on the idea that traditional divides between primary and acute care or between health care and social care needed to be dissolved. It provided support for what were termed new models of care, or "Vanguards," involving care homes, primary and community care, and acute hospital services.

These new models of care drew on examples at home and from further afield. In Spain, the Alzira Model (de Rosa Torner, 2012), originating in Valencia, operated as a collaboration between the public and private sectors with an integrated IT system across health and social care. The Gesundes Kinzigtal Model (Zanon, 2015), a regional integrated care management system in Germany, emphasized self-care and population health. In 2007, the Canterbury Health System in New Zealand (Charles, 2017) started out on a more integrated pathway in the wake of the Christchurch earthquake. By 2017, the health system was supporting more people in their homes and communities, using new delivery models that involved better integration of care. In England, a number of local initiatives to integrate services began around the same time. For example, in Birmingham, the Rapid Assessment, Interface and Discharge (RAID) set up in 2009 was an innovative service started by clinicians in community and acute hospital settings that transformed mental health care across the city (Dougall et al., 2018). From 2013, Integrated Health and Social Care Pioneers (NHS England, 2021) developed innovative ways to integrate care around people's needs. Some of these places met with real success. In Wakefield, for example, the Connecting Care initiative led to extended access, including through better use of technology and more care delivered at home or in the community, such as through Connecting Care Hubs, with staff from across health and social care working together at one site (NHS Wakefield Clinical Commissioning Group, 2020).

At the same time, many of the on-the-ground projects supported by the Systems Leadership–Local Vision initiative were also demonstrating that system approaches could work—sometimes with unforeseen benefits. In Plymouth, work to reduce alcohol abuse in the city contributed to measurable impacts, including a reduction in alcohol-related hospital admissions and joint commissioning across the NHS and the local authority for services to support people with complex needs related to alcohol abuse. The council was also able to reduce the number of children going into foster care because of their parents' alcohol problems (Dalton et al., 2015).

However, there has been a lack of connection between these different initiatives in England, and the economic case for the Vanguards, in terms of financial savings, has been questionable. Not all examples of integrated working have stood the test of time: the Torbay Health and Care Trust, a pioneer of integrated health and social care for older people lauded by the House of Lords (2012), was subsumed into a local NHS Foundation Trust in 2012–13. Moreover, as studies from the Health Foundation (2020) show, they tend to take time to deliver financial savings. However, there is an evidence base for what these exercises in collaborative leadership have achieved. The six Enhanced Health in Care Homes Vanguards that were built enhanced primary care support, with linked GP practices, pharmacy services, and nurse specialists; developed multidisciplinary team support; promoted reablement and independence; fostered better end-of-life care; and significantly reduced hospital admissions for ambulatory care conditions (NHS England and NHS Improvement, 2020).

The movement toward integration is clear. In Scotland, where law and policy make integration not just an aspiration but a requirement, more than half the total NHS and adult social care budget is now delegated to Integration Joint Boards, with Chief Officers in place to ensure a steady focus on collaborative working and service transformation. In Wales, local health boards are required to produce integrated health and social care plans for each local authority area, including identifying strategic priorities for multi-agency working. In Northern Ireland, integrated care partnerships are playing a key role in bringing together health and social care. Finally, for NHS England (2019a), the NHS Long-Term Plan is predicated on the idea of integrated care systems, empowered to make system-wide decisions to strengthen the health of their local populations.

If anything, the COVID-19 pandemic appears to have accelerated the trend toward integrated working, with the NHS People Plan (NHS England, 2020), for example, noting how distributed leadership has proven

more critical than ever in the fight against the virus. This is one leadership innovation that is not going away.

## SUMMARY POINTS

- Innovations in leadership, grounded in behaviors and combined with system approaches, have been used to address troubling and complex issues in health and social care, especially relating to changing demographics and/or health inequalities.
- Innovations have often been linked in practice to integrating services around an individual, especially away from acute hospital settings.
- There are numerous examples from within and outside the United Kingdom, with projects and programs often having beneficial outcomes.
- In the English context, there has been a lack of connection between initiatives and not all examples have stood the test of time.
- An evidence base has developed, showing what these exercises in collaborative leadership have achieved.
- The movement toward integrated services is clear.

## COMPASSIONATE LEADERSHIP

Compassionate leadership, also touched on in other chapters, is worth mentioning in the context of innovation. On the one level, it seems bizarre to have to single out compassion when talking about caring professions but calls for more compassionate leadership have become increasingly common over the last decade, especially in relation to the NHS. Compassion usually relates to ideas around helping others in some form of distress, or at least understanding what it might be like to be in another person's shoes, together with notions such as justice, kindness, fairness, and interdependence. In other words, it is about behaviors and is thereby an intrinsic part of leadership.

In a health context, compassionate leadership has been used as a tool to push back against behaviors that have had scant regard for justice, fairness, or kindness. Bullying, for instance, has been an endemic problem. Kline (2013) notes that a quarter of NHS staff felt they were bullied and that the rate of reported bullying had doubled in just four years. Even in 2018, the NHS staff survey showed that 19% and 13% of staff had experienced bullying and harassment in the past year from colleagues and their manager, respectively.

Moreover, whistle-blowers have not always been treated with compassion. Dr Steve Bolsin raised concerns about mortality in the Bristol pediatric heart surgery scandal, which resulted in a public inquiry (Department of Health, 2001); he reported being ostracized and eventually left the United Kingdom to work in Australia. In the Mid Staffordshire Foundation Trust inquiry, Sir Francis (2013) highlighted both a culture of bullying and of fear, in which staff did not feel able to report concerns. Thus the shift toward compassionate leadership has recognized that it can have significant benefits, not only for patient care but also for innovation and improvement, neither of which can flourish in a culture of fear.

There have been concerted attempts to address these issues and encourage compassionate leadership to become the norm. For example, the NHS Social Partnership Forum (2016) launched its Tackling Bullying Call to Action, inviting leaders across the NHS to commit to making a difference by promoting supportive cultures. Additionally, the NHS Improvement and Leadership Development Board's (2016, p. 2) national framework for leadership development has as one of its five key areas for actions to build just cultures, "compassionate, inclusive leadership skills at all levels." Over the past five years, health think tanks have consistently argued for compassion. Indeed, in the joint report, "Closing the gap," the Health Foundation, the Nuffield Trust, and the King's Fund (Beech et al., 2019, p. 49) state explicitly: "Compassionate and inclusive leadership.... enables teams to deliver better patient care and value for money while also delivering continuous improvements to population health."

Is it making a difference? Definitive answers are hard to come by. On the one hand, the bullying figures in the 2018 NHS National Survey showed an increase over the previous 12 months. On the other hand, that might actually be a good sign if it means that more staff were willing to call it out. Early in the COVID-19 pandemic, Bailey and West (2020, para. 3) announced renewed calls for compassionate leadership, emphasizing its importance: "It is vital that, as the NHS responds to COVID-19 challenges, leaders and managers model and promote compassion in an enduring way including

self-compassion." NHS England (2020) also had compassionate leadership as one of its key themes.

Yet another reason for the focus of the People Plan (NHS England, 2020) on compassion and inclusion was that Public Health England (2020) discovered that institutional racism and bullying had made nurses from minority ethnic backgrounds afraid to speak up about issues that put them at higher risk of contracting COVID-19. Discombe (2020) reports on health care professionals having been "gagged" by hospitals and NHS bodies, with some reports of threats of disciplinary action if staff raised concerns about PPE shortages or testing shortfalls. Consequently, the jury is still out. The hope has to be that new ways of working, informed by compassionate leadership, gradually become the norm.

## SUMMARY POINTS

- The drive toward compassionate leadership in health care services, seen in the context of a pushback against bullying, poor service quality, and cultures of fear, is another example of innovation in 21st century approaches to leadership.
- There have been concerted attempts to bring compassionate leadership to center stage.
- The COVID-19 pandemic has seen renewed calls for compassionate leadership
- In the English context, we are still some distance from seeing compassionate leadership embedded in practice.

## LEADERSHIP IN THE COMMUNITY: INNOVATIONS IN DELIVERING CARE

Not all innovation has begun in the context of national bodies or been centered on acute hospitals. There have also been new approaches to people's roles, how they work, and what they do, and these are important indicators of changes in 21st century leadership.

A key development has been the advent of self-managed health and social care teams, supporting people in their own homes. One of the most well-known examples is Buurtzorg, a nurse-led model of holistic community care founded by Jos de Blok in the Netherlands in 2006 (Gray et al., 2015). De Blok's founding principle was that teams of nurses, working from their intrinsic motivation, could lead and manage themselves and hold each other to account to provide high quality care. By 2018, the organization had grown from a single team of four community nurses to some 10,000 nurses and nursing assistants, working in approximately 900 independent teams and providing care to more than 70,000 people. More than half of all district nurses in the Netherlands now work for Buurtzorg. The organization also has bases in Sweden, Japan, the United States, France, and the United Kingdom, with pilot sites in London, Kent, and Suffolk and three in Wales.

Buurtzorg nurse teams provide a range of services, reflecting the drive toward health and social care integration described earlier in this chapter. A Buurtzorg team can provide not only nursing and medical services but also personal care and support that would (in a UK setting) be provided by social care, such as help with dressing and bathing, alongside health coaching or supporting people's management of their own health to improve their quality of life and prevent or minimize further illness. The emphasis is on autonomy and coaching rather than on traditional management, with a small group of staff (still around 50 at the time of writing) providing administration and with the operation underpinned by a bespoke IT system designed to enable coordinated care. Outcomes have included better quality of care; reduced costs; fewer hospital admissions; and consistently high levels of satisfaction for patients, families, and staff. Buurtzorg is rated as having the most satisfied workforce of any Dutch company with more than 1000 employees.

There are analogous models of nursing and care teams developing elsewhere in the United Kingdom. Scotland, for example, has established its own Neighbourhood Care program, initially in seven pilot areas and now being more widely expanded (Health Improvement Scotland, 2020). Neighbourhood Care teams look to provide person-centered and holistic care to enable people to live well in the community for longer. In England, Sanderson (2018) established Wellbeing Teams in 2016 to demonstrate what personalized and person-centered care could look like in a home-care setting. Like Buurtzorg, there have been positive outcomes: Wellbeing Teams is currently rated "Outstanding" by the Care Quality Commission, the national regulator for social care (Law, 2018).

The second area of change has been expansion within traditional roles and development of new roles, often spanning the boundary between sectors or professions. For example, both in the NHS and in local authorities in England, Care Navigators—who can double as administrative staff—guide people to sources of help, advocacy, and support, and help people play an active role in managing their own health (Walker, 2019). The NHS England (2019a) Long-Term Plan highlights the potential value of these roles, particularly in relation to primary care and mental health, noting how new roles, such as GP Associates, Nursing Associates, Allied Health Professional Associates, and Advanced Clinical Practitioners, can be an important part of meeting current and future workforce demand. The evidence for these approaches is strong—introducing mental health peer support workers to acute settings has been shown to reduce readmissions.

There is a strong link to another role: social prescribing. In York, for example, the Ways to Wellbeing service uses social prescribers to connect patients via their GP to non-medical activities, services, and groups in their community that can support their health and well-being needs (York, 2020). The Long-Term Plan aims for more than 900,000 people to be able to be referred to social prescribing schemes by 2023–24.

Multi-disciplinary hubs, such as the Connecting Care Hubs in Wakefield mentioned earlier, provide a flavor of what integration could look like (NHS Wakefield Clinical Commissioning Group, 2020). They will need time and money, not to mention the people to resource and develop them. They offer a potential step change in the capacity of systems to deliver more effective care and rely on individuals stepping up to their leadership roles.

## SUMMARY POINTS

- Not all innovation has been initiated in national bodies or centered on acute hospitals. There have been new approaches to people's roles, how they work, and what they do, and these are important indicators of change in 21st century leadership.
- A key development has been the advent of self-managed health and social care teams, supporting people in their own homes.
- Buurtzorg is an example of a nurse-led model of holistic community care.

- Buurtzorg approaches have resulted in better quality of care, reduced costs, and consistently high reported levels of satisfaction among service users and their families.
- There are analogous services now operating in England and Scotland.
- There has also been innovation through expansion within traditional roles and the development of new roles, often spanning the boundary between sectors or professions.
- New roles offer a potential step change in the capacity of systems to deliver more effective care.

## DOING IT FOR THEMSELVES: PERSONALIZED CARE AND PATIENT LEADERS

This chapter has focused mainly on leadership innovation related to staff and professionals in health and social care systems. Nonetheless, one of the most heartening developments in recent years has been the encouragement of patient leadership (NHS England, 2019b), both through personalized care and through individuals using their expertise in their own conditions and experiences. Personalized care describes a way of working that enables individuals and clinicians to work together to design and deliver care that is appropriate for and tailored to the person. In the UK context, it has been a thread running through the NHS, starting with Principle 4 of the NHS Constitution (NHS England, 2015a).

Personal health budgets were piloted in England in 2009, with independent evaluations identifying clear benefits from the approach. This led to the NHS Comprehensive Model of Personalised Care and a further roll-out of the program. By September 2018, more than 200,000 people had joined. The NHS England (2019a) Long-Term Plan aims for 2.5 million people to be able to obtain personalized care by 2025.

Beyond personalized care, there has been an increasing commitment to and evidence of patient leadership. The Keogh Review (2013) of hospital quality and care called on NHS organizations to harness the leadership potential of patients, and the Berwick Review (2013) welcomed the idea of patient partnership. The idea is slowly gaining traction. The Centre for Patient Leadership (2013, para. 2) was set up to help enable

patients, service users, and caregivers "to become influential leaders and effective agents of change." The NHS has commissioned studies to bring together examples of good practice in patient leadership, with key recommendations including investing in patient leaders and making them an integral part of formal and informal decision-making. There have been local and national development programs for patient leaders; Care Quality Commission inspection teams now routinely include Experts by Experience, and the current NHS England's (2019a, p. 25) Long-Term Plan commits to "a systematic approach to engaging patients in decisions about their health and wellbeing."

In the community, the award-winning Bromley-by-Bow Centre in the East End of London is an example of developing leadership capacity in people who use services. The Centre is an innovative community organization based in one of the most deprived areas of the United Kingdom. It aims to improve the lives of local people by addressing their social needs, building services with and around them, rather than *doing to* (NHS England, 2015b; Stocks-Rankin et al., 2018). As with Buurtzorg, it has brought together holistic support. The Centre uses social prescribing to link people across health care and other sectors and also provides support with education, training, and advice. The key factor in its success has been local and community leadership, starting from the belief that everyone has something to offer, and everyone can play a leadership role. As with other innovations in health care leadership, it will take time; it has taken Bromley-by-Bow, for example, more than 20 years. However, the take-home message is the growing understanding that if we want person-centered care, we need to involve patients in leading it.

### SUMMARY POINTS

- A key innovation in 21st century leadership has been encouraging patient leadership, both through personalized care and through individuals using their expertise in their own conditions and experiences.
- Personal health budgets have delivered benefits for patients and reduced costs, and the NHS Long-Term Plan aims to significantly expand the service.
- Beyond personalized care, there has been an increasing commitment to and evidence of patient leadership.

- There are examples in the community of developing leadership capacity in people who use services.
- If we want person-centered care, we need to involve the people at the center of it—the patients themselves—as leaders in their own right and recognize that it will take time to evolve.

## CONCLUSION

Innovations in leadership have grown in response to wider changes in society, such as demographic shifts or growth in health inequalities. Currently, a sudden emergency such as a global pandemic can accelerate changes already underway. For the past decade, there has been an increasing focus on behaviors and actions and on "getting off the dancefloor and onto the balcony" to take a system-wide view, especially where complex and "wicked" issues/ problems are involved.

There is now recognition that "leadership" is not synonymous with "leader." We can all do something to model leadership, whether that is ceding leadership to others who might be in a better position to make progress on an issue, giving people autonomy where it might lead to better outcomes, supporting people to experiment and try a new way of working, or practicing compassionate leadership with the people around us. Leadership is not confined to particular professional settings: it can happen in and with communities.

Not all progress to date has been linear and steadily upwards; however, it would be equally untrue to say there has been no progress at all. An evidence base of research and real-world examples in leadership innovation is now available to draw upon. Starting out, even in a small way, and taking action can be beneficial. Leading with others and across sectors and professional boundaries is helpful to experience leadership in practice and coach others so that they can work their way through problems rather than settling into fixed positions. If we want to see more innovation and better care in our health and caring systems, we need to be compassionate with ourselves and with others; there has never been a better time to put this into practice.

## REFERENCES

Bailey, S., & West, M. (2020). *Covid-10: Why compassionate leadership matters in a crisis*. The Kings Fund. <https://www.kingsfund.org.uk/blog/2020/03/covid-19-crisis-compassionate-leadership>.

Barker, K. (2014). *A new settlement for health and social care: final report*. Commission on the Future of Health and Social Care in England. <https://www.kingsfund.org.uk/publications/new-settlement-health-and-social-care>.

Beech, J., Bottery, S., Charlesworth, A., Evans, H., Gershlick, B., Hemmings, N., … Palmer, B. (2019). *Closing the gap: Key areas for action on the health and care workforce*. The Health Foundation, The King's Fund, the Nuffield Trust. <https://www.nuffieldtrust.org.uk/files/2019-03/heaj6708-workforce-full-report-web.pdf>.

Berwick, D. (2013). *A promise to learn – A commitment to act: Improving the safety of patients in England*. National Advisory Group on the Safety of Patients in England. <https://assets.publishing.service.gov.uk/government/uploads/system/uploads/attachment_data/file/226703/Berwick_Report.pdf>.

Charles, A. (2017). *Developing accountable care systems: Lessons from Canterbury*. New Zealand: The King's Fund. <https://www.kingsfund.org.uk/sites/default/files/2017-08/Developing_ACSs_final_digital_0.pdf>.

Dalton, M., Jarvis, J., Powell, B., & Sorkin, D. (2015). *The revolution will be improvised part II. Insights from places on transforming systems*. The Leadership Centre. <https://www.thinklocalactpersonal.org.uk/_assets/News/The_Revolution_will_be_Improvised_Part_II.pdf>.

de Rosa Torner, A. (2012). *Lessons from Spain: The Alzira Model*. The King's Fund International Integrated Care Summit. <https://www.kingsfund.org.uk/sites/default/files/alberto-roso-torner-integrated-care-spain-alzira-model-kings-fund-may12.pdf>.

Department of Health. (2001). https://webarchive.nationalarchives.gov.uk/20090811143810/http://www.bristol-inquiry.org.uk/final_report/report/index.htm.

Department of Health, Northern Ireland. (2014). *The health and social care collective leadership strategy*. <https://www.health-ni.gov.uk/sites/default/files/publications/health/hsc-collective-leadership-strategy.pdf>

Department of Health and Skills for Care. (2014). *The leadership quality framework for adult social care*. <https://www.skillsforcare.org.uk/Documents/Leadership-and-management/Leadership-Qualities-Framework/Leadership-Qualities-Framework.pdf>

Discombe, M. (2020, 21 April). Hancock: Staff should be free to speak out over coronavirus concerns. *Health Service Journal* <https://www.hsj.co.uk/hancock-staff-should-be-free-to-speak-out-over-coronavirus-concerns/7027467.article>.

Dougall, D., Lewis, M., & Ross, S. (2018). *Transformational change in health and care: Reports from the front line*. The King's Fund. <https://www.kingsfund.org.uk/publications/transformational-change-health-care>.

Francis, R. (2013). Report of the Mid Staffordshire NHS Foundation Trust Public Inquiry. <https://www.gov.uk/government/publications/report-of-the-mid-staffordshire-nhs-foundation-trust-public-inquiry>

Ghate, D., Lewis, J., & Welbourn, D. (2013). *Systems leadership: Exceptional leadership for exceptional times*. The Virtual Staff College. <https://thestaffcollege.uk/wp-content/uploads/VSC_Synthesis_exec_complete.pdf>.

Gray, B. H., Sarnak, O., & Burgers, J. S. (2015). *Home care by self-governing nursing teams: The Netherlands' Buurtzorg Model*. The Commonwealth Fund. <https://www.commonwealthfund.org/

publications/case-study/2015/may/home-care-self-governing-nursing-teams-netherlands-buurtzorg-model>.

Healthcare Improvement Scotland. (2020). Neighbourhood Care: Working with health and social care organisations to test the principles of a holistic model of care in the community. <https://ihub.scot/improvement-programmes/living-well-in-communities/our-programmes/neighbourhood-care/>

Health, Quality and Safety Commission New Zealand (HQSCNZ). (2016). From knowledge to action: A framework to build quality and safety capability in the New Zealand health system. <https://www.hqsc.govt.nz/assets/Quality-Improvement/PR/From-knowledge-to-action-Oct-2016.pdf>

Health Workforce Australia. (2013). Health LEADS Australia: The Australian health leadership framework. <https://www.aims.org.au/documents/item/352>

Heifetz, R. (1994). *Leadership without easy answers*. Harvard University Press. <https://www.hup.harvard.edu/catalog.php?isbn=9780674518582>.

House of Lords Select Committee on Public Services and Demographic Change. (2012). Ready for ageing? <https://publications.parliament.uk/pa/ld201213/ldselect/ldpublic/140/140.pdf>

Keogh, B. (2013). Review into the quality of care and treatment provided by 14 hospital trusts in England: Overview report. <https://www.nhs.uk/nhsengland/bruce-keogh-review/documents/outcomes/keogh-review-final-report.pdf>

Kline, R. (2013). *Bullying: The silent epidemic in the NHS*. Public World, Democracy at Work. <http://publicworld.gridhosted.co.uk/blog/bullying_the_silent_epidemic_in_the_nhs>.

Law, R. (2018). Public service mutuals in social care. *Care Management Matters*, June, 26–28. <https://issuu.com/carechoices/docs/cmm_15.4_june_2018_lr?e=7472320/61617535>.

LEADS Collaborative. (2015). *Health leadership capabilities framework*. Canadian College of Health Leaders. <http://leadscollaborative.ca/uploaded/web/Resources/LEADS_Brochure_2015.pdf>.

Marmot, M. (2010). *Fair society, healthy lives: The Marmot review*. Strategic Review of Health Inequalities in England post-2010. <https://www.parliament.uk/globalassets/documents/fair-society-healthy-lives-full-report.pdf>.

Marmot, M., Allen, J., Boyce, T., Goldblatt, P., & Morrison, J. (2020). *Health equity in England: The Marmot review ten years on*. The Institute for Health Equity, commissioned by the Health Foundation. <https://www.health.org.uk/publications/reports/the-marmot-review-10-years-on>.

NHS England. (2014). Five year forward view. <https://www.england.nhs.uk/wp-content/uploads/2014/10/5yfv-web.pdf>

NHS England. (2015a). The NHS constitution: The NHS belongs to us all. <https://assets.publishing.service.gov.uk/government/uploads/system/uploads/attachment_data/file/480482/NHS_Constitution_WEB.pdf>

NHS England. (2015b). Improving experience of care through people who use services. <https://www.england.nhs.uk/wp-content/uploads/2013/08/imp-exp-care.pdf>

NHS England. (2019a). The NHS long-term plan. <https://www.longtermplan.nhs.uk/wp-content/uploads/2019/08/nhs-long-term-plan-version-1.2.pdf>

NHS England. (2019b). Comprehensive model of personalised care. <https://www.england.nhs.uk/publication/comprehensive-model-of-personalised-care/>

NHS England. (2020). We are the NHS: People plan for 2020–21 – Action for us all. <https://www.england.nhs.uk/wp-content/uploads/2020/07/We_Are_The_NHS_Action_For_All_Of_Us_FINAL_24_08_20.pdf>

NHS England. (2021) Integrated Care Pioneers. https://www.england.nhs.uk/integrated-care-pioneers/

NHS England and NHS Improvement. (2020). The framework for enhanced health in care homes version 2. <https://www.england.nhs.uk/wp-content/uploads/2020/03/the-framework-for-enhanced-health-in-care-homes-v2-0.pdf>

NHS Improvement and Leadership Development Board. (2016). Developing people – Improving care: A national framework for action on improvement and leadership development in NHS-funded services. <https://improvement.nhs.uk/documents/542/Developing_People-Improving_Care-010216.pdf>

NHS Leadership Academy. (2013). NHS healthcare leadership model: The nine dimensions of leadership behaviour. <https://www.leadershipacademy.nhs.uk/wp-content/uploads/2014/10/NHSLeadership-LeadershipModel-colour.pdf>

NHS Scotland. (2009). Delivering quality through leadership: The NHS Scotland leadership qualities framework. <https://www.gov.scot/binaries/content/documents/govscot/publications/strategy-plan/2010/01/delivering-quality-through-leadership-nhsscotland-leadership-development-strategy/documents/0088790-pdf/0088790-pdf/govscot%3Adocument/0088790.pdf>

NHS Social Partnership Forum. (2016). Creating a culture of civility, compassion and respect. <https://www.socialpartnershipforum.org/priority-areas/creating-a-culture-of-civility,-compassion-respect/>

NHS Wakefield Clinical Commissioning Group. (2020). Connecting care hubs. <https://www.wakefieldccg.nhs.uk/home/patient-in-wakefield/connecting-care/about-connecting-care/connecting-care-programmes/connecting-care-hubs/>

Office for National Statistics. (2015). How has life expectancy changed over time? <https://www.ons.gov.uk/peoplepopulationandcommunity/birthsdeathsandmarriages/lifeexpectancies/articles/howhaslifeexpectancychangedovertime/2015-09-09>

Office for National Statistics. (2020). Leading causes of death in the UK, 2001-18. <https://www.ons.gov.uk/releases/leadingcausesofdeathuk>

Public Health England. (2020). Beyond the data: Understanding the impact of COVID-19 on BAME groups. <https://assets.publishing.service.gov.uk/government/uploads/system/uploads/attachment_data/file/892376/COVID_stakeholder_engagement_synthesis_beyond_the_data.pdf>

Sanderson, H. (2018). (Editorial) Wellbeing teams: Making self-managing homecare a reality. *Care Management Matters*, June, 30. <https://issuu.com/carechoices/docs/cmm_15.4_june_2018_lr?e=7472320/61617535>.

Senge, P., Hamilton, H., & Kania, J. (2015). The dawn of system leadership. Stanford Social Innovation Review. <https://ssir.org/articles/entry/the_dawn_of_system_leadership>

Snowden, D. (2020). The Cynefin framework. <https://www.cognitive-edge.com/the-cynefin-framework/>

Stocks-Rankin, C., Seale, B., & Mead, N. (2018). Unleashing healthy communities. Full report. Bromley By Bow Insights. <https://www.bbbc.org.uk/wp-content/uploads/2018/07/BBBC-UnleashingHealthyCommunities-FullReport-June2018.pdf>

Stoye, G. (2017, May 3). UK health spending. Institute for Fiscal Studies. <https://www.ifs.org.uk/publications/9186>

The Centre for Patient Leadership. (2013). The engagement cycle. <http://engagementcycle.org/about-us/centre-for-patient-leadership/>

The Health Foundation. (2020). The long-term impacts of new care models on hospital use: An evaluation of the Integrated Care Transformation Programme in Mid-Nottinghamshire. <https://www.health.org.uk/publications/reports/the-long-term-impacts-of-new-care-models-on-hospital-use-midnotts>

Timmins, N. (2015). The practice of system leadership: Being comfortable in chaos. The King's Fund. <https://www.kingsfund.org.uk/sites/default/files/field/field_publication_file/System-leadership-Kings-Fund-May-2015.pdf>.

Walker, S. (2019). Plotting the right path with care navigators. NHS England (blog, 4 February). <https://www.england.nhs.uk/blog/plotting-the-right-path-with-care-navigators/#:~:text=Care%20Navigators%20can%20have%20a,in%20managing%20their%20own%20health>

Weir, B. (2019). Space-based leadership: The real challenge in systems: *Centre for Health and Social Care Leadership*. University of Birmingham. <https://www.birmingham.ac.uk/research/health-and-social-care-leadership/news/2019/space-based-leadership.aspx>.

York, C.V.S. (2020). Ways to wellbeing: Growing social prescribing. https://www.yorkcvs.org.uk/ways-to-wellbeing/

Zanon. E. (2015). *Germany's approach to integrated care is delivering a trio of achievements*. NHS Confederation, European Office. <https://www.nhsconfed.org/blog/2015/07/improving-health-integrating-services-and-reducing-costs>.

## REFLECTIVE QUESTIONS

- Based on your own experiences, how far is the idea of leadership as being grounded in behaviors and actions understood and practiced in your organization? How far do you practice it?

- How do you work with colleagues to come to a collective understanding of whether you are facing a complex, as opposed to complicated, issue?

- How do you practice leadership with your team so that they understand how to work in complexity? How much space do you give them to experiment and innovate? Are they—are you—allowed to shut down what is not working?

- If you think of someone you respected who practiced compassionate leadership in a difficult situation, how did they act, and what did they do? What were the outcomes?

- If you are working in and with communities, how might you support them to develop their leadership?

- How might you capture and sustain what you are learning about leadership?

- How might you enable others to share their learning about leadership to strengthen leadership capacity across a team, organization, community, or system?

# 3

# CRAFTING POSITIVE ORGANIZATIONAL CULTURE AND BEHAVIOR IN 21ST CENTURY HEALTH AND SOCIAL CARE: FUTURE IMPLICATIONS FOR LEADERSHIP

CAROL L. HUSTON

## OBJECTIVES

*After reading this chapter, you should be able to:*

- Describe the four organizational models (clan, hierarchy, adhocracy, and market) commonly found in organizations.
- Discuss why positive work cultures are critical for organizational success.
- Identify at least three potential threats to creating and maintaining positive organizational cultures.
- Explore the role leaders play in creating and then actively sustaining a positive organizational culture.
- Identify at least four strategies both leaders and workers can use to create work cultures that encourage excellence, productivity, innovation, and ethical behavior.

## INTRODUCTION

We have likely all worked in organizations where the work was stimulating, desired outcomes were achieved, innovation and risk-taking were encouraged, co-workers were supportive, and workers felt empowered by management. We have also likely worked in organizations where the opposite was true. What factors contributed to the difference? In all probability, it was the intentional efforts of organizational leaders to create a positive organizational culture and shape behavior expectations accordingly.

Huston (2020, p. xi) notes that "positive work cultures don't happen by accident. They happen because of the hard work of many people, but especially the individuals who hold both formal and informal leadership roles in that culture." Indeed, "culture is everything to a team, and while everyone on the team plays a part in the ongoing development of the culture, it's the leader's responsibility to create and mold it" (Eades, 2018, para. 4). Culture, then, should not be taken for granted; it must be actively created and maintained.

This chapter defines organizational culture; describes culture types; suggests why positive work culture matters; identifies threats to creating positive work cultures; explores the role leaders play in shaping positive cultures; and suggests strategies that both leaders and workers can use to create work cultures that encourage excellence, productivity, innovation, and ethical behavior. It should be noted that while this book specifically targets workers in health and social care organizations, this chapter generally refers to organizations in the broadest sense. This is because health and social care organizations represent a wide range of diverse entities globally, from professionals leading and managing care independently in client's own homes or connected collaboratively in widely spread interprofessional teams, to institutions where formal leadership and management occur in overt hierarchical structures. For this reason, "organizational culture" in this chapter should be applied whenever possible to each reader's own work setting.

In addition, while organizational culture is recognized as a global phenomenon, it should be acknowledged that the description of what constitutes positive organizational culture and behavior differs around the world. For example, a recent study undertaken by Yo-Jud Cheng and Groysberg (2020) finds that caring is a global organizational value, while authority is one of the least salient cultural attributes. Moreover, the cultural attributes that explain how people can and should respond to change (more specifically, organizations' tendencies toward stability versus flexibility) significantly vary worldwide.

Additionally, research by Steelcase of 100 workspaces in China, France, Germany, Great Britain, India, Italy, Morocco, Spain, Russia, the Netherlands, and the United States found that the notion of hierarchy, collaboration, and mobility, and the different ways that these can manifest, can vary significantly according to cultural values (Cagnol, 2013). Thus, coworking and "alternative workspaces" should take cultural differences into consideration. Certainly, it should be recognized that the literature used to support the arguments in this chapter primarily reflects the values and beliefs of western cultures.

## ORGANIZATIONAL CULTURE

The Business Dictionary (2020, para. 1) defines an organizational culture as:

> the values and behaviors that contribute to the unique social and psychological environment of an organization. Organizational culture includes an organization's expectations, experiences, philosophy, and values that hold it together, and is expressed in its self-image, inner workings, interactions with the outside world, and future expectations. It is based on shared attitudes, beliefs, customs, and written and unwritten rules that have been developed over time and are considered valid.

Wagner (2020, para. 1) defines an organizational culture simply as "how things are done around here," which dictates the core values, underlying beliefs, processes, and standards that thrive in an organization. Both definitions suggest that culture provides an organization's "feel" and determines what is right or wrong, important or unimportant, and workable or unworkable. In other words, culture is everywhere and affects everything (Huston, 2020).

### Culture Types

Quinn and Cameron (Organizational Culture Assessment Instrument (OCAI), 2010) developed the Competing Values Framework Model, which maps out four organizational models or cultural types commonly found in organizations. These types are clan, hierarchy, adhocracy, and market (Fig. 3-1)

- **Clan cultures** are exemplified in small companies or businesses and are intimate in nature. Thus, interpersonal connections are close and the focus on affiliation needs is strong. Communication is simple and direct, and the organization is bound by commitment and tradition.
- **Hierarchy cultures** are more formalized and structured. Adherence to policies and procedures create efficiency and predictability; therefore, productivity is usually high.

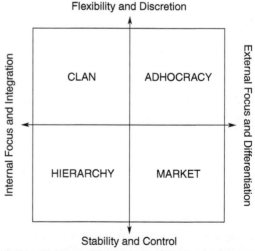

**Fig. 3-1** ■ Quinn and Cameron's typology of cultures commonly found in organizations. (Source: Organizational Culture Assessment Instrument (OCAI). (2010). Organizational Culture Assessment Instrument (OCAI) explained. https://ocai.wordpress.com/2010LeadCla/05/21/organizational-culture-assessment-instrument-ocai-explained/. Reproduced with permission from Kim Cameron.)

- **Adhocracy cultures** are energetic and creative, encouraging risk-taking and innovation. The focus is on establishing a preferred future by creating new resources; thus individual ingenuity and risk-taking are rewarded.
- **Market cultures** focus on achieving desired outcomes through competition. Workers must strive to meet the high expectations of organizational leaders and ensure that organizational reputation and success are secured.

Typically, organizations have one leading culture style, but Quinn and Cameron (OCAI, 2010) suggest that most organizations have more than one culture type. Indeed, many organizations have a mix of the four organizational cultures and these differing cultures can compete against each other. Leaders then must work to suppress or control the competing cultures that threaten the desired culture style while recognizing there are positive qualities inherent in each culture that may contribute to organizational well-being.

While there is no one best culture style for all organizations, the determination of which culture style leaders want to promote depends on the organization's primary values. The Society for Human Resource Management (SHRM, 2020) suggests that the common organizational values that should be considered in selecting the best culture for an organization include but are not limited to those listed in as follows:

- **Outcome orientation:** Emphasizing achievements and results
- **People orientation:** Insisting on fairness, tolerance, and respect for the individual
- **Team orientation:** Emphasizing and rewarding collaboration
- **Attention to detail:** Valuing precision and approaching situations and problems analytically
- **Stability:** Providing security and following a predictable course
- **Innovation:** Encouraging experimentation and risk-taking
- **Aggressiveness:** Stimulating a fiercely competitive spirit

Once organizational leaders have clarity about which organizational values are held most highly, the desired leading culture becomes more apparent, and these values can be made transparent in everything the organization does and the behaviors it encourages.

## WHY DOES CULTURE MATTER?

Culture affects nearly every aspect of an organization, whether positively or negatively. Indeed, Morgan (2017) suggests that an organization's culture determines how employees are treated, the products or services that are created, the partnerships that are established, and even how employees get their jobs done. Thus, organizational culture can both catalyze and undermine organizational success (Corritore et al., 2020). Research by Deloitte finds that 94% of executives and 88% of employees in their US sample believed a positive work culture was important to organizational success (Kohll, 2018).

Not unexpectedly, a positive work culture is considered a common denominator among successful organizations globally. This is because, in positive work cultures, employees not only enjoy their work, they also perform at high levels and develop a feeling of loyalty and attachment to their employing organization (Juneja, 2020). In addition, employees who work in positive work cultures feel more encouraged to get to know their coworkers and team members. When everyone is interested in getting to truly know the people they spend each day with, collaboration in the work environment is more likely to occur (Craig, 2017). Positive work cultures also inspire creativity. When employees feel that they can speak up about new ideas for solving problems or improving services, creativity increases, and fresh perspectives play an important role in increasing productivity (Craig, 2017).

In addition, research has found a strong correlation between a positive work culture and US employees who claim to feel happy and valued at work. Positive cultures also improve employee retention; foster a sense of employee loyalty; facilitate social interaction, teamwork, and open communication; boost employee morale; reduce workplace stress; and increase productivity (Kohll, 2018).

By contrast, negative or toxic work environments almost always either lead to or are indicative of organizational culture failure. Tynan (2020, para. 2) defines a toxic workplace as "any job where the work, the atmosphere, the people, or any combination of those things cause serious disruptions in the rest of your life." Indicators of a toxic or negative workplace culture include high levels of employee burnout, fatigue, and illness; narcissistic leadership; little to no enthusiasm in the work environment; a lack of communication or negative communication; high turnover; and the overwhelming presence of infighting, cliques, gossip, and rumors (Tynan, 2020).

One example of organizational culture failure occurred at a small district general hospital in Staffordshire, United Kingdom, over a 50-month period (January 2005–March 2009), when somewhere between 400 and 1,200 patients died as a result of poor care (Francis, 2013). The hospital was run by the Mid Staffordshire NHS Hospital Trust, which in 2008 acquired Foundation Trust status, making it semi-independent of Department of Health (DH) control. Public inquiries chaired by Robert Francis QC noted that poor decision-making and a focus on extreme cost-cutting were key reasons why poor care took hold and was allowed to persist for so long (Campbell, 2013; Francis, 2013). The inquiries also revealed a profound crisis of culture at every level of the health service (Holmes, 2013, para. 8), including

> a deep rooted, pernicious cult of management, obsessed with achieving ill-conceived targets yet isolated and willfully oblivious to day-to-day operational reality, and fixated on image management and cultivating positive publicity while demonstrating little or no interest in acknowledging or addressing problems.

In addition, an oppressive culture existed in which intimidation and bullying were rife, preventing staff from raising concerns or when they were raised, sweeping them under the carpet (Holmes, 2013). In parallel, the multiplicity of bodies with regulatory and oversight responsibilities in the NHS seemed to be either unaware or complacent in terms of oversight and response (Francis, 2013). Indeed, the report suggested that the solution to this cultural crisis was nothing short of a cultural revolution that called for re-founding the current system to reemphasize what was truly important: establishment of a strong commitment to common values throughout the system;

zero tolerance of noncompliance with fundamental standards of care; a revision of the NHS Constitution to ensure transparency and candor in all of the system's business; strong leadership in nursing and other professional values; more support and training for those in leadership roles; true accountability; and accessible information to enable comparison of performance by individuals, services, and organizations (Francis, 2013; Holmes, 2013). The report concluded that a common and positive culture could be created but only if all these interventions were implemented.

## THREATS TO POSITIVE WORK CULTURES

There are many threats to creating and maintaining a positive work culture. Only four are detailed in this chapter: a lack of vision, bullying and incivility, negative attitudes and big egos, and mergers and acquisitions.

### Lack of Vision

Purpose or meaning is a fundamental human need. "Leaders who understand, engage in, and effectively communicate a shared vision build positive workplace cultures where employees know why they are turning up to work every day, and what their role is in the shared vision" (Cridland, 2014, para. 25). Theodore Hesburgh, President of the University of Notre Dame, agrees, suggesting that the very essence of leadership is having a vision; moreover, it must be a vision that can be articulated clearly and forcefully on every occasion (Heathfield, 2019a). This is why vision is one of the hallmarks of leadership; it is about movement toward a goal, betterment, growth, or success. Thus, it communicates possibilities and solutions to both current problems and future challenges.

Unfortunately, some people in leadership positions lack either the capacity or risk-taking necessary to be visionary. Instead, they simply accept their current circumstances with few questions or ideas for betterment. Without the drive to find a better way, forge a new path, or change the world around them in any way, complacency can result in defeat (Strategic Manipulation, 2018). There is nothing more demoralizing than a leader who cannot clearly articulate why he or she is doing what they are doing (Kouzes & Posner, 2017).

There must also, however, be an action component to vision. Visions that are carefully developed but not implemented are pointless. Leadership expert Warren Bennis notes that leadership is the capacity to translate vision into reality (Leadership, 2020). When leaders develop and share their vision, a road map is created of what needs to happen next, and workers feel more secure that their efforts are directed at achieving a higher goal.

## Bullying and Incivility

Bullying and incivility in the workplace are recognized globally as threats to workplace culture. Indeed, recent research with samples from Australia, Canada, China, Korea, the Philippines, Singapore, the United Kingdom, Sweden, South Africa, and Japan finds that 77% of respondents reported experiencing at least one uncivil behavior in the past year, and one-third experienced uncivil behavior at least once a month (Chen et al., 2019). The Workplace Bullying Institute (2019) defines bullying as repeated, health-harming mistreatment of one or more persons (the targets) by one or more perpetrators. Even a series of seemingly trivial actions added up over time can constitute bullying (Heathfield, 2019a). Black (2018) defines bullying as repeated and unreasonable behavior directed toward a worker or a group of workers that creates a risk to health and safety, while the American Nurses Association defines bullying as "repeated, unwanted, harmful actions intended to humiliate, offend, and cause distress in the recipient" (Civility Best Practices, 2018, para. 1). All three definitions imply bullying is abusive conduct that is threatening, humiliating, or intimidating in nature. When it occurs between coworkers, it is known as horizontal bullying.

Incivility is another term used to describe mistreatment or discourtesy to another person. Clark (2017) sees incivility as a continuum, with disruptive behaviors such as eye-rolling and other nonverbal behaviors and sarcastic comments on one end of the spectrum and threatening behaviors such as intimidation and physical violence on the opposite end. In addition, bullying can manifest as mobbing, when employees "gang up" on an individual. The degree of harm a worker experiences from bullying or mobbing often depends on the frequency, intensity, and duration of the behavior and/or tactic used (Hockley, 2020).

Moreover, what one person considers to be a harmful experience, another may not. Therefore, every person's experience with or perceptions about bullying and incivility are unique to that person (Hockley, 2020).

When bullying, incivility, and mobbing occur in the workplace, it is known as workplace violence. Hockley (2020) maintains that while workplace violence can include physical violence, it can also involve various antisocial behaviors and incidents that lead a person to believe that they have been harmed by the experience. It includes, but is not limited to, such behaviors as engaging in favoritism, being verbally abusive, sending abusive correspondence, bullying, pranks, and setting workers up for failure. Workplace violence can extend to economic aggression, such as denying workers promotional opportunities

While workplace violence occurs in all sectors, health care has been noted to be one where it is most prevalent. Indeed, Edmonson and Zelonka (2019) suggest the problem is endemic in nursing, noting that it typically begins well before nursing school and continues throughout a nurse's career. This bullying culture contributes to the significant percentage of nurses who leave their first job and results in increased risk to patients, lower patient satisfaction scores, and greater nurse turnover.

Research by Cassie and Crank (2018) suggests that workplace bullying also impacts social workers in the United States at a higher rate than the general population. In their study, characteristics associated with bullying included emotional exhaustion, depersonalization, dedication, absorption, and race. Unfortunately, bullying and incivility are common in organizations with negative work cultures; this negatively impacts everyone and what is trying to be achieved. Hockley (2020) maintains that the responsibility for dealing with workplace violence should initially lie with frontline workers, but organizational leaders must become involved if the problem is not immediately resolved. In addition, organizations must have a workplace violence policy in place that clearly describes zero tolerance as the expectation, because bullying and incivility should never be a part of workplace culture.

## Negative Attitudes and Big Egos

Juneja (2020) suggests that negative attitudes and big egos are two of the biggest threats to organization culture. Indeed, having just a few disengaged or incompetent employees can sow the seeds of a negative culture and potentially ruin the performance of an entire organization (McCarthy, 2019) This is because disgruntled, unhappy, constantly complaining individuals demoralize everyone around them and create a culture where no one even wants to come to work. Productivity plummets and employees withdraw. In contrast, positive attitudes at work generally lead to positive outcomes. In fact, happy individuals are more successful in many areas of their lives, especially at work, compared with those who struggle to find happiness or think positively (Mind Tools Content Team, 2020).

Effective organizational leaders recognize that the root cause of negative employee attitudes may be personal problems, so exploring the cause of the bad behavior and offering support to the employee is often an effective first step. It is important, however, not to excuse or minimize the bad behavior. Remember, too, that it does not help anyone if you focus on everything that is wrong or negative about a worker's actions and outlook (Sodexo, 2019). If anything, it will only cause more negative feelings and deeper resentment. Instead, focus on the solution by using effective coaching skills. Give employees with negative attitudes a goal and explain why it matters (Sodexo, 2019). Include them in the process of finding a solution for their negative attitude. "Be firm about establishing a reasonable timeline for behavioral change and make a well-documented record of their progress. That way, your judgment toward their attitude will always be objective" (Sodexo, 2019, para. 14).

Sometimes, however, all the coaching in the world will not deter the unhappy worker and continuing to employ them threatens the stability of the positive culture you are working so hard to create. Their attitude and behaviors simply do not fit with your work culture. In those cases where a worker cannot or will not modify their behaviors to fit the organization's desired culture, that employee must be terminated. Failure to do so reduces other employees' trust in management to protect them from repeated negativity and sends a message that unacceptable behavior will be tolerated.

Similarly, individuals who bring their egos to work make it difficult to establish a positive work culture because it is difficult for ego-driven individuals to work well in teams or relate to fellow workers. Martin (2019,

para. 9) notes that, "Typically, egomaniacs manifest themselves in the workplace as those individuals who refuse to admit when they are wrong and may diminish other's achievements or attempt to undermine their co-worker's accomplishments by sabotaging or derailing projects through passive-aggressive behavior."

Martin (2019) notes, however, that there is a difference between having a big ego (or weak ego) and a strong ego or strong personality. "The person with the 'big' or 'weak' ego needs constant validation and feels threatened by anyone whom they perceive to be more intelligent, more attractive or having more of any desirable trait than they perceive themselves to have. A strong ego, on the other hand, is often described as having a strong personality" (Martin, 2019, paras. 2–3). Like employees with negative attitudes, employees with big egos generally need to have their behavior addressed. These interpretations, however, may vary globally. Organizations with positive work cultures must have employees who can function effectively within teams and who can focus on what is best for the organization instead of themselves.

## Mergers and Acquisitions

SHRM suggests that mergers and acquisitions pose specific challenges to work cultures, even when work cultures have historically been positive. Indeed, two out of three mergers fail because of cultural problems (SHRM, 2020). This is because there is typically a need to blend and redefine the culture, reconcile the differences between them, and build a shared vision for the future.

When cultures are merged, organization leaders have three choices: attempt to destroy the existing cultures, nurture the existing cultures, or evolve them (Solomon, 2018). The most appropriate response depends on the situation. Destroying the existing cultures and replacing them with something new is both the most ambitious and riskiest, although it may be necessary if failure to achieve it will mean the ultimate death of the organization. Surrendering to the existing cultures is easier, although the ability to successfully steward/sustain an existing culture depends on that culture's strength and viability. If the existing cultures are strong, then stewardship is easy, but if they are weak, it becomes much harder. Evolving a new culture is frequently the best choice for leaders who want to effectively make changes (Solomon, 2018). Evolving the culture involves embracing what is good and replacing what is bad.

## SUMMARY POINTS

- Building and sustaining a positive culture requires a leader's interpersonal, teambuilding, and communication skills.
- The *Competing Values Framework Model* maps out four organizational models or cultural types commonly found in organizations. These types are clan, hierarchy, adhocracy, and market.
- Typically, organizations have one leading culture style, but most also have more than one culture type. These culture types can compete.
- There is no one best culture style for all organizations.
- The determination of which culture style leaders want to promote depends on the organization's primary values.
- Organizational culture can both catalyze and undermine organizational success.
- A positive work culture is endemic to successful health and social care organizations.
- Threats to positive work cultures include a lack of vision by the organization's leaders, bullying and incivility, negative attitudes and big egos, and mergers and acquisitions.

## STRATEGIES FOR CREATING POSITIVE WORK CULTURES THAT PROMOTE DESIRED BEHAVIORS

There are almost limitless strategies for creating positive work cultures in health and social care organizations to promote desired behaviors; eight are detailed in this chapter.

1. Know who you are/have a clear brand
2. Remember that people matter; recognize and appreciate them
3. Give workers a voice
4. Seek cultural fit and cultural adaptability in hiring
5. Foster diversity, inclusion, and cultural humility
6. Build effective teams
7. Identify and address organizational conflict in its early stages
8. Communicate endlessly

### Know Who You Are/Have a Clear Brand

SHRM (2020, para. 1) notes that the key to a successful organization is having a culture based on a strongly held and widely shared set of beliefs that are supported by strategy and structure. "When an organization has a strong culture, three things happen: Employees know how top management wants them to respond to any situation, employees believe that the expected response is the proper one, and employees know that they will be rewarded for demonstrating the organization's values."

Indeed, a clear brand is needed to unify an organizational culture and give workers a theme or concept to rally behind for every touchpoint along the way, big and small (McCarthy, 2019). Patterson (2020) suggests, however, that despite all the talk about "purpose" in organizations, many of the people practices (the symbols, stories, and rituals that organizations have in place) are outdated or, even worse, fly in the face of the organization's stated purpose. Organizations cannot get away with random or disconnected people practices, so leaders must ensure that these practices are reviewed periodically and designed in a way that links them to the organization's purpose (Patterson, 2020).

When an organization has clarity about its purpose and the actions taken are consistent with its mission and goals, employees feel secure about what their organization is trying to achieve and the role they play in making that happen. "When employees have a real sense of purpose, they feel connected to the organization and are more likely to put in their best work because they want to, not just because they need to" (Morgan, 2017, para. 6). They also are more apt to stay in their jobs. Using nationally representative data on US public school teachers, Hayes and Stazyk (2019) find that the teachers were at least 11% more likely to remain at their current school if they agreed that most of their colleagues shared their beliefs and values about what the school's central mission should be, compared with teachers who did not agree. In addition, the positive relationship between mission congruence among staff and employee turnover was quite robust, given that all types of teachers responded similarly when mission congruence among staff was high.

## Remember that People Matter; Recognize and Appreciate Them

Cridland (2014) notes that the most important part of any organization is its people, which is why organizations that focus on people are better able to create positive workplace cultures. When employees are treated as people, not as assets, they are happier and more engaged (Sullens, 2018). Indeed, Cridland (2014, para. 21) notes John C. Maxwell's famous saying that "People don't care how much you know until they know how much you care." Since caring involves thought, foresight, and consistency, when people know you care, they are likely to go out of their way to also show care in what they do (Cridland, 2014). Simply put, when it comes to human interaction, empathy is important. "Engaging employees and having empathy for them and their lives is fundamental to creating relationships as well as culture" (6Q, 2020, para. 21).

Also important is having appropriate employee rewards. Appreciation can be shown in many formal ways, including awards, promotions, and pay increases (Cridland, 2014). Having a transparent policy for progression and promotion is also important for creating a positive work culture because when goals are positively reinforced and achievements are recognized and celebrated, employees feel valued, creating pride and ownership (Agarwal, 2018). They are then willing to invest their future in the organization and work hard to create opportunities that will benefit the organization. These formal ways of showing appreciation, however, should occur in addition to daily acts of gratitude and appreciation such as regularly and sincerely saying "thank you."

The reality is that people feel good about doing business with companies that treat their people well, and employees who are treated well do good work. Southwest Airlines, a US-based airline, is an example of a company that has actively worked to create an "employee-first" organizational culture. The Southwest mantra is that: "If we treat our employees right, they will treat our customers right, and in turn that results in increased business and profits that make everyone happy" (McCarthy, 2019, para. 16).

## Give Workers a Voice

Fortunately, most employees want to be part of something bigger than themselves. "They no longer work for companies just to have the company name on their resume. Employees, particularly the younger generations, want to know why they are doing what they are doing. It is not enough to just know how, they want to know the impact of their efforts. They want to feel intimately connected to the goal and to their part in reaching that goal" (Work Points Play, 2019, para. 2).

Since people have options in terms of where they work, they also want a say in shaping work cultures from the ground up (Patterson, 2020). This trend toward increasing employee activism, which is defined as employees coming together to make their voices heard to effect change within organizations, includes giving workers a voice in designing that change. Patterson noted that it is not a new concept to include those affected by change in the conversation, but a shift has occurred from a "push" model to more of a "pull" model. This has allowed workers to be part of solving the important issues organizations face and suggest solutions that might not have been identified from the "ivory tower."

When employees are highly engaged (the term used to describe an employee's emotional commitment to the organization and its goals), they enjoy their work, find it meaningful, and work hard to achieve shared goals (Huston, 2020). They are also excited about the future because they know where they are headed and feel they can play a role in reaching important organizational goals. Feeling valued, being treated fairly, receiving feedback and direction, and generally having strong working relationships between employees and their managers that are based on mutual respect, all contribute to employee engagement and the creation of a positive work culture (Custom Insight, 2020).

In addition, organizations in the United States with engaged employees outperform those without by up to 202%, and highly engaged employees are 87% less likely to leave the company they work for (McCarthy, 2019). Similarly, a study in Sweden found that as co-workers perceived an increase in their ability to participate in the organization, pride increased (Ingelsson et al., 2018). This resulted in enhanced involvement and ownership of the organization as a collective. These findings suggest implications for health care settings that seek to alter the traditional silo structure model and move to a participatory model based on caregiver teams.

## SUMMARY POINTS

- A clear brand is needed to unify an organizational culture.
- When organizations have clarity about their purpose and the actions taken are consistent with their mission and goals, employees feel secure about what their organization is trying to achieve and the role they play in making that happen.
- Employees who feel valued and are consistently shown respect and appreciation typically work harder to meet organizational goals.
- Feeling valued; being treated fairly; and receiving honest, constructive feedback and direction contribute to high levels of employee engagement.
- An increasing trend toward employee activism and promoting employee engagement includes giving workers a voice in designing the work culture and participating in organizational change.

### Seek Cultural Fit and Cultural Adaptability in Hiring

Cridland (2014) notes that hiring the right people is essential to positive workplace cultures globally. People with aligned values and behaviors create positive workplace cultures. Consequently, successful organizations spend much time and money on attracting, retaining, and developing people with the right values, cultural fit, and attitude.

To increase the likelihood of a cultural fit, employers should try to hire employees who share the organization's values, norms, and behaviors. Indeed, recent research has found that a high level of cultural fit leads to more promotions, more favorable performance evaluations, higher bonuses, and fewer involuntary departures (Corritore et al., 2020). Cultural adaptability—the ability to rapidly learn and conform to organizational cultural norms as they change over time—is also important and may in fact be even more important for success than cultural fit (Corritore et al., 2020). Research suggests that employees who can quickly adapt to cultural norms as they change over time are more successful than employees who exhibited high cultural fit when

first hired. "These cultural 'adapters' were better able to maintain fit when cultural norms changed or evolved, which is common in organizations operating in fast-moving, dynamic environments" (Corritore et al., 2020, para. 7). This suggests that cultural alignment does not end at the point of hire. Instead, most employees must continually adapt to the behavioral norms of their peers, and those who have long employment tenure at an organization tend to exhibit increasing cultural fit over time.

### Foster Diversity, Inclusion, and Cultural Humility

Positive organizational cultures foster diversity, inclusion, and cultural humility. Indeed, a positive workplace "is one where all the employees are valued, supported and nurtured irrespective of gender, sexual orientation or color" (Agarwal, 2018, para. 5). An inclusive workplace is one that values individual differences in the workforce and makes individuals feel welcome and accepted (Agarwal, 2018). When people from diverse backgrounds, religions, races, sexual orientations, and generations are encouraged to mix and work well together, employees feel freer to be themselves and share their unique points of view (Morgan, 2017).

When significant diversity exists, however, there is greater potential for culture clash. Diversity requires workers to try to better understand culture differences and make efforts to support the rights of others to have cultural values different than their own. Cultural humility exists when someone recognizes that they may have knowledge deficits or biases about other cultures. This recognition occurs as a result of deliberative self-reflection about personal values that may lead to failure to recognize and respond appropriately to significant cultural issues others may be experiencing.

Stewart (2019) suggests that cultural humility gives us a better understanding of cultures different from our own and helps us recognize each patient's unique cultural experiences. Through these efforts, we can promote accessible, affordable, culturally proficient, and high-quality care. Culturally humble people try to continue learning throughout their lives and be humble about their level of knowledge regarding the beliefs and values of others, are aware of their own assumptions and prejudices, and recognize the importance of institutional accountability (Stewart, 2019).

In addition, proponents of cultural diversity often suggest it leads to cognitive diversity, that is, diversity in thoughts and ideas (Corritore et al., 2020). This diversity of thought can contribute to greater creativity and innovation in the organization.

Yet, conventional wisdom suggests that organizations must choose between a homogeneous, efficient culture and a diverse, innovative culture (Corritore et al., 2020). In homogeneous cultures, employees tend to agree about the norms and beliefs guiding their work, which can improve efficiency and coordination, but innovation and creativity may be limited in such an environment. In contrast, a heterogeneous culture sacrifices the benefits of consensus for healthy disagreement among employees, often promoting greater adaptability and innovation. Corritore et al. (2020) suggest, however, that organizations may be able to resolve the trade-off by encouraging diverse cultural ideas while fostering agreement among employees about the importance of a common set of organizational norms and beliefs.

In addition, while managers can increase retention by hiring candidates with a cultural fit, too much emphasis on this can lead to overlooking promising candidates with unique perspectives. Again, cultural adaptability is ultimately a better predictor for creating and maintaining positive work cultures.

## Build Effective Teams

Scudamore (2016, para. 1) suggests that "team building is the most important investment you can make for your employees. That is because teambuilding builds trust, mitigates conflict, encourages communication, and increases collaboration." This makes sense. Cultures are created by people who must come together to achieve organizational goals, so it seems clear that team building is a critical leadership skill in creating positive work cultures. When people work in teams, the chances of confusion and misunderstanding are reduced because communication is more streamlined. In addition, teams understand and believe that thinking, planning, decisions, and actions are better when done cooperatively. When work cultures value collaboration and discourage competition, employees are better able to work together and use all available resources and skills to reach organizational goals (Heathfield, 2019b).

Teambuilding, however, often requires deliberate and sustained effort on the part of organizational leaders. However, while people in every workplace talk about the importance of building teams, many people do not understand the experience of teamwork or how to develop effective teams. Since organizations consist of individuals with different world views, values, fears, and confidence levels, while each employee may understand how their job fits within the hierarchy, they may not recognize that they are a part of a larger team (Huston, 2020). In addition, effective team building as part of creating a positive work culture requires fundamentally rethinking how the organization is structured, from management styles to compensation strategies (Heathfield, 2019b). Work cultures that celebrate individual performance and contributions do not encourage teamwork; they encourage competition.

Consequently, Heathfield (2019b) suggests that to build a positive work culture, leaders must model teamwork and collaboration and be open and receptive to ideas and input from others. In addition, the organization must openly talk about and identify the value of team work, including sharing the organization's stories and folklore that emphasize teamwork. Heathfield also notes that teamwork must be rewarded and recognized, and that the performance management system used must place emphasis and value on teamwork.

In addition, arranging time for specific team-building activities can improve internal communication and encourage employees to work together more comfortably and successfully (Heathfield, 2019b). Scott (2021) agrees, noting that communication and team building are intertwined, since team building activities encourage trust, cooperation, and communication within a group and improving communication enhances how workers interact with one another.

## Identify and Address Organizational Conflict in its Early Stages

Conflict can result anytime there are differences in ideas, values, or feelings between two or more people and should be an expected occurrence in all organizations (Marquis & Huston, 2021). Conflict is also created when there are differences in economic and professional values and when there is competition among professionals for scarce resources.

Restructuring and poorly defined role expectations are also frequent sources of conflict in organizations (Marquis & Huston, 2021).

Conflict, however, is not always negative; it can lead to new ideas or changes that need to be made. Too much conflict (qualitative or quantitative), however, can become a problem since it can disrupt working relationships and result in lower productivity if not managed appropriately. It is imperative, then, that organizational leaders identify the origin of conflict when it first occurs and intervene as necessary to promote cooperative, if not collaborative, conflict resolution (Huston, 2020). Unfortunately, leaders sometimes procrastinate in addressing conflict, even at the risk of the conflict aftermath becoming greater than the original conflict.

Marquis and Huston (2021) also note that at times, organizational leaders must facilitate conflict resolution between others. This occurs when employees simply cannot or will not resolve their differences, and these issues can then escalate and begin to negatively affect work and other employees. While leaders want to give individuals a chance to resolve minor situations informally, it may be wise to address these conflicts early, before resentments develop and the conflict escalates (Browne, 2017). The goal of this conflict resolution should always be a "win-win" situation.

Organizations should also establish written conflict resolution policies for the workplace, and these policies should be reviewed at least annually by a trained human resource professional (Browne, 2017). They must include, at a minimum, an emphasis on respectful communication between all interested parties, the specific steps to be taken in the conflict resolution process, and who to contact to begin the process. In addition, Browne suggests that job descriptions and individual responsibilities must be clear to avoid ambiguity and that the organizational culture should focus on organizational goals rather than individual goals to minimize conflicts of interests.

## Communicate Endlessly

Watson Wyatt (2006, p. 1) notes that "effective communication is the lifeblood of a successful organization. It reinforces the organization's vision, connects employees to the business, fosters process improvement, facilitates change and drives business results by changing employee behavior." Thus effective communication is critical for establishing positive work cultures.

Indeed, organizational leaders have the formal authority and responsibility to communicate endlessly with many people in the organization. Managers must ensure productivity and continuity by appropriately sharing information, and leaders must ensure that communication channels are developed that encourage an open flow of ideas and concerns (Marquis & Huston, 2021). In addition, both leaders and managers must use clear communication to clarify organizational goals and work with teams to reach those goals. Indeed, Agarwal (2018) suggests that leadership and management styles that encourage teamwork and open and honest communication are vital to creating positive workplaces. Communication has always been an important skill for all clinicians and teams (Melnyk et al., 2020).

It is a responsibility of the leader or manager to use communication in such a way that it builds team relationships for mutual goal attainment. "Open and honest communication also means that regular audits are taken to evaluate how people are interacting with each other, feedback is welcomed and taken on board, and opportunities for social interaction are enabled" (Agarwal, 2018, para. 4).

## SUMMARY POINTS

- To increase the likelihood of a cultural fit, employers should seek to hire employees who share the organization's values, norms, and behaviors.
- The need for cultural alignment does not end at the time of hire, which is why cultural adaptability—the ability to rapidly learn and conform to organizational cultural norms as they change over time—is important.
- Positive organizational cultures foster diversity, inclusion, and cultural humility.
- Team building is a critical leadership skill in creating positive work cultures.
- For a positive work culture to exist, organizational leaders must identify the origin of conflicts when they first occur and intervene as necessary to promote cooperative, if not collaborative, conflict resolution.
- Poor internal communication is an undeniable sign of a negative culture
- (6Q, 2020)

## CONCLUSION

Positive attitudes and behaviors in the workplace are the direct result of effective leadership and a positive management style (Agarwal, 2018). Employees want to feel valued at work and know their work is appreciated, their presence is noticed, their ideas are listened to, and they will be compensated appropriately for the work they contribute (Morgan, 2017). Unfortunately, many organizations have work cultures that suggest workers do not matter or that do little to encourage excellence, productivity, innovation, and ethical behavior. Indeed, "toxic behavior, distrust, and resentment, as well as egregious conduct like harassment, discrimination, and bullying are prevalent in today's workplace" (Facility Executive, 2019, para. 1). This is often because organizational leaders lack either the skill or the courage to attempt a culture change. In fact, recent research notes that only 38 percent of US respondents felt that leaders in their organization took proactive steps to create a positive workplace culture (Facility Executive, 2019).

Regrettably, the more entrenched a negative work culture is, the more challenging the change process for a leader. This is when leadership matters most. "Courage is a critical leadership skill and risk taking is a big part of courage. Negative or toxic work cultures will not change on their own. They require the skills of a dedicated and courageous change champion" (Huston, 2020, p. 11). Leaders must recognize the threats or barriers that exist to creating and maintaining positive work cultures, and then consciously and systematically employ strategies to overcome those obstacles. They must then build teams with common values and create a plan that will let workers know they are valued, heard, and appreciated.

Bradberry (2018) suggests it may be helpful to remember that the first step in leading change is always the hardest. Once you take that step, anxiety and fear often dissipate in the name of action. "People who dive headfirst into taking that brutal first step aren't any stronger than the rest of us; they've simply learned that it yields great results… and that procrastination only prolongs their suffering" (para. 7). "No one wants to work in an organization with a negative culture; isn't it better to take the risk to make things better than to sit back and accept a situation where you might have made a difference?" (Huston, 2020, p. 14).

## REFERENCES

6Q. (2020). 10 warning signs of a negative corporate culture. <https://inside.6q.io/10-warning-signs-negative-corporate-culture/>

Agarwal, P. (2018, August 29). How to create a positive workplace culture: *Forbes* <https://www.forbes.com/sites/pragyaagarwaleurope/2018/08/29/how-to-create-a-positive-work-place-culture/#41d3ad174272>

Black, S. E. (2018). Finding strength after bullying in the workplace: A reflective account. *MIDIRS Midwifery Digest*, *28*(1), 23–27.

Bradberry, T. (2018, January 27). 10 harsh lessons that will make you more successful. *Huffington Post* <http://www.huffingtonpost.com/dr-travis-bradberry/10-harsh-lessons-that-wil_b_14422346.html>

Browne, C. (2017, September 26). How to address conflict in the workplace. <https://bizfluent.com/how-7557497-address-conflict-workplace.html>

Business Dictionary. (2020). Organizational culture (definition). <http://www.businessdictionary.com/definition/organizational-culture.html>

Cagnol, R. (2013, March 22). The differences between work cultures found in eleven countries. <http://www.deskmag.com/en/steel-case-maps-work-cultures-among-11-countries>

Campbell, D. (2013, February 6). Mid Staffs hospital scandal: The essential guide. *The Guardian* <https://www.theguardian.com/society/2013/feb/06/mid-staffs-hospital-scandal-guide>

Cassie, K. M., & Crank, A. K. (2018). Bullies in our midst: Workplace bullying among social service workers in long term care facilities. *Human Service Organizations: Management, Leadership & Governance*, *42*(4), 417–431.

Chen, Y., Wang, Z., Peng, Y., Geimer, J., Sharp, O., & Jex, S. (2019). The multidimensionality of workplace incivility: Cross-cultural evidence. *International Journal of Stress Management*, *26*(4), 356–366.

Civility Best Practices for Nurses. (2018). Violence, incivility & Bullying October, November, December. *Kentucky Nurse*, *66*(4), 12–13.

Clark, C. (2017). *Creating and sustaining civility in nursing education* (2nd ed). Sigma Theta Tau International.

Corritore, M., Goldberg, A., & Srivastava, S. B. (2020, January/February). The new analytics of culture. *Harvard Business Review* <https://hbr.org/2020/01/the-new-analytics-of-culture>

Craig, W. (2017). 3 reasons why positive work cultures are more productive: *Forbes* <https://www.forbes.com/sites/williamcraig/2017/07/25/3-reasons-why-positive-work-cultures-are-more-productive/#7d282cc11ede>

Cridland, C. (2014). How you can build a positive workplace culture?: *Mindful Mediation* <http://www.mindfulmediation.com.au/building-positive-workplace-cultures/>

Custom Insight. (2020). What is employee engagement? <http://www.custominsight.com/employee-engagement-survey/what-is-employee-engagement.asp>

Eades, J. (2018, December 11). Want to become a great leader in 2019? Look for these 7 signs. <https://www.inc.com/john-eades/7-signs-you-are-on-your-way-to-becoming-a-great-leader-in-2019.html>

Edmonson, C., & Zelonka, C. (2019). Our own worst enemies: The nurse bullying epidemic. *Nursing Administration Quarterly*, *43*(3), 274–279.

Facility Executive. (2019, November 20). Toxic cultures, negative behaviors prevalent in the workplace. <https://facilityexecutive.com/2019/11/toxic-cultures-negative-behaviors-prevalent-in-the-workplace/>

Francis, R. (2013). Report of the Mid Staffordshire NHS Foundation Trust Public Inquiry. <https://assets.publishing.service.gov.uk/government/uploads/system/uploads/attachment_data/file/279124/0947.pdf>

Hayes, M. S., & Stazyk, E. C. (2019). Mission congruence: To agree or not to agree, and its implications for public employee turnover. *Public Personnel Management*, *48*(4), 513–534.

Heathfield, S.M. (2019a, Nov. 30). Leadership vision. You can't be a real leader who people want to follow without vision. *The Balance Careers*. <https://www.thebalancecareers.com/leadership-vision-1918616>

Heathfield, S.M. (2019b, Nov. 29). Build teamwork into your company culture. *The Balance Careers*. <https://www.thebalancecareers.com/how-to-build-a-teamwork-culture-1918509>

Hockley, C. (2020). Violence in nursing: The expectations and the reality. In C. J. Huston (Ed.), *Professional issues in nursing: Challenges & opportunities* (5th ed). Wolters Kluwer.

Holmes, D. (2013, February 16). Mid Staffordshire scandal highlights NHS cultural crisis. *The Lancet*, *381*(9866), 521–522. https://doi.org/10.1016/S0140-6736(13)60264-0.

Huston, C. J. (2020). *The road to positive work cultures*. Sigma Theta Tau International.

Ingelsson, P., Bäckström, I., & Snyder, K. (2018). Strengthening quality culture in private sector and health care. *Leadership in Health Services*, *31*(3), 276–292.

Juneja, P. (Reviewed by the Management Study Guide Content Team) (2020). Threats to organizational culture. <https://www.managementstudyguide.com/threats-to-organization-culture.htm>

Kohll, A. (2018, August 14). How to build a positive company culture. *Forbes* <https://www.forbes.com/sites/alankohll/2018/08/14/how-to-build-a-positive-company-culture/#49b2447c49b5>.

Kouzes, J. M., & Posner, B. (2017). The leadership challenge: *How to make extraordinary things happen in organizations* (6th ed.). Wiley.

Leadership. (2020). *Psychology Today*. <https://www.psychologytoday.com/us/basics/leadership>

Marquis, B., & Huston, C. (2021). *Leadership roles and management functions* (10th ed.). Wolters Kluwer.

Martin, K. (2019, June 19). Dealing with ego in the workplace. <https://medium.com/the-bad-influence/dealing-with-ego-in-the-workplace-4ddd4f6ddecc>

McCarthy, M. (2019). Why organizational culture matters (and 6 success factors to make it work). <https://www.itagroup.com/insights/why-organizational-culture-matters-and-success-factors>

Melnyk, B., Malloch, K., & Gallagher-Ford, L. (2020). Developing effective leaders to meet 21st century health care challenges. In C. Huston (Ed.), *Professional issues in nursing. Challenges and opportunities* (5th ed.). Chapter 3. Wolters Kluwer.

Mind Tools Content Team (2020). Building a positive team. Helping your people to be happy and engaged. Retrieved Feb. 12, 2020 from <https://www.mindtools.com/pages/article/building-positive-team.htm>

Morgan, J. (2017, December 29). Why culture matters at work. <https://www.inc.com/jacob-morgan/why-culture-matters-at-work.html>

Organizational Culture Assessment Instrument (OCAI). (2010, May 21). Organizational Culture Assessment Instrument (OCAI) explained. <https://ocai.wordpress.com/2010LeadCla/05/21/organizational-culture-assessment-instrument-ocai-explained/>

Patterson, J. (2020, January). 2020 emerging trends in organizational culture. <https://www.augustjackson.com/post/2020-trends-organizational-culture/>

Scott, S. (2021). Team building activities focusing on communication. <https://smallbusiness.chron.com/team-building-activities-focusing-communication-10561.html#:~:text=Team%20building%20activities%20encourage%20trust%2C%20cooperation%20and%20communication,on%20verbal%2C%20nonverbal%20and%20visual%20forms%20of%20communication>

Scudamore, B. (2016, March 9). Why team building is the most important investment you'll make. *Forbes* <https://www.forbes.com/sites/brianscudamore/2016/03/09/why-team-building-is-the-most-important-investment-youll-make/#2a51eaeb617f>

Society for Human Resource Management. (SHRM). (2020). Understanding and developing organizational culture. <https://www.shrm.org/ResourcesAndTools/tools-and-samples/toolkits/Pages/understandinganddevelopingorganizationalculture.aspx>

Sodexo. (2019, Sept. 19). Negative employee attitudes and how to manage them. <https://www.sodexo.ph/blogs/negative-employee-attitudes-and-how-to-manage-them/>

Solomon, M. (2018, October 5). Does culture really eat strategy for lunch? How leadership and company culture interact. *Forbes* <https://www.forbes.com/sites/micahsolomon/2018/10/05/does-culture-really-eat-strategy-for-lunch-how-leadership-and-company-culture-interact/#1fde31903f0d>

Stewart, A. (2019, April 18). Cultural humility is critical to health equity. <https://www.aafp.org/news/blogs/leadervoices/entry/20190418lv-humility.html>

Strategic Manipulation. (2018, November 19). The importance of vision to leadership. <https://strategicmanipulation.wordpress.com/2018/11/19/the-importance-of-vision-to-leadership/>

Sullens, C. (2018). Making the link between wellbeing and culture change. *Occupational Health & Wellbeing*, *70*(4), 9.

Tynan, L. (2020). Signs you're in a toxic work environment — and how to handle it. Top Resume. <https://www.topresume.com/career-advice/how-to-handle-toxic-work-environment>

Wagner, M. (2020, January 27). What is organizational culture? Types of culture models for creating a winning company. <https://blog.walkme.com/what-is-organizational-culture/>

Watson Wyatt. (2006). Effective communication: A leading indicator of financial performance. White Paper from Watson Wyatt Worldwide. <https://www.worldcat.org/title/effective-communication-a-leading-indicator-of-financial-performance-20052006-communication-roi-study/oclc/70910620> <https://www.sociabble.

com/publications/employee-communications/?utm_source=
google&utm_medium=paidsearch&utm_campaign=uk-
ec-textads-icdlwp&gclid=Cj0KCQjw--GFBhDeARIsACH_
kdYnOOt5ggPh9KI-iN5YRr1uxwIQhsatdiAnCzKzSbY-
iv3DEAaspJKMaAsAREALw_wcB> <https://www.sociabble.com/
publications/employee-communications/?utm_source=google&utm_
medium=paidsearch&utm_campaign=uk-ec-textads-
icdlwp&gclid=Cj0KCQjw--GFBhDeARIsACH_kdYnOOt5gg-
Ph9KI-iN5YRr1uxwIQhsatdiAnCzKzSbYiv3DEAaspJKMaAsA-
REALw_wcB>

Workplace Bullying Institute. (2019). Definition of workplace bullying. <http://www.workplacebullying.org/individuals/prob-lem/definition/>

Work Points Play. (2019). The five trends that will impact employee recognition in 2019. <https://workpointsplay.com/blog/2019-employee-recognition-trends>

Yo-Jud Cheng, J., & Groysberg, B. (2020, January 8). How corporate cultures differ around the world. *Harvard Business Review* <https://hbr.org/2020/01/how-corporate-cultures-differ-around-the-world>

## REFLECTIVE QUESTIONS

- In applying the Competing Values Framework Model, what is the leading culture style in the organization in which you are currently employed? What values drove the selection of that cultural style?

- Think about both positive and negative work cultures you have experienced in your past or present employment. What were the most important factors in each situation that determined whether you felt the culture was positive or negative?

- Have you ever attempted to change a negative culture to become more positive? How difficult was it to be a change agent in this role? What were the greatest barriers to this change?

- Does your current employer have clear policies regarding workplace violence, and does your employer enforce a culture of zero tolerance in terms of bullying and incivility? If so, does this negate or minimize the problem?

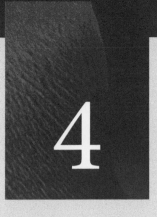

# 4

# STRATEGIC AND EXECUTIVE LEADERSHIP IN HEALTH AND SOCIAL CARE: THROUGH POLITICS AND POWER

SUZIE BAILEY

*"If you find it in your heart to care for somebody else, you will have succeeded."*
**Maya Angelou**

## OBJECTIVES

*After reading this chapter, you should be able to:*

- Describe what is meant by executive/strategic leadership.
- Explain the core duties of the board of directors and the responsibilities of executives and non-executives.
- Describe how politics and national policy help shape the leadership and structure of local systems.
- Outline the range of strategic, operational, and financial issues that board leaders are required to decide.
- Identify how the link between leadership and culture affects the quality of care.
- Summarize the changing role of leaders over time toward greater system leadership.

## INTRODUCTION

To understand some of the complexity faced by those in strategic leadership positions, this chapter explores executive and board leadership in health and social care, identifies core duties and responsibilities, and looks at the changing landscape. The health and social care sector relies on the effective management of millions of people, and the World Health Organization (2016) calculates a future shortage of approximately 18 million health workers, one-fifth of the workforce needed to keep health care systems going. Given the size of this global workforce crisis, executives and board leaders not only have the legal responsibility, but also a moral duty, to create healthy workplace cultures in which staff can do their best work. Therefore, this chapter also

addresses the critical relationship between leadership, culture, and the role of the board. The context, as outlined in Chapter 1, and the global challenges to population health necessitate ever greater collaboration and integration of health and social care services, relying on effective system leadership that goes beyond single institutions. Fundamentally, however, the role of leaders in this sector concerns the care of those in need. The reader is therefore asked to keep in mind that the work of executive/strategic leaders should be in the service of caring for patients, communities, and staff.

The chapter focuses on the health and care system in England in the context of the UK National Health Service (NHS) which was founded over 70 years ago; the NHS is the United Kingdom's largest employer and one of the biggest employers globally. Dixon (2017, para. 6) describes the NHS as "the most complex, risky, and expensive single industry in Europe with the most educated (and intrinsically motivated) staff."

The NHS works in close partnership with social care, where the need for reform and greater investment in England is well known. The context for leadership and management in social care in England differs from that of the NHS. While most social care services are commissioned by local authorities, data show that in 2018, there were 18,500 primarily private sector enterprises involved in providing or organizing adult social care in England (Skills for Care, 2019). These range from large national employers, large charities, and local authority adult social service departments to small independent care services but

41

do not include individuals employing their own care and support staff or the millions of unpaid caregivers. To appreciate the scale, approximately 40 percent of the organizations that currently provide adult social care have one to four employees and about 85 percent have fewer than 50 employees. Most staff work in residential homes and in care and support services provided to people at home, known as domiciliary care. In the past decade, there have been a series of government consultations and proposals for legislative changes related to social care, but none of these proposed reforms have been implemented (Jarrett, 2019). This has resulted in a wider health and social care landscape with unwarranted variation in quality and outcomes for the communities they serve.

While there will be differences from health and social care services in other countries, including the legal, structural, and policy approaches, the principles and challenges of strategic and executive leadership can also be used to explore the context in differing geographical areas.

## STRATEGIC/EXECUTIVE LEADERSHIP

To explore the nature of strategic and executive leadership in the United Kingdom's health and social care sector, it is important to understand a little of both the history that has led to the current leadership arrangements and the context that today's leaders face. The frequent structural changes that have been made to the health and social care sector by successive UK governments have direct implications for the leaders, who must manage and adapt services and ways of working according to those policy changes. The ongoing legislative, structural, and cultural changes continue to impact the delivery of health and social care in England. The reader is encouraged to reflect on the key changes that such legislation has brought about and some of the potential unintended consequences of often well-intended policy changes. Doing so will enable a better understanding of the links and potential tensions that arise when implementing health and social care legislation and national policies.

This analysis begins with the major review of NHS management undertaken by Sir Roy Griffiths in 1983, which resulted in the most significant change

in the management structure of the NHS since its inception in 1948 (Gorsky, 2013). Griffiths concluded that the problems with the NHS were due to the lack of a general management structure, and stated in the accompanying letter to the Secretary of State (Griffiths, 1983, General Observations, para. 5) that, "if Florence Nightingale was carrying her lamp through the corridors of the NHS today, she would almost certainly be searching for the people in charge." He proposed that there should be regional and district managers and a central management board of the NHS within the Department of Health and Social Security. This was based on a business model from industry, which added a new layer of leadership to the NHS to supplement its traditional clinical roots, where doctors and matrons had been the organizational decision-makers. A new business model was introduced with executive and non-executive directors; day-to-day decisions were intended to be made at the hospital and unit levels and doctors would remain closely involved in management decisions. Pollitt et al. (1991) explore the impact of these changes through interviews with over 300 leaders and argue that Griffiths failed to address the powerful relationship and tensions between the NHS and the political system. These tensions remain today, and the NHS is often referred to as a "political football" due to the multiplicity of issues that are of interest and relevance to local and national politics. The authors also criticize Griffiths' view of managers as technicians, failing to recognize the complexities in health care, where managers have to work with greater ambiguity than do business leaders.

The next wide-ranging legislative change to the NHS in England was the Health and Social Care Act (2012). This Act made fundamental changes to every level of the NHS structure, creating an independent NHS Board. Its goal was to promote greater patient choice and reduce NHS administration costs by one-third, including abolishing regional structures and introducing the concept of providing competitively priced NHS care by "any qualified provider." The Act also introduced legal duties for national health bodies regarding health inequalities, which led the way for greater emphasis on population health and the policy drive toward greater integration of health and social care, which is explored later in the chapter.

*It will require leadership of the highest order to manage further organisational change, ensure that the quality of care is kept centre stage and balance budgets. The NHS in 2013 is no place for the faint hearted.*

*(Ham, 2013, para. 9)*

Bevan et al. (2014) highlight the major contrast between the NHS in England and the NHS in Scotland; England has a model based on choice and competition, while there has been a hierarchical yet integrated model in Scotland since 2004. They suggest that the stability of the system in Scotland "is the envy of all who have suffered from the successive 're-disorganisations' in the NHS in England" (Bevan et al., p 34).

It must therefore be asked: What are the main roles of organizational boards in these complex health and social care settings? An NHS board has a duty to ensure effective governance consistent with the Seven Principles of Public Life (Box 4-1), also known as the Nolan Principles (Nolan, 1995), to ensure the organization's long-term vision and strategy. Public office-holders are servants of the public and stewards of public resources and therefore should abide by these principles.

Structurally, a board chair leads the board, and the chief executive leads the organization with a team of executive directors. The executive directors, who include clinical leaders (e.g., a medical director or chief nurse), have operational responsibility for delivering care and performance management. The non-executives on the board have a different role and bring external and independent expertise and judgement regarding strategy, performance, and accountability. Boards hold the organization to account for delivery of the strategy, ensuring value for money, and assuring that risks to the organization and the public are effectively managed and mitigated.

A chair in the NHS (NHS Improvement, 2019) has five responsibilities, which help illustrate the core functions of a board: strategic, people, professional acumen, outcomes focus, and partnerships. Executive and non-executive directors come together as a board to shape the organization's strategic vision and organizational approach and to make decisions. The purpose of NHS boards is to govern effectively, and in so doing, build patient, public, and stakeholder confidence that

---

**BOX 4-1**
## THE SEVEN PRINCIPLES OF PUBLIC LIFE

1. **Selflessness:** Act solely in terms of the public interest.
2. **Integrity:** Avoid placing themselves under any obligation to people or organizations that might try to inappropriately influence them in their work. They should not act or make decisions to gain financial or other material benefits for themselves, their family, or their friends. They must declare and resolve any interests and relationships.
3. **Objectivity:** Act and make decisions impartially, fairly, and on merit, using the best evidence and without discrimination or bias.
4. **Accountability:** Accountable to the public for decisions and actions and must submit to the scrutiny necessary to ensure this.
5. **Openness:** Act and make decisions in an open and transparent manner. Information should not be withheld from the public unless there are clear and lawful reasons for doing so.
6. **Honesty:** Be truthful.
7. **Leadership:** Exhibit these principles in their own behavior. They should actively promote and robustly support the principles and be willing to challenge poor behavior wherever it occurs.

Nolan, L. M. P. (1995). Standards in public life: First report of the Committee on Standards in Public Life. HM Stationery Office. https://assets.publishing.service.gov.uk/government/uploads/system/uploads/attachment_data/file/336919/1stInquiryReport.pdf

---

their health and health care is in safe hands. This may sound like a very technical task, but, to be successful, it relies on the executive and non-executive directors having considerable relational capabilities. Griffin and Stacey (2005) describe how organizations can be understood as processes of humans relating to each other where behaviors range from cooperation/consensus to conflict and competition. These behavioral patterns are also experienced at the board table, so the relationship and level of trust between a CEO and the board chair is an important factor in effective organizational leadership.

## SUMMARY POINTS

- Leading health and social care systems is complex and requires both technical and relational skills.
- The role of leaders is constantly changing and is impacted by national policy and politics.

- Boards must combine the skills and expertise of executive and non-executive leaders to provide effective strategic leadership.
- Boards have a duty to govern well and ensure patient, public, and stakeholder confidence.

## DEVELOPING THE STRATEGIC DIRECTION

Developing the strategic direction of any organization involves a set of choices and principles that support achieving its long-term goals. The development of any strategy in health or social care should also draw on the expertise of staff, patients/clients, communities, and a wide range of stakeholders. Dixon-Woods et al. (2014) conducted the largest multi-method study to date into the culture and behaviors in the English NHS and found that despite many examples of high-quality care, consistently achieving this was hampered by unclear objectives or goals, overlapping priorities, and bureaucratic management that focused too strongly on compliance. They described these as *"priority thickets"* (Dixon-Woods et al., 2014, p. 109). Their study also shows that despite being fundamental to workplace culture and directly related to patient experience, safety, and quality of care, good staff support and management are highly variable within organizations.

As noted in Chapter 3, the critical link between board leadership and quality of care was highlighted by a public inquiry into the serious failings in care at the Mid Staffordshire NHS Foundation Trust. This remains an enduring and powerful illustration of deficiencies in the leadership of health and care services. The litany of failings at the hospital and what led to these continues to be a profound lesson for health leaders in the United Kingdom and beyond. The public inquiry led in 2013 by Sir Robert Francis QC made 290 recommendations and concluded that there had been warning signs that the Board and leadership of the organization had "failed to appreciate the enormity of what was happening, reacted too slowly, if at all, to some matters of concern of which they were aware, and downplayed the significance of others" (Francis, 2013, p. 43). Francis was clear that the Board had prioritized finances over the quality of care and had failed to put patients at the center of their work. Francis drew attention to the board's important role in creating and maintaining culture and identifying the negative cultural aspects (Box 4-2) present in the Mid Staffordshire system. These characteristics offer a clear illustration of how power can be used and abused at the board table, leading to tragic consequences.

An independent review of failings in another UK hospital (Kirkup, 2018, p. 60) concluded that the substantial changes in the NHS underway at the time, including regulatory systems, "impacted significantly the ability to detect developing problems in the Trust and its service provision through external scrutiny." The lead investigator was clear in his conclusion that the constant reorganization of the health and care system may have unintended and harmful consequences.

During this period, another review of leadership in the NHS was undertaken in 2015 by Lord Rose for the Secretary of State for Health (Rose, 2015). While the focus of his review was on leaders in NHS provider organizations and clinical commissioning groups, he concludes that his findings and recommendations are applicable to the whole of the service. He states that the "NHS performs an extraordinary service and is staffed by some extraordinary people, but the whole organization could and should be made more effective by the application of some common-sense tactical and strategic thinking" (Rose, 2015, p. 4).

Various tools can assist with reviews to detect shortcomings in health and social care organizations.

---

**BOX 4-2**

## THE NEGATIVE ASPECTS OF CULTURE IN THE SYSTEM

- Lack of openness to criticism
- Lack of consideration for patients
- Defensiveness
- Looking inward, not outward
- Secrecy
- Misplaced assumptions about the judgements and actions of others
- Acceptance of poor standards
- Failure to put the patient first in everything that is done

---

Francis, R. (2013). Report of the Mid Staffordshire NHS Foundation Trust Public Inquiry: Executive summary. The Stationery Office (Vol. 947). https://assets.publishing.service.gov.uk/government/uploads/system/uploads/attachment_data/file/279124/0947.pdf

The Care Quality Commission has used the Well-Led Framework (NHS Improvement, 2017) to administer a well-led assessment of organizations as part of their inspection regime. The framework is also used by boards to help them review their own effectiveness, including commissioning independent reviews of their leadership. The key lines of enquiry, known by the abbreviation KLOEs (Fig. 4-1), illustrate the range of leadership responsibilities of NHS Boards. The well-led framework is structured around eight KLOEs, and there are more detailed review questions under each KLOE.

Given the scale of the failings at Mid Staffordshire, there were national policy attempts post Francis to help the NHS become a learning organization. Professor Don Berwick, former health advisor to President Obama, President Emeritus, and Senior Fellow, Institute for Healthcare Improvement, led a subsequent review of patient safety in the NHS (Berwick, 2013) in which he discovered an explicit link between leadership, culture, and quality improvement. Jacobs et al. (2013) also provide evidence of the link between culture and organizational performance in hospitals.

Berwick was clear that the NHS needed to establish a culture of learning and placed considerable emphasis on the role modeling and behavior of senior leaders as being critical for sustaining the necessary cultural changes.

*Leadership requires presence and visibility. Leaders need first-hand knowledge of the reality of the system at the front line, and they need to learn directly from and remain connected with those for whom they are responsible. Culture change and continual improvement come from what leaders do, through their commitment, encouragement, compassion and modelling of appropriate behaviours.*

(*Berwick, 2013 p.15*)

*Don Berwick: A promise to learn – a commitment to act: Improving the safety of patients in England (Berwick, 2013 p.15)*

While there has been considerable change and learning in the United Kingdom since the Mid Staffordshire Public Inquiry, the introduction of the systematic

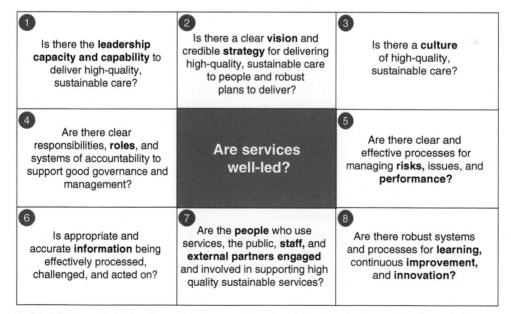

**Fig. 4-1** ■ Well-led framework for key lines of enquiry. (Adapted with permission from NHS Improvement. Developmental reviews of leadership and governance using the well-led framework: Guidance for the NHS trusts and NHS foundation trusts. NHS Improvement, 2017.)

use of the KLOEs, and growth in the use of quality improvement methods, there is also evidence from a mixed methods study (Chambers et al., 2018) that increasing performance pressures, including financial and workforce pressures, may threaten a board's focus on quality. From their research on what changes boards had made since the publication of the Francis Inquiry, the authors suggest that more work is required on the roles of boards as "conscience, as sensor, as diplomat, as coach and as shock absorber" (Chambers et al., 2018, p. 183). They also state that "NHS boards are odd creatures of corporate governance—even Foundation Trusts are not autonomous—the government role of central control is very powerful, and this has also arguably got tighter over recent years" (Chambers et al., 2018, p. 43).

## LEADERSHIP AND CULTURE

*The notion that a few extraordinary people at the top can provide all the leadership needed today is ridiculous and it's a recipe for failure.*

*(Kotter, 2013)*

While Chapter 3 considered organizational culture, this issue is also examined here, particularly in relation to an organization's board and strategic leaders. The King's Fund (2011) initiated a commission to look at the state of management and leadership in the NHS. The commission suggests that the NHS needs to move beyond "heroic" leadership and value leadership that is shared, distributed, and adaptive. There has been growing recognition that "post-heroic" leadership (McCrimmon, 2010) is required, where followers have a key role to play and leaders are required to be skilled facilitators. This represents a shift in emphasis to participative decision-making and a change from more traditional leadership approaches that typically focus on the role of individual leaders. Collective leadership is described by West et al. (2014, p. 4), as "everyone taking responsibility for the success of the organisation as a whole—not just for their own jobs or area." Developing collective leadership within organizations requires strategic leadership commitment to creating enabling cultures and greater emphasis on supporting and developing effective teams.

Health care is complex and no single person can know everything needed to make well-informed leadership decisions. Stacey (2007) calls this the "Zone of Complexity," where people are far from certainty and agreement about the solutions needed to address issues. Gobillot (2007, p. 5) argues that the "real" organization as opposed to the "formal" organization is made up of networks of relationships between people. Within these networks, the best leaders are those who are connected and "channel the vitality of the 'real' organisation to achieve the goals of the 'formal' organisation." This view of leadership is echoed by Hamel and LaBarre (2013, para 2), who describe how true leaders assume no power but have an ability to "mobilise others and accomplish amazing things." They outline the following qualities found in these leaders: "passion, curiosity, compassion, daring, generosity, accountability and grit" (Hamel & LaBarre, 2013, para. 2). Block (1993) also writes of the importance of ownership at every level of the organization and advocates stewardship over leadership as an alternative way to govern institutions, arguing for distributed leadership where employees may be considered partners in serving communities. Bennis and Thomas (2002) discover something novel in their research on leaders: the importance of a quality of neoteny, which is retention of youthful qualities by adults, including curiosity, energy, and fearlessness. They suggest that leaders who can remain open to possibility, learning, and taking risks are much more likely to have the necessary adaptive capacity to thrive in a changing environment.

West et al. (2014a,b), highlight themes that successful health care organizations commonly prioritize; each has an implication for leaders of improvement and for boards. These include how to create a compelling strategic narrative, practice inclusive leadership, empower staff to lead service change, and lead with strong values and integrity. Edmondson (2018) suggests that leaders should create psychological safety in workplaces so people can speak up and be candid about ideas or concerns and colleagues respect and trust one another. However, she argues that most workplaces are not achieving this for their staff.

There is a critical link between culture, leadership, staff health and well-being, and organizational performance. A review by Boorman (2009) into NHS staff health and well-being shows that organizations that focus on staff health and well-being perform better. However, the review team also concludes that the issues were not given enough priority or seen as central to the work of NHS provider organizations, and that the connections were not being made between improving staff health and well-being and organizational performance. The interim report demonstrates the business case for action on staff health and well-being, including an estimate that cutting one-third of NHS staff sickness could generate 3.4 million additional working days a year, equivalent to 14,900 full-time equivalent staff. Boorman's final comment in the foreword to the report (Boorman, 2009) is therefore poignant for a service that is about health and well-being: "the cobbler's children do not deserve bad shoes!"

## INCLUSIVE AND COMPASSIONATE LEADERSHIP

Arguably, diversity and inclusion should be strategic, operational, and moral priorities for all health and care organizations to create inclusive cultures for delivering high-quality health care. However, on equal opportunities and diversity in the workplace, three policy think tanks in the United Kingdom (Beech et al., 2019) are clear in their conclusion that the NHS has failed its workforce. The NHS Staff Survey in England has been conducted since 2013, and the key finding relating to equality, diversity, and inclusion shows a decline since 2015. The results from 2019 (Picker Institute Europe, 2020) demonstrate that, compared with White staff, people from ethnic minority groups experience continued discrimination and higher levels of bullying, harassment, or abuse from other staff.

Health care staff are also subjected to racism by patients and other members of the public during their work, with predictable harmful consequences for their health and well-being. It is critical that executive and non-executive leaders prioritize addressing equality, diversity, and inclusion as a core business. This requires being willing to confront difficult and uncomfortable questions in their individual and collective roles in systemic racism and a relentless commitment to learn and do better regarding race inequality. Cultural change will not be fast or easy to achieve and requires action at every level of any health and social care system.

### Developing People and Leaders

The national strategic framework for the NHS in England, Developing People, Improving Care (NHS Improvement, 2016) recognizes that distributed, inclusive, and compassionate leadership is increasingly essential for delivering high-quality health care (NHS Improvement, 2016).

The framework's aim was to develop a critical set of leadership and improvement capabilities within the workforce, including executive leadership. The framework drew on global research and evidence to set out commitments and actions necessary at the national, regional, and local levels of the health and social care system to develop capabilities in systems leadership, quality improvement methods, inclusive and compassionate leadership, and talent management. The framework was developed by national organizations, including the Department of Health and Social Care, and contained commitments from several of the main arm's length government bodies, such as NHS England, NHS Improvement, and the Care Quality Commission, to ensure its implementation. The framework states the importance of action at every level of the health and social care system to create five conditions (Box 4-3) to develop the leaders and skills necessary for both today's challenges and those up to 20 years in the future.

However, the interim People Plan (National Health Service England (NHS England), 2019a, p. 14) states that Developing People, Improving Care "has

---

**BOX 4-3**
**FIVE CONDITIONS COMMON TO HIGH-QUALITY SYSTEMS**

1. Leaders equipped to develop high-quality local health and care systems in partnership
2. Compassionate, inclusive, and effective leaders at all levels
3. Knowledge of improvement methods and how to use them at all levels
4. Support systems for learning at local, regional, and national levels
5. Enabling, supportive, and aligned regulation and oversight

NHS Improvement. (2016). Developing people improving care. NHS Improvement. https://improvement.nhs.uk/resources/developing-people-improving-care/

not led to the widespread culture change it set out to deliver," admitting that this is in part due to the failure of the national bodies to demonstrate the framework's value. However, it restates the ambition to develop inclusive and compassionate cultures within the NHS. Ten years after the recommendations of the Boorman Review (2009), it is evident there is still a long way to go to create the necessary healthy workplaces for NHS staff.

## SUMMARY POINTS

- Boards must balance strategic, operational, and financial issues to lead successfully.
- The board has a significant role in and responsibility for ensuring delivery of high-quality care.
- There are potentially tragic human consequences if organizations are not led well.
- Culture and leadership are core responsibilities of board directors.
- There is a link between staff health and well-being and organizational performance.
- Health and social care system leadership requires a shift from heroic to collective, inclusive, and compassionate approaches.

## SYSTEM LEADERSHIP AND THE INTEGRATION OF CARE

*Systems leadership recognizes that leadership is not vested in people solely through their authority or position; so it involves sharing leadership with others, coming together on the basis of a shared ambition.*

*(Vize, 2014, p. 2)*

The increasing global emphasis on system integration in the health and social care systems requires health and care leaders to adapt to different ways of working and influencing. Integrated Care Systems (ICSs) are part of the NHS Long-Term Plan (NHS England, 2019b) and are intended to achieve transformation in how health and care services are delivered. The core roles for an ICS are identified as system transformation and collective management of system performance. Such transformation requires effective partnerships between local providers and commissioners and between the NHS and

local authorities, involving the voluntary, community, and social enterprise (VCSE) sector and importantly, citizens and communities.

NHS England has committed to moving to a "system by default" model and to supporting every health care system in every part of the country becoming an ICS by April 2021. Approximately half the population in England is now covered by an ICS, but the current system architecture, including regulation and payment for services in the NHS, is on an institutional, that is, hospital, basis rather than a system basis. The more recent White Paper (DHSC 2021) sets out legislative proposals for a health and care Bill to move more firmly to establish ICSs as statutory bodies across all parts of England (The Kings Fund 2021).

Transitioning the NHS to more integrated ways of working will require significant strategic leadership capability and capacity, and sufficient time for leaders to develop trusting local relationships. Vize (2014, p. 9) also describes the experience of leaders in 25 different geographies where they were addressing a policy, service, or system leadership challenge: "strong, trusting relationships will not be built in formal meetings. The different parties need to get together in ways which allow them to have conversations rather than negotiations, where listening and understanding are just as important as talking." Timmins (2019) suggests that while there has been progress in integrating care in England, it is not easy work and is slow. One of the interviewees, an ICS lead, describes the importance of humility and curiosity and how "the exhausting bit, as a system leader, is that you are managing everyone's fear of loss of control, loss of authority and power" (Timmins, 2019, p. 12).

One of the ambitions is that ICSs will become responsible for quality, financial, and workforce planning and for the transformation of local care. However, despite strong support for the vision in the NHS Long-Term Plan (NHS England, 2019b), there is also growing concern about how "load bearing" ICSs can or should become and the leadership capacity and capability required to manage this. How far can or should they take on responsibility for quality and financial performance as opposed to planning and implementing the "transformation" of care? In other words, what will their relationship eventually be with the center, region, and regulators? There are also concerns about the lack of a pipeline of future leaders for ICSs.

NHS organizations also have the size and assets to be used for wealth building in the local community (Reed et al., 2019). Social determinants of health, such as housing and education, are outside the direct control of the NHS; however, the NHS has considerable influence within local communities in both social and economic terms. The Health Foundation recommends that NHS organizations adopt an "anchor mission," which will require the NHS boards to balance several tensions in their local priorities.

Another model worth viewing and that contrasts with the more typical and dominant centralist approach to management of health and social care is an experiment in the formal devolution of power from the central government to Greater Manchester. Walshe et al. (2016) suggest that Manchester may be in a unique position due to having the history, geography, and local leaders to make this experiment work. They acknowledge the significant courage of local leaders in this pioneering work but also highlight their track record in successful collaboration. Heimans and Timms (2014) describe "old power" as being held by a few whereas "new power" is owned by many; moreover, the aim of "new power" is not to hold on to it. Thus a very important consideration for modern health and care services is how to harness ways of working with "new power." This represents opportunities to radically challenge and change existing paradigms of power and control in health and social care for social justice and equity. However, in addition to the considerable benefits this could bring, it requires radical leadership transformation in how health and social care services are led, co-designed, and delivered, including greater emphasis on the roles of citizens and communities.

## LEADERSHIP LESSONS FROM THE COVID-19 PANDEMIC

The world is currently experiencing a COVID-19 global pandemic; in time, there is likely to be much written about the international experiences of leaders, staff, and systems in health and social care during this period. For now, a brief reflection on health and social care leadership in an unparalleled and yet significant period in our lifetime is provided by the Health Systems Innovation Lab at London South Bank University (Malby & Hufflett, 2020). They conducted a survey of staff from across the NHS, including those involved in direct patient care, and middle, senior, and board leaders, and asked them to reflect on their experiences working in the active phase of the pandemic in England. In their words, the authors describe the results of the survey as "astounding," given some people's descriptions of the positive changes that have been possible through shared purpose, innovations in service delivery, evidence of more engaged leadership, and a flattening of hierarchy. However, there is also concern that, despite some positives, the NHS still needs to change the dominant command-and-control leadership approach.

## SUMMARY POINTS

- There is growing policy emphasis on the need to integrate health and care services for population health.
- System leadership requires a significant shift in leadership and governance approaches, including the roles of citizens and communities.
- Devolution of power from central to local governments is an alternative model to the traditional centralist approach of health and care systems.
- There is considerable learning to be harnessed from the experiences of leading health and social care services throughout the COVID-19 pandemic.

## CONCLUSION

This chapter has outlined the role of executive/strategic leaders and described the main responsibilities of organizational boards in health and social care. Given the demands placed on leaders in the NHS, including constant policy changes and the scrutiny and involvement of national government and politicians, these roles are not for the fainthearted. The task of strategic leadership is also evolving, with greater emphasis on system leadership to transform services and improve the health and well-being of local populations. Post-heroic leaders require good relational skills and the ability to develop collective, inclusive, and compassionate leadership cultures where leadership is distributed. The health and social care sector is, at its heart, a people business and relies on the effective management of millions of staff. Despite all the complexities of leadership today and the demands placed upon it, the role of health and social care executive/strategic leaders is fundamentally about caring for people: patients/clients, staff, and wider communities. Leaders should remain open to feedback and challenge to ensure their personal leadership and behaviors are truly in the service of that moral duty to care for people.

## REFERENCES

Beech, J., Bottery, S., Charlesworth, A., Evans, H., Gershlick, B., Hemmings, N., ... Palmer, W. (2019). *Closing the gap: Key areas for action on the health and care workforce*. The Health Foundation, Nuffield Trust, The King's Fund. <https://www.kingsfund.org.uk/sites/default/files/2019-03/closing-the-gap-health-care-workforce-full-report.pdf>.

Bennis, W. G., & Thomas, R. J. (2002). *Geeks and geezers: How era, values, and defining moments shape leaders*. Harvard School Press.

Berwick, D. (2013). A promise to learn, A commitment to act: Improving the safety of patients in England. National Advisory Group on the Safety of Patients in England. <https://assets.publishing.service.gov.uk/government/uploads/system/uploads/attachment_data/file/226703/Berwick_Report.pdf>

Bevan, G., Karanikolos, M., Exley, J., Nolte, E., Connolly, S., & Mays, N. (2014). The four health systems of the United Kingdom: How do they compare? Summary report. <https://researchonline.lshtm.ac.uk/id/eprint/1649072/1/140411_four_countries_health_systems_full_report.pdf>

Block, P. (1993). *Stewardship: Choosing service over self-interest*. Berrett-Koehler Publishers.

Boorman, S. (2009). NHS health and well-being review: Interim report. <https://webarchive.nationalarchives.gov.uk/20130103004910/http://www.dh.gov.uk/en/Publicationsandstatistics/Publications/PublicationsPolicyAndGuidance/DH_108799>

Chambers, N., Thorlby, R., Boyd, A., Smith, J., Proudlove, N., & Kendrick, H. (2018). *Responses to Francis: Changes in board leadership and governance in acute hospitals in England since 2013*. University of Manchester. <https://www.birmingham.ac.uk/Documents/college-social-sciences/social-policy/Publications-HSMC/2018/Responses-to-Francis-report-January-2018.pdf>.

Dixon, J. (2017). The NHS Five Year Forward View—the task now is delivery. <https://blogs.bmj.com/bmj/2017/04/03/jennifer-dixon-the-nhs-five-year-forward-view-the-task-now-is-delivery/>

Dixon-Woods, M., Baker, R., Charles, K., Dawson, J., Jerzembek, G., Martin, G., ... West, M. (2014). Culture and behaviour in the English National Health Service: Overview of lessons from a large multimethod study. *BMJ Quality and Safety, 23*(2), 106–115.

Edmondson, A. C. (2018). *The fearless organization: Creating psychological safety in the workplace for learning, innovation, and growth*. John Wiley & Sons.

Francis, R. (2013). *Report of the Mid Staffordshire NHS Foundation Trust Public Inquiry: Executive summary* (Vol. 947). The Stationery Office. <https://assets.publishing.service.gov.uk/government/uploads/system/uploads/attachment_data/file/279124/0947.pdf>.

Gobillot, E. (2007). *The connected leader: Creating agile organizations for people, performance and profit*. Kogan Page Publishers.

Gorsky, M. (2013). "Searching for the people in charge": Appraising the 1983 Griffiths NHS Management Inquiry. *Medical History, 57*(1), 87–107. <https://www.ncbi.nlm.nih.gov/pmc/articles/PMC3566753/>.

Griffin, D., & Stacey, R. D. (Eds.). (2005). *Complexity and the experience of leading organizations*. Taylor & Francis.

Griffiths, R. (1983). Letter to Secretary of State for Social Security on NHS Management Inquiry. <https://www.sochealth.co.uk/national-health-service/griffiths-report-october-1983/>

Ham, C. (2013). The NHS in 2013: No place for the faint hearted. <https://www.kingsfund.org.uk/blog/2013/04/nhs-2013-no-place-faint-hearted>

Hamel, G., & LaBarre, P. (2013). How to lead when you're not in charge. *Harvard Business Review* <https://hbr.org/2013/05/how-to-lead-when-youre-not-in>.

Health and Social Care Act. (2012). Stationery Office. <http://www.legislation.gov.uk/ukpga/2012/7/part/1/enacted>

Heimans, J., & Timms, H. (2014). Understanding 'new power'. *Harvard Business Review, 92*(12), 48–56. <https://hbr.org/2014/12/understanding-new-power>.

Jacobs, R., Mannion, R., Davies, H. T., Harrison, S., Konteh, F., & Walshe, K. (2013). The relationship between organizational culture and performance in acute hospitals. *Social Science and Medicine, 76*(1), 115–125.

Jarrett, T. (2019). Adult social care in England: Possible reforms? <https://commonslibrary.parliament.uk/social-policy/health/adult-social-care-in-england-possible-reforms/>

Kirkup, B. (2018). Report of the Liverpool Community Health independent review. *NHS Improvement* <https://improvement.nhs.uk/documents/2403/LiverpoolCommunityHealth_IndependentReviewReport_V2.pdf>.

Kotter, J. P. (2013). Management is (still) not leadership. *Harvard Business Review* <https://hbr.org/2013/01/management-is-still-not-leadership>.

Malby, B., & Hufflett, T. (2020). *10 leaps forward - Innovation in the pandemic*. London South Bank University. <https://www.lsbu.ac.uk/__data/assets/pdf_file/0019/264340/Back-to-better-7.pdf>.

McCrimmon, M. (2010). Is heroic leadership all bad? *Development and learning in Organizations: An International Journal* <https://iveybusinessjournal.com/publication/is-heroic-leadership-all-bad/>.

National Health Service England (NHS England). (2019a). *Interim NHS people plan*. NHS Improvement. <https://www.longtermplan.nhs.uk/wp-content/uploads/2019/05/Interim-NHS-People-Plan_June2019.pdf>.

National Health Service England (NHS England). (2019b). The NHS long-term plan. <https://www.longtermplan.nhs.uk/>

NHS Improvement. (2016). *Developing people improving care. NHS Improvement*. <https://improvement.nhs.uk/resources/developing-people-improving-care/>.

NHS Improvement. (2017). *Developmental reviews of leadership and governance using the well-led framework: Guidance for NHS trusts and NHS foundation trusts. NHS Improvement*. <https://improvement.nhs.uk/documents/1259/Well-led_guidance_June_2017.pdf>.

NHS Improvement. (2019). The role of the NHS provider chair – a framework for development. <https://improvement.nhs.uk/resources/the-role-of-the-nhs-provider-chair-a-framework-for-development/>

Nolan, L. M. P. (1995). *Standards in public life: First report of the Committee on Standards in Public Life.* HM Stationery Office. <https://assets.publishing.service.gov.uk/government/uploads/system/uploads/attachment_data/file/336919/1stInquiryReport.pdf>.

Picker Institute Europe. (2020). NHS staff survey results. <https://www.nhsstaffsurveys.com/Page/1085/Latest-Results/NHS-Staff-Survey-Results/>

Pollitt, C., Harrison, S., Hunter, D. J., & Marnoch, G. (1991). General management in the NHS: The initial impact 1983–88. *Public Administration, 69*(1), 61–83.

Reed, S., Göpfert, A., Wood, S., Allwood, D., & Warburton, W. (2019). *Building healthier communities: The role of the NHS as an anchor institution. The Health Foundation.* <https://aace.org.uk/wp-content/uploads/2019/08/HF-Building-healthier-communities-Aug-19.pdf>.

Rose, L. (2015). *Better leadership for tomorrow: NHS leadership review. Department of Health.* <https://www.gov.uk/government/publications/better-leadership-for-tomorrow-nhs-leadership-review>.

Skills for Care. (2019). *The state of the adult social care sector and workforce in England. Skills for Care.* <https://www.skillsforcare.org.uk/adult-social-care-workforce-data/Workforce-intelligence/documents/State-of-the-adult-social-care-sector/State-of-Report-2019.pdf>.

Stacey, R. D. (2007). *Strategic management and organisational dynamics: The challenge of complexity to ways of thinking about organisations.* Pearson Education.

The King's Fund. (2011). The future of leadership and management in the NHS: No more heroes: *Report from The King's Fund Commission on Leadership and Management in the NHS. The King's Fund.* <https://www.kingsfund.org.uk/sites/default/files/future-of-leadership-and-management-nhs-may-2011-kingsfund.pdf>.

The Kings Fund. (2021). Integrated care systems explained: making sense of systems, places and neighbourhoods. <https://www.kingsfund.org.uk/publications/integrated-care-systems-explained#legislative-change Integrated care systems explained | The King's Fund (kingsfund.org.uk) >

Timmins, N. (2019). *Leading for integrated care.* The King's Fund. <https://www.kingsfund.org.uk/publications/leading-integrated-care>.

Vize, R. (2014). The revolution will be improvised. Stories and insights about transforming systems. <http://leadershipforchange.org.uk/wp-content/uploads/Revolution-will-be-improvised-publication-v31.pdf>

Walshe, K., Coleman, A., McDonald, R., Lorne, C., & Munford, L. (2016). Health and social care devolution: The Greater Manchester experiment. *BMJ, 352* <https://www.bmj.com/content/352/bmj.i1495.long>.

West, M., Eckert, R., Steward, K., & Pasmore, B. (2014). *Developing collective leadership for health care.* The King's Fund. <https://www.kingsfund.org.uk/publications/developing-collective-leadership-health-care>.

World Health Organization. (2016). Working for health and growth. Investing in the health workforce. <https://apps.who.int/iris/bitstream/handle/10665/250047/9789241511308-eng.pdf;jsessionid=5C4762460C2C0D2AC937385DF78802A5?sequence=1>

## REFLECTIVE QUESTIONS

- From your own experience as a leader, how do you try to balance all the demands that you face?
- How would you ensure that you remain open to challenges from your colleagues to avoid collective collusion?
- From the description of collective leadership, how can you encourage a distributed leadership culture and still have a clear line of sight and authority as a leader?
- Being a compassionate leader includes being able to give difficult feedback and manage poor performance. Thinking of your own experience, how might you challenge poor behaviors and what do you need to develop within your leadership style to be compassionate?
- Thinking of a leader you respect, reflect on how they manage to be an authentic leader when actions are under scrutiny.
- What will a board need to look like in 5 to 10 years, given greater emphasis on integration and population health?

# 5

# STRONG LEADERSHIP: QUALITY CARE, SAFETY, AND SAFEGUARDING

LEE-ANN FENGE

## OBJECTIVES

*After reading this chapter, you should be able to:*

- Identify what is meant by strong leadership and its importance in health and social care.
- Identify the challenges facing health and social care leaders in the context of dealing with "wicked" problems.
- Recognize the importance of strategic partnerships to strengthen leadership and the role of the human factor in learning from past mistakes.
- Critically analyze the importance of patient/client safety in health and social care and the challenges this presents.
- Identify the importance of measures required to ensure effective safeguarding of vulnerable citizens.

## INTRODUCTION

This chapter explores strong leadership and its importance in the context of health and social care. Globally, health and social care leaders are confronted with "wicked" problems (Rittel & Webber, 1973), which are characterized by their complexity, long-standing origin, and lack of an easy solution. "A 'wicked' problem is complex, rather than just complicated—that is, it cannot be removed from its environment, solved, and returned without affecting the environment" (Grint, 2010, pp. 169–170). This means that leaders need an appreciation of the wider historical and structural origins of long-standing issues which beset contemporary health and social care practice. This helps contextualize the origins of "wicked" problems and how different sectors make sense of them.

Strong leadership is essential to navigate the challenges posed by "wicked" problems, particularly as these problems may be understood and approached differently across different stakeholders. Health and social care systems are in a constant state of flux and change; leaders therefore require resilience to deal with these challenges and the ability to work collaboratively within and across systems to create a shared vision. Strong leadership attributes, including integrity, accountability, empathy, humility, resilience, vision, influence, and positivity, are important at all levels of an organization to uphold quality of care, patient safety, and best practices in safeguarding patients and service users.

Strong leaders are accountable first and foremost to the public to ensure appropriate levels of service delivery to those that use health and social care and to the staff that work within those services. However, behind this is a complex system of accountability to a range of key stakeholders, including professional bodies, funders, and internal and external governance and review mechanisms. Leaders need to continually review outcomes and the most appropriate measurements of impact to ensure that shared visions are developed and sustained to uphold quality of care. Within the context of integrated care, health and social care leaders must be comfortable working across blurred boundaries. They need to understand the wider cultural and sociopolitical dimensions that influence the organizational context of health and social care provision, including requirements to provide person-centered compassionate care within a context where patient safety and safeguarding practices are central concerns.

## STRONG LEADERSHIP

Strong leadership is essential for establishing the vision and values that support high-quality care within health and social care organizations. Strong leadership promotes and sustains a culture of care underpinned by a clear value base, which enables each individual worker within the organization to uphold best practices. In developing and embedding a clear vision, leaders should focus on where the service is heading and what it will look like once it has arrived. Research in England suggests that healthcare leaders in the best performing organizations "prioritised a vision and developed a strategic narrative focused on high quality, compassionate care" (West et al., 2015, p. 5).

Developing a strategic vision cannot be achieved in isolation; it should be developed in collaboration with key stakeholders and should be reinforced by clear and effective communication. Effective communication skills involve the ability to clearly share vision and values while listening to and engaging with the views of patients, service users, and staff. Good communication is built on the ability to demonstrate integrity and empathy while building trust with key stakeholders. It is also important that leaders ensure that their communication strategy is inclusive of diverse voices.

Good communication means ensuring that communication strategies are accessible for everyone, including within and outside the organization. This is particularly important when considering the inclusion of patient and service user perspectives. Within the United Kingdom (UK), those who may have English as a second language may require translation of materials or specialist translation services during their interactions with professionals. Similarly, those individuals with communication difficulties may need specialist formats for communication, such as Makaton. It is important to consider how patient and public involvement (PPI) is embedded as a central element in service development and delivery. Attention needs to be given to ensure that this does not become tokenistic but acts as a highly valued driver within the organization. Strategies for effective PPI should consider the diversity of voices represented and ways of ensuring that seldom heard groups are included, for example those from black and ethnic minority communities, those with cognitive impairment, and those from lesbian, gay, bisexual, transgender, transsexual, queer, and questioning + (LGBTQ+) communities.

To demonstrate integrity, leaders in health and social care should adopt an ethical approach that promotes ethical conduct within professional practice. An authentic style of leadership can model high standards of ethical and moral conduct to build cultures of trust and respect within the working environment (Wong & Cummings, 2009). Leaders should be mindful that trust is something that develops over time but can be destroyed very quickly. Integrity and ethical leadership are key elements identified in the Leadership Qualities Framework for Adult Social Care (The National Skills Academy for Social Care, 2014, p. 14), which states that "acting with integrity means behaving in an open, honest and ethical manner—of equal importance is a willingness to take appropriate action when ethics are breached by others." Ethical leaders are therefore central in establishing an organization's ethical tone (Mayer et al., 2012) and have an important role to play in establishing organizational resilience and adaptability to respond to the "wicked" problems that beset health and social care. (Trevino et al., 2003) suggest that ethical leadership is linked to concern for people and fair treatment of employees, and this may be important in terms of promoting staff retention. In a study of ethical leadership in social work, Choi (2014) finds an ethical approach to leadership was an important preceding factor that influences trust in the organization and organizational commitment. This is particularly important for health and social care organizations where retention of a skilled workforce is a primary concern.

Ethical leadership should be reinforced by an approach in which leaders take time to think critically and reflectively about the decisions they make as they learn from their practice. A communicative style is important, as a leader needs to engage in collaborative conversations that extend and build trust to shape the organization's vision and context. Strong ethical leadership is therefore underpinned by a commitment to support the development of staff within an overarching learning culture. It is about co-operative learning where mistakes are used as catalysts for change rather than tools to blame. Key tasks for ethical leaders are included in Box 5.1:

Strong leadership can promote cohesive team environments, which promote organizational resilience.

- Effective and inclusive communication approaches are essential in developing a shared strategic vision.
- Strong leaders demonstrate integrity underpinned by ethical practice, which promotes ethical conduct within the wider organization
- It is important to create a culture of trust in which mistakes can be accepted and used as a basis for review and learning rather than attributing blame.
- A commitment to a culture of co-operative learning is important to support reflective practices and leadership skills across the organization.

Collaborative and inclusive approaches are important to develop and cascade organizational vision and values; this can create a working environment that promotes employee satisfaction and job retention. A recent American (US) study of strong leadership within the armed forces suggests that junior officers who experienced immediate bosses with strong leadership abilities in their first four years in the Army were more likely to remain on active duty at eight years of service (Carter et al., 2019).

Strong leadership skills are important to leaders as they deal with the challenges involved in contemporary health and social care delivery. Strong leadership is about supporting a responsive organization that communicates effectively with all stakeholders and works co-operatively with them to create solutions. It is built on integrity and trusting relationships that enable everyone in the organization to reach their full potential.

## SUMMARY POINTS

- Health and social care leaders worldwide are confronted with "wicked" problems, which are complex, long standing, and have no easy solutions.
- Leaders require resilience to deal with these challenges and the ability to work collaboratively within and across systems to create a shared vision.

## THE CHALLENGES FACING HEALTH AND SOCIAL CARE

Chapter 1 referred to the "wicked" problems that face the contemporary health and social care sector. These challenges are entrenched and complex and are identified in Box 5.2:

Globally, a key challenge for health and social care agencies as they grapple with "wicked" problems is the rise of "new managerialism" and modernizing services in the image of an efficiently run corporation to increase efficiency (Cope et al., 2016). The rise of managerialism has been identified as a risk to person-centered services as the focus is on cost-cutting and performance measures in which service users "are viewed as sources (or hindrances) of revenue, and are re-labelled as consumers or customers" (Hasenfeld, 2015, p. 2). This is the antithesis of "person-centered practice" and can be seen as a challenge to the professional value base of health and social care professionals. Such approaches also undermine professional autonomy as systems become increasingly bureaucratic, intensifying the stress for those working on the frontline (Cope et al., 2016).

Such "new managerial" approaches can be viewed as "a defensive response" to deal with the complexity and uncertainty inherent in public service provision (Haworth et al., 2018, p. 4). However, top-down bureaucracy can stifle the creativity required to address the challenges posed by "wicked" problems. The task for leaders in public service is therefore a balancing act between managing efficiencies driven by top-down managerialism and meeting the requirements of upholding an approach rooted in strong professional values that enhance human dignity and compassion, challenge discrimination, and counteract social inequality (Hasenfield, 2015).

Compared to relatively wide literature and empirical research concerning leadership in health care, leadership in social work has been poorly defined globally and under researched (Hafford-Letchfield et al., 2014). As a result, leadership has not received the attention that it does in other professions, leading to a "cycle of missing leadership" in social work (Haworth et al., 2018) (Box 5-3). Leadership in social work is poorly defined and absent across a range of core domains within practice.

Despite a lack of clarity about leadership practice in social work, it is important to remember that the core elements of leadership are similar across health and social care (Sullivan, 2016). An early study of leadership in social work in the United States (US) and the United Kingdom (UK) finds that social work leaders were particularly guided by professional values and the code of ethics and were more likely to adopt a participatory leadership style (Rank & Hutchison, 2000). As we move toward more integrated ways of working, social work and social care have much to offer in terms of enhancing a "strengths-based" approach to leadership practice (SCIE, 2019). This includes a focus on a systems approach to leadership, which develops a culture of distributed leadership and influence at all levels within an organization. A strengths-based approach supports staff development through good supervision, mentoring, and coaching and by providing a safe space for reflexive conversations. It is also built

> ### BOX 5-3
> ### ASPECTS OF THE "CYCLE OF MISSING LEADERSHIP" IN SOCIAL WORK.
>
> - A lack of leadership content in qualifying social work programs
> - A lack of practice leaders contributing to qualifying social work programs
> - Lack of leadership role models during novice practice experience
> - No professional advancement without management
> - Lack of social work leadership CPD qualifications
> - Problems improving practice standards without clear leadership
>
> From Haworth, S., Miller, R. and Schaub, J. (2018) Leadership in Social Work: and can it learn from clinical healthcare. https://www.birmingham.ac.uk/Documents/college-social-sciences/social-policy/Misc/leadership-in-social-work.pdf. University of Birmingham p. 31

upon a commitment to coproduction with patients and service users to support people with lived experiences as equal partners in the design of the services, care, and support they receive. Within increasingly integrated systems of health and social care, it is vital that leaders act collectively in strengths-based approaches to promote best practices and quality services for their local populations.

At the time of writing, the current COVID-19 pandemic has brought the deep-rooted differences in health and social care services in England into the spotlight. Historically, health care in England has been universally free and delivered through the National Health Service (NHS), whereas social care has been provided through a decentralized quasi-market model of provision through means-tested eligibility. This has resulted in a two-tier system that works against seamless patient transition across health and social care provision. The pandemic has placed huge pressure on public services and on the ability of the NHS to deliver safe, high-quality care. Although there have been amazingly quick transformations of service provision to cope with the demands caused by the pandemic, the position of social care in England as the poor relation of health care has been all too obvious. As we look to the future, the value of social care in supporting some of the most vulnerable members of society must not be forgotten; hopefully, the

COVID-19 Pandemic will bust the myth forever that low pay means low skill and low value (Humphries, 2020). Integrated provision can only succeed if the essential role of social care is recognized by the leaders of integrated services.

## THE IMPACT AND CONSEQUENCES OF LEADERSHIP DECISIONS

The decisions made by leaders are pivotal in making sense of the risk and uncertainty produced by "wicked" problems in health and social care. These decisions set the strategic vision and tone of an organization and influence the ways others embrace leadership at different levels within the organization. The leadership culture and relationships within an organization can be an important source of informal support for staff members and can support a culture of learning in which individuals are encouraged to share ideas and best practices.

Within the context of integrated health and social care in England, it is important for leaders to build trust and collaborative working to facilitate shared decision-making with key stakeholders, including those who are experts by experience. This links to the discussion earlier in this chapter about good communication and inclusive approaches that support shared decision-making with patients, service users, and caregivers. This approach depends on clear and effective communication and a commitment to listen to the experiences and concerns of patients, service users, and staff. Collaborative approaches to decision-making are essential to uphold the quality of care for person-centered service provision. Shared decision-making is increasingly evident in strengths-based approaches within social work and nursing practice across the world (Barker & Thomson, 2015; Truglio-Londrigan & Slyer, 2018).

To achieve successful shared decision-making, it is important for the strategic leader to establish a culture where other stakeholders feel able to be actively involved in co-creating the strategic vision and the decisions behind it. This is about establishing a clear expectation that others have a key role to play in the decisions that are made and that their contributions will be valued. As part of a decision-making process, it is vital that leaders are reflexive about the process

to counteract potential bias that might undermine the decisions made.

Decision-making is affected by the way information is framed, by our values and beliefs, and the influence of relationships with others and the wider environment. Leaders need to be aware of the influence of prejudicial notions, which can creep into professional practice and create tunnel vision. For example, ageist practices can work to silence older people in society based on assumptions linked to negative views of aging and reduced mental capacity. It is therefore important that leaders are alert to and challenge systems that reinforce bias in decision-making and remember that "the lens we use to view the world creates the field of vision we see" (Fenge & Lee, 2020, p. 6).

### SUMMARY POINTS

- New managerial approaches can be a defensive response to deal with the complexity and uncertainty inherent in health and social care provision.
- Leaders need to balance managerial efficiencies while upholding person-centered humanized services.
- Compared to healthcare, leadership in social work is poorly defined and under researched, leading to a cycle of "missing leadership" within the social work profession.
- Social work and social care contribute a "strengths-based" approach to leadership practice, which has a positive influence within integrated teams.
- A systems approach to leadership supports a culture of distributed leadership and influence at all levels within an organization and supports collective responses in partnership with other organizations.
- Leaders need to maintain a reflexive stance about the potential of bias within decision-making.

## THE IMPORTANCE OF STRATEGIC PARTNERS FOR PROMOTING PATIENT/CLIENT SAFETY IN HIGH QUALITY SOCIAL CARE

Health and social care organizations are increasingly required to work effectively together to develop and deliver services through strategic partnerships. In England, The NHS Long-Term Plan (NHS England, 2019a) sets out key objectives over the next 10 years, including a commitment to improve the delivery of care outside hospital settings through integrated community-based health and social care. For those leading the transformation to integrated services, a key requirement is supporting the workforce across health and social care to work in different ways and across traditional boundaries

Research in England finds that effective leadership in integrated teams has a significant and consistently strong impact on both team and individual staff level dynamics (Smith et al., 2018); this is essential as the workforce is required to adapt and change to new roles and ways of working. A move toward integrated provision requires "different people in different professions working in different ways" (NHS England, 2019b, p. 2), and this demands new ways of thinking about partnerships working across health and social care. Leaders of integrated services must therefore adopt a more holistic understanding of strategic care delivery that recognizes the integral part played by social care (Burdett & Fenge, 2019). The recent COVID-19 pandemic has highlighted the central role that social care plays in supporting the health and wellbeing of people within a community, and it is essential for health care services to recognize and value this vital contribution that social care partners make to support the health and well-being of local populations.

Promoting and sustaining good-quality health and social care remains a challenge for leaders. A recent report by the Care Quality Commission (CQC, 2019, p. 7), the independent regulator of health and adult social care in England, suggests that "leaders need to have a more urgent focus on delivering care in innovative, collaborative ways." Strong leadership should therefore embrace strategic partnerships to develop innovative and creative ways of working differently. Innovation may include technological advances and the use of digital tools and resources to promote patient/service user safety and quality of care. Research by Maguire et al (2018) suggests that successful digital innovations often depend on finding a leader with specific interests and skills in technology who is motivated by improving outcomes for patients/service users rather than just reducing costs for the organization. Leading digital transformations is not without its challenges, and some organizational cultures may

be unfamiliar with and suspicious of technological innovations. When working collaboratively across traditional health and social care boundaries, it may be difficult to bring different organizations together, particularly when they may have a long history of using different IT systems or mistrust of working in partnerships with other organizations.

Innovation in workforce planning should see strategic partnerships used to develop new roles and new ways of working across health and social care that support people living independently in their community longer. Workforce redesign will need to occur across health and social care to establish new ways of working. For example, the development of new nursing associate roles provides staff development opportunities across adult services in health and social care (Maguire et al., 2018). The development of new roles may provide opportunities for improving the retention of skilled staff through opportunities to provide progression pathways and upskilling for existing staff.

It is clear from the earlier discussion that to cope with the "wicked" nature of problems, it is important for leaders to think beyond the usual leadership and management approaches to break with the constraints of the past. Strong leadership is not top-down and requires individuals who can facilitate a collaborative approach to harness creativity across both internal and external stakeholders. Creative leadership solutions can be nurtured to sustain new approaches to collaborative working, developing new roles and seamless person-centered provision through effective system leadership. Leaders of integrated services need to work with the resources within their own workforce by adopting "the moral resourcefulness" to engage in challenging conversations (Hutchinson et al., 2015, p. 3022).

## Promoting patient safety and high-quality care

Promoting patient/service user safety is a key concern for health and social care leaders globally. The World Health Assembly (WHA) (2019) has declared that patient safety is a global health priority, and one that requires global leadership to tackle. The WHA, (2019) resolution has firmly put patient safety center stage on the global agenda by endorsing the establishment of World Patient Safety Day to be observed annually on September 17. This action promotes a global commitment that no one should be harmed by health care. Alongside adequate infrastructure and access to appropriate clinical resources, this approach highlights the importance of promoting continued staff education and training to ensure that they have the necessary skills and competencies to safely undertake their professional roles.

Following the public inquiry into poor quality of care at the Mid Staffordshire NHS Foundation Trust in England (Francis, 2013), a lack of compassionate care was identified that occurred while the organization was focused on creating efficiencies and financial savings. The findings of the Francis Report (2013) suggested that changes to the organizational culture were required to create a focus on patient safety and wellbeing. Unsurprisingly, poor leadership within the Mid Staffordshire Foundation Trust was highlighted as the root of the inadequate care provided. The report concluded that concerns raised by patients and staff members were ignored by the organization's leaders and Trust Board. Silencing the concerns of key stakeholders, including patients and their relatives, resulted in a system that failed to tackle poor standards of care and lacked any clear responsibility to ensure patient safety and quality of care. A Care Quality Commission investigation into Southern Health NHS Foundation Trust in England (CQC, 2016) also found a lack of responsiveness to patient and caregiver concerns and found that the trust did not effectively respond to concerns about safety raised by patients, their caregivers, and staff.

Leaders have a pivotal role in establishing a positive safety culture that is embedded in a culture of learning, which promotes patient safety across the organization. Organizations that embed a positive safety culture build this on mutual trust, confidence in preventative measures, and a shared commitment to the centrality of patient safety within the organization (Health and Safety Commission, 1993). Good communication is a clear element in an effective system that upholds patient safety. This includes communicating effectively to reduce incidences that undermine patient safety, communicating learning from such incidences across the organization, and communicating with candor with patients and families when things go wrong.

---

### BOX 5-4
### FIVE KEY CULTURAL ELEMENTS

1. An inspiring vision cascaded through every level of the organization
2. Clearly communicated and aligned objectives for all staff members, teams, and departments
3. Supportive leadership that promotes high levels of staff engagement
4. The creation of a learning culture that embeds learning, innovation, and quality improvement for all staff
5. Effective team working

From West, M.A., Eckert, R., Steward, K. and Pasmore, B. (2014) Developing collective leadership for healthcare. London: The King's Fund. https://www.kingsfund.org.uk/sites/default/files/field/field_publication_file/developing-collective-leadership-kingsfund-may14.pdf

---

A duty of candor for health care providers was introduced in England in 2014 (Health and Social Care Act 2008 (Regulated Activities), Regulations 2014, Regulation 20) to ensure that they are open and honest with patients and their caregivers when things go wrong with their care. This puts open and honest communication with those that use services at the heart of patient safety and high-quality care.

In the UK, West et al (2014) suggest that five key cultural elements are necessary to sustain cultures that ensure high-quality compassionate care with patient/service user safety at its heart (Box 5-4). These elements echo the description of strong leadership described earlier in this chapter.

More than ever before, strong leadership and collaboration are crucial to delivering good-quality care. It is important that leaders instill a culture that learns from preventable incidents to create a culture of learning that can support a proactive approach to improving patient care and safety.

### SUMMARY POINTS

- Strong and effective leadership in integrated teams has a significant and consistently strong effect on both team and individual staff level dynamics.
- Leaders of integrated services are required to adopt a more holistic understanding of strategic care delivery that recognizes the integral part played by social care.

- Successful digital innovations often depend on finding a leader with specific interest and skills in technology who is motivated by improving outcomes for patients/service users.
- Innovation in workforce planning should see strategic partnerships used to develop new roles and new ways of working across health and social care.
- Leaders have a pivotal role in establishing a positive safety culture underpinned by an embedded culture of learning that promotes patient safety across the organization.

## THE IMPORTANCE OF MEASURES REQUIRED TO ENSURE EFFECTIVE SAFEGUARDING OF VULNERABLE CITIZENS

The task for those leading effective safeguarding activities is to ensure "joined up" working and shared decision-making to protect the most vulnerable members of society. Decades of evidence from serious case reviews (SCRs) have highlighted that poor information sharing between agencies has resulted in negative outcomes for vulnerable citizens experiencing harm or abuse (Preston-Shoot, 2017). For example, one particular Serious Case Review suggested that a multi-agency strategy meeting "… may well have resulted in a more holistic and coordinated approach being taken, involving all relevant agencies" (Cornwall Safeguarding Adults Board, 2008, p. 6). This particular review concerned the death of TS, a woman aged 43 years who died after being admitted to hospital with a broken femoral neck. She had a history of alcohol misuse and died in the hospital from complications linked to liver failure, alcohol cirrhosis, renal failure, and septicemia, in addition to the infected fracture. While many professionals had been involved over a number of years with TS (e.g., police, health and social care), they did not use the procedures available to them to safeguard TS, and there was a lack of strategic leadership in dealing with her complex array of problems.

The issues identified in the case example above are illustrative of the wider issues highlighted by a review of SCRs, which suggests that "in many cases, agencies tended to work on parallel lines, lacking a joint or shared approach, or any sense of shared ownership"

(Preston-Shoot, 2017, p. 43). A lack of clear strategic leadership concerning inter-agency safeguarding practices can lead to fragmented systems, resulting in inadequate risk assessment and failure to recognize and act upon persistent and escalating risks.

To facilitate improved safeguarding practices, Multi-Agency Safeguarding Hubs (MASH) were introduced in England in 2010 to facilitate improved inter-agency communication and joint decision-making (Home Office, 2014). These hubs set out to improve information sharing and shared decision-making across agencies and offer a first point of contact for new safeguarding concerns. Enabling agencies to work more effectively together to safeguard those at risk of abuse is important, as this may help facilitate improved intelligence concerning patterns of abuse, repeat offenders, and joined-up ways of protecting those vulnerable to abuse. The Statutory Guidance accompanying the Care Act 2014 (DHSC, 2020, para 14.12) reinforces the requirement of multi-agency working to provide effective coordinated assessments and interventions to safeguard those at risk of abuse and neglect.

The 2014 Care Act (Department of Health and Social Care [DHSC] 2020) expects service delivery to be informed by six safeguarding principles to facilitate and personalize safeguarding processes (Box 5-5).

This legislation and the guidance around Making Safeguarding Personal (MSP) (Local Government Association, 2014) puts the individual at the center of the safeguarding process. This represents a culture shift from a process supported by conversations to a series of conversations supported by a process. It is

---

**BOX 5-5**
**SIX SAFEGUARDING PRINCIPALS**

1. Empowerment
2. Partnership
3. Protection
4. Prevention
5. Proportionality
6. Accountability

From Care act (2014) Department of Health and Social Care (DHSC) (2020) Care Act Guidance: care and support statutory guidance. https://www.gov.uk/government/publications/care-act-statutory-guidance/care-and-support-statutory-guidance

about having conversations with people about how we might better respond to the safeguarding situations that affect their lives and about seeing people as experts in their own lives and working alongside them. Prior to this change in policy, vulnerable adults tended to be excluded from safeguarding processes and decision-making. Research suggests that MSP supports consideration by agencies and practitioners of the outcomes of safeguarding interventions from a "user" perspective (Manthorpe et al., 2014).

These changes can be seen to echo the elements of strong leadership identified earlier in the chapter, which emphasized a "strengths-based" approach to leadership practice (SCIE, 2019). MPS is a strengths-based approach to safeguarding practice and "it is about having conversations with people about how we might respond in safeguarding situations in a way that enhances involvement, choice and control as well as improving quality of life, wellbeing and safety" (LGA, 2014, p. 4).

In terms of safeguarding vulnerable children at risk of harm and abuse, similar concerns have been expressed about a lack of clear strategic leadership to work effectively across agency boundaries. The Department for Education (DfE) is responsible for child protection in England and setting out policy, legislation, and statutory guidance. Local authority Children's Services teams have the responsibility of investigating child protection referrals, working alongside two other statutory safeguarding partners—the clinical commissioning group (health) and the police. Child protection, like many areas of public service provision, is beset by "wicked" problems, including high caseloads, rapid staff turnover, underfunding, and "compliance-focused bureaucratic cultures" ("Cortis et al., 2019, p. 55).

SCRs over several decades have highlighted systemic failings in protecting children at risk of harm and abuse. For example, a recent SCR concerning a 14-year-old young person who died from an aggressive malignant tumor identified failures to understand and act upon the child's voice. The child had presented at the GP twice and at the hospital Accident and Emergency department on five occasions. The child was convinced that it was seriously ill and shared this with the foster caregivers and various professionals on more than one occasion. The foster caregivers thought the child had made up the illness as the result of a previous trauma.

In addition to not engaging with the child's voice, the review found evidence of poor interagency communication and information sharing (NSPCC, 2019). Many of these failings mirror issues identified in SCRs concerning safeguarding adults practices including a lack of "professional curiosity" and poor inter-professional partnership working (Brandon et al., 2012).

A key requirement for those leading safeguarding adults and children's services is involving all agencies in the strategic development of safeguarding practices. This includes facilitating joint training across multi-agency partnerships and exploring creative methods to engage and support service user voice within safeguarding processes. Leaders need to drive a transparent process of information sharing and analysis to promote best practices, underpinned by effective systems for tracking the outcomes of review recommendations and embedding these within a shared culture of learning.

Strong leadership in safeguarding is about creating a shared culture of understanding safeguarding practices, including clarity about roles, expectations, and responsibilities in terms of the policies, procedures, and frameworks of safeguarding interventions. It is built on strong values and ethics around delivering person-centered care and a commitment to engage with those at the center of the safeguarding process. This can be facilitated by a shared culture of learning, which enables practitioners and agencies to critically reflect upon what is known and what is unknown in terms of safeguarding referrals and within which discrepancies and lack of clarity can be challenged. Effective safeguarding can only occur within clearly communicated and accountable processes and procedures that work seamlessly across agency boundaries.

## SUMMARY POINTS

- Evidence from serious case reviews highlight that poor information sharing between agencies has resulted in negative outcomes for vulnerable citizens experiencing harm or abuse.
- Poor safeguarding practices occur when agencies lack a joined-up or shared approach and work on parallel lines.
- To facilitate improved safeguarding practice, Multi-Agency Safeguarding Hubs (MASH) were introduced in England in 2010 to facilitate improved inter-agency communication and joint decision-making.

- Making Safeguarding Personal (MSP) puts the individual at the center of the safeguarding process. Safeguarding practices should be person-centered to support service user voices within safeguarding processes.
- Those who lead safeguarding processes should involve all agencies in the strategic development of safeguarding practices. This includes facilitating joint training across multi-agency partnerships, working according to agreed procedures and frameworks, and open and clear communication.

## CONCLUSION

Leaders in health and social care need to demonstrate strong leadership skills to deal with the "wicked" problems inherent in contemporary practice. Integrity, resilience, and the ability to work collaboratively within and across systems is vital, as leaders are required to think beyond the usual leadership and management approaches. Strong leaders need to demonstrate an ability to break with the constraints of the past as they establish creative visions for the future of health and social care in the context of increasingly integrated provision.

The ability to facilitate meaningful collaborative working across a range of health and social care stakeholders is required to ensure best practices and uphold patient safety and safeguarding outcomes. This should be underpinned by a commitment to person-centered practices where the voice and experience of patients/service users is valued and central to service delivery and improvement.

## REFERENCES

Barker, J., & Thomson, L. (2015). Helpful relationships with service users: linking social capital. *Australian Social Work*, 68(1), 130–145.

Brandon, M., Sidebotham, P., Bailey, S., Belderson, P., Hawley, C., Ellis, C., & Megson, M. (2012). New learning from serious case reviews: A two-year report for 2009-2011 Department for Education. *Research Brief*. https://www.basw.co.uk/system/files/resources/basw_113140-1_0.pdf.

Burdett, T., & Fenge, L. (2019). Achieving the NHS Long-Term Plan through integrated care provision: rhetoric or reality? *Journal of Community Nursing*, 33(6), 61–64.

Care Quality Commission (CQC) (2016) CQC tells Southern Health NHS Foundation Trust to take urgent action to improve governance arrangements to ensure patient safety. https://www.cqc.org.uk/news/releases/cqc-tells-southern-health-nhs-foundation-trust-take-urgent-action-improve-governance

Care Quality Commission (CQC). (2019). State of health care and adult social care in England 2018/19. https://www.cqc.org.uk/sites/default/files/20191015b_stateofcare1819_fullreport.pdf

Carter, S. P., Dudley, W., Lyle, D. S., & Smith, J. Z. (2019). Who's the boss? The effect of strong leadership on employee turnover. *Journal of Economic Behavior & Organization*, 159, 323–343.

Choi, S. Y. (2014). The effects of leadership on social workers' organizational commitment: Focusing on ethical leadership, organizational trust, and supervisor trust. *Information. International Information Institute: Tokyo*, 17(10A), 4771, ISSN 1343-4500.

Cornwall Safeguarding Adults Board. (2008). *Executive Summary of a Serious Case Review in Respect of an Adult Female Who Died 12th March 2007*. Truro: Cornwall Safeguarding Adults Board.

Cope, V., Jones, B., & Hendricks, J. (2016). Resilience as resistance to the new managerialism: portraits that reframe nursing through quotes from the field. *Journal of Nursing Management*, 24(1), 115–122.

Cortis, N., Smyth, C., Wade, C., & Katz, I. (2019). Changing practice cultures in statutory child protection: practitioners' perspectives. *Child & Family Social Work*, 24(1), 50–58.

Department of Health and Social Care (2020), Care Act Guidance: care and support statutory guidance (DHSC). https://www.gov.uk/government/publications/care-act-statutory-guidance/care-and-support-statutory-guidance

Fenge, L., & Lee, S. (2020). Reflecting on values and bias within mental capacity decision making. In S. Lee, L. Fenge, B. Brown, & M. Lyne (Eds.), *Demystifying mental capacity. Learning Matters A Sage Publishing Company: London*.

Francis, R. (2013). Report of the mid Staffordshire NHS Foundation trust public inquiry. https://assets.publishing.service.gov.uk/government/uploads/system/uploads/attachment_data/file/279124/0947.pdf

Grint, K. (2010). Wicked problems and clumsy solutions: the role of leadership. In Brookes, S., & Grint, K. (Eds.), *The new public leadership challenge* (pp. 169–186). Basingstoke: Palgrave MacMillan.

Hasenfeld, Y. (2015). What exactly is human services management? *Human Service Organizations: Management, Leadership & Governance*, 39(1), 1–5.

Hafford-Letchfield, T., Lambley, S., Spolander, G., & Cocker, C. (2014). *Inclusive leadership in Social work and social care*. Policy Press: Bristol.

Haworth, S., Miller, R. & Schaub, J. (2018). Leadership in Social Work: and can it learn from clinical healthcare. https://www.birmingham.ac.uk/Documents/college-social-sciences/social-policy/Misc/leadership-in-social-work.pdf. University of Birmingham

Health & Safety Commission. (1993). *ACSNI human factors study group: third report: organising for safety*. HMSO: London.

The Health and Social Care Act. (2008). *Regulated Activities Regulations*. HMSO: London, 2014, Regulation 20: Duty of Candour.

Home Office (2014). Multi Agency Working and Information Sharing Project: Final Report. https://assets.publishing.service.gov.uk/government/uploads/system/uploads/attachment_data/file/338875/MASH.pdf

Humphries, R. (2020). Integrating Health and Social Care in the COVID-19 (coronavirus) response. https://www.kingsfund.org.uk/blog/2020/04/health-social-care-covid-19-coronavirus

Hutchinson, M., Daly, J., Usher, K., & Jackson, D. (2015). Editorial: leadership when there are no easy answers: applying leader moral courage to wicked problems. *Journal of Clinical Nursing, 24*(21-22), 3021–3023.

Local Government Association (LGA). (2014). Making Safeguarding Personal: Guide 2014. https://documents/Making%20Safeguarding%20Personal%20-%20Guide%202014.pdf.

Maguire, D., Evans, H., Honeyman, M. & Omojomolo, D. (2018). Digital change in health and social care. https://www.kingsfund.org.uk/sites/default/files/2018-06/Digital_change_health_care_Kings_Fund_June_2018.pdf. The King's Fund

Manthorpe, J., Klee, D., Williams, C., & Cooper, A. (2014). Making Safeguarding Personal: developing responses and enhancing skills. *The Journal of Adult Protection, 16*(2), 96–103.

Mayer, D. M., Aquino, K., Greenbaum, R. L., & Kuenzi, M. (2012). Who displays ethical leadership, and why does it matter? An examination of antecedents and consequences of ethical leadership. *Academy of Management Journal, 55*(1), 151–171.

NHS England (2019a). The NHS long-term Plan. https://www.england.nhs.uk/long-term-plan/. *NHS England: London*

NHS England (2019b). Interim NHS people Plan. https://www.longtermplan.nhs.uk/wp-content/uploads/2019/05/Interim-NHS-People-Plan_June2019.pdf. NHS England: London

Preston-Shoot, M. (2017) What difference does legislation make? Adult safeguarding through the lens of serious case reviews and safeguarding adult reviews. A report for south west region safeguarding adults' boards. *report for South West Region Safeguarding Adults Boards*. https://ssab.safeguardingsomerset.org.uk/wp-content/uploads/SW-SCRs-SARs-Report-Final-Version-2017.pdf. South West ADASS: Bristol

Rank, M. G., & Hutchison, W. S. (2000). An analysis of leadership within the social work profession. *Journal of Social Work Education, 36*(3), 487–502.

Rittel, H. W. J., & Webber, M. M. (1973). Dilemmas in a general theory of planning. *Policy Sciences, 4*(2), 155–169.

Social Care Institute for Excellence (SCIE) (2019). Leadership in strengths-based social care. https://www.scie.org.uk/strengths-based-approaches/leadership

Smith, T., Fowler-Davis, S., Nancarrow, S., Ariss, S. M. B., & Enderby, P. (2018). Leadership in interprofessional health and social care teams: A literature review. *Leadership in Health Services, 31*(4), 452–467.

Sullivan, W. P. (2016). Leadership in social work: where are we? *Journal of Social Work Education, 52*(sup1), S51–S61.

The National Skills Academy for Social Care. (2014). *The Leadership Qualities Framework for Social Care.* https://www.skillsforcare.org.uk/Documents/Leadership-and-management/Leadership-Qualities-Framework/Leadership-Qualities-Framework.pdf

Treviño, L. K., Brown, M., & Hartman, L. P. (2003). A qualitative investigation of perceived executive ethical leadership: Perceptions from inside and outside the executive suite. *Human Relations, 56*(1), 5–37.

Truglio-Londrigan, M., & Slyer, J. T. (2018). Shared decision-making for nursing practice: An integrative review. *The Open Nursing Journal, 12*, 1–14.

West, M.A., Eckert, R., Steward, K. & Pasmore, B. (2014). Developing collective leadership for healthcare. https://www.kingsfund.org.uk/sites/default/files/field/field_publication_file/developing-collective-leadership-kingsfund-may14.pdf. The King's Fund: London

West, M., Armit, K., Loewenthal, L., Eckert, R., West, T. & Lee, A. (2015) Leadership and leadership development in healthcare: the evidence base. https://www.kingsfund.org.uk/sites/default/files/field/field_publication_file/leadership-leadership-development-health-care-feb-2015.pdf. Faculty of Medical Leadership and Management: London. The King's Fund

Wong, C., & Cummings, G. (2009). Authentic leadership: A new theory for nursing or back to basics? *Journal of Health Organization & Management, 23*(5), 522–538.

World Health Assembly (WHA) (2019). Global action on patient safety. *Agenda ITEM, 12*, 5. https://apps.who.int/gb/ebwha/pdf_files/WHA72/A72_R6-en.pdf?ua=1

## REFLECTIVE QUESTIONS

- From your own experience, what are the particular "wicked" problems within your own agency setting?
- What are the characteristics of strong leadership that you have observed in the leaders in your field of practice?
- How are patient/service users involved in strategic decision-making in your own organization? How might they be included further in meaningful partnerships?
- What learning can you apply in terms of best practices in patient safety and safeguarding to your own practice?

# 6

# MANAGING AND LEADING PEOPLE AND TEAMS: BUILDING STRONG TEAMS

TONY SMITH

## OBJECTIVES

*After reading this chapter, you should be able to:*

- Identify what is meant by a team in relation to leadership and its importance in health and social care.
- Understand the challenges facing health and social care leaders in the context of teams and teamwork.
- Recognize that there are different types of teams.
- Critically analyze the importance of group dynamics within teams in health and social care and the challenges they present.
- Identify key elements of effective team leadership.
- Understand the importance of leading interdisciplinary health and social care teams.

## INTRODUCTION TO TEAMWORKING IN HEALTH AND SOCIAL CARE

Over the last two to three decades, health and social care organizations, professionals, and researchers have become increasingly preoccupied with teamworking and leadership. The seeds of the focus on these phenomena in the United Kingdom and other Organisation for Economic Co-operation and Development (OECD) countries lay in a perceived need to reform the public health and social care systems, which have been seen as poorly managed and too focused on the concerns and interests of professionals. In the United Kingdom, commercial management techniques were introduced in the National Health Service (NHS) to attempt to modernize practices, reduce fragmentation of care, and provide greater focus on patients' interests.

The "New Public Management" movement, which assumes that private sector management techniques and the introduction of market forces are the key to public sector improvement, has resulted in numerous reforms. One of the key innovations has been the adoption of a systematic engineering approach for designing operational disease/care pathways for patients. Within this approach, care is organized around patients, who receive a range of inputs depending on their needs at different stages of their journey along a pathway. These structural changes in service configuration require forming interprofessional networks that span service-user pathways to form groupings based around particular disease intervention points rather than professional expertise. The changes have resulted in an increasing emphasis on teamworking as a universal means of efficiently and safely improving service-user outcomes (Department of Health, 2008).

This is not straightforward, however, as it conflicts with autonomy, one of the fundamental tenets of professionalism (Reeves et al., 2010). Professions place exclusive claims on areas of knowledge and practice and seek closed licensing from nation states to protect their ability to practice autonomously (Freidson, 1970). Requiring professionals to share responsibility for care delivery and outcomes blurs the boundaries of expertise, which often leads to challenging renegotiations of professional boundaries. Significantly, leadership has been found to be instrumental in successfully developing and implementing care pathways (Currie & Harvey, 2000).

According to Xyrichis and Lowton (2008), a wide range of pronouns are used to describe teamworking arrangements between professionals. Terms such as interprofessional and multi-professional are often used interchangeably in the literature to refer to different types of teams and different processes within them (Leathard, 2003). Another issue is that non-professionals deliver increasing amounts of care, particularly in community and social care settings (Moran, 2008). However, Pollard, Ross et al. (2005) find that nonprofessional staff and students are largely passive in interprofessional interactions; they are also omitted from much interprofessional literature. According to Nancarrow et al. (2012), there is a subtle difference between the terms interprofessional and interdisciplinary. Interdisciplinary is often used when the focus of the literature is on sharing specialist knowledge in work collaborations, while the term interprofessional is often used when the focus is on professional boundaries and roles.

## UNDERSTANDING TEAMWORK AND LEADING TEAMS (GENERIC LITERATURE)

To fully understand the role of leadership in teams, it is first necessary to define the concept of a team. While there may be contention over the constituent elements of teamworking, there appears to be a wider consensus on the definition of a team. A review of a number of key texts on teamworking reveals that definitions center around three common characteristics (Cohen & Bailey, 1997; Katzenbach & Smith, 2005; Lafasto & Larssen, 2002; Larssen & Lafasto, 1989; Staniforth & West, 1995) (Box 6-1).

There is an almost universal assertion in management literature that, compared to other modes of organizing, teamworking offers superior performance and outcomes. The central tenet is that the synergies that develop in teamworking lead to superior outcomes. According to Sennett (1998), the development of the discourse on teams in health and social care in the last decade is similar to its development in the generic management literature, where it led to an almost ubiquitous deployment of teamworking in management practice in the late 1980s and 1990s. Today, "team" has become a term that is almost universally applied to all sorts of work groups with the assumption that it has positive effects.

However, the reality about teamwork in health and social care may not be as clear cut as the discourses within management theory and health policy would suggest. The potential gains that teamworking appears to offer may not be easy to realize for a number of reasons (Staniforth & West, 1995) (Box 6-2). Team decision-making is costly, and these costs may mitigate any superior overall performance and goal achievement; in other words, "teams are not easy to form, straightforward to manage, or immediately capable of producing both efficient and effective outcomes" (Staniforth & West, 1995, p. 33). The authors conclude that without appropriate leadership, whether from one person or several members of a group, it is unlikely that teams will offer significant performance improvements compared to other ways of working.

---

### BOX 6-1
### THREE COMMON CHARACTERISTICS OF TEAMWORKING

1. A team is made up of two or more people. Most authors do not specify a maximum limit; however, there is debate about the optimum number of people in a team.
2. A team has specific performance objectives or common goals to attain.
3. Completing the tasks the team must undertake requires interdependence and coordinated action by the members.

Staniforth & West (1995), Cohen & Bailey (1997), and Katzenbach & Smith (2015).

---

### BOX 6-2
### REASONS WHY GAINS FROM TEAMS ARE DIFFICULT TO IDENTIFY

1. The assumption that group decisions are better than individual ones may be erroneous. Staniforth and West (1995, p. 28) assert that while "the quality of team decisions is likely to be less than that of the best individual team member, it is however likely to be better than that of the average team member."
2. Group decision-making can be a much slower process than individual decision-making.
3. Group decision-making can lead to role conflict and lack of clarity about goals.

Staniforth, D., & West, M. A. (1995). Leading and managing teams. *Team Performance Management, 1*, 28–33.

## TYPES OF TEAMS

A further issue that requires clarification relates to the nature of the teams being discussed. According to Yukl (2019), a team contrasts with a work group, which may perform the same type of work but whose members do not rely on and are not interdependent on each other. In terms of leadership, this distinction between teams and groups is important, as team leadership requires more complex leadership processes, particularly in contexts where leadership needs to be shared to some extent among team members. A further complication is that there are various types of teams. Yukl (2019) identifies four basic team types (Table 6-1). I have added inter-agency/organizational teams to this table, as teams are increasingly being formed of members from different organizations/services. The team types are roughly arranged within the table according to level of autonomy. However, what determines whether a group is a team or vice-versa relates to how the members work together and interact.

In the literature on health and social care teams, the term team seems to be used ubiquitously. However, the terms used by Yukl, which are commonplace in wider organizational literature, are less often used in that literature. All five types of teams described in the table are found in health and social care, but types of teams are often unacknowledged in interprofessional teamwork literature.

Nonetheless, understanding the types of teams health and social care workers operate in is vital to understanding team dynamics. Cross-functional or inter-agency teams are significantly different from functional or uni-professional in-service teams.

## GROUP DYNAMICS AND TEAM DEVELOPMENT

When work groups undertake work tasks, three levels of issues need to be dealt with simultaneously.

- **Content** issues are related to the specific activity the group is faced with completing.
- **Process** issues can be divided into two categories:

  - **Task** issues relate to how the group is to work together to accomplish the task, not to what task is being attempted.
  - **Maintenance** issues are those related to how a group is functioning with regard to meeting group members' psychological and emotional needs (Osland et al., 2000).

According to Schein (2016), the main determinant of work group effectiveness is process. Groups that are not able to recognize the difference between content and process issues or to openly discuss the

| | **TABLE 6-1** | | | | |
|---|---|---|---|---|---|
| **Common Characteristics of Four Types of Teams (Yukl, 2019) with Inter-agency Team Type Added** | | | | | |
| Defining Characteristic | Functional Operating Team | Cross-functional Team | *Inter-agency Team* | Self-managed Operating Team | Top Executive Team |
| Autonomy to determine mission and objectives | Low | Low to moderate | *Low to moderate* | Low to moderate | High |
| Autonomy to determine work procedures | Low to moderate | High | *High* | High | High |
| Authority of internal leader | High | Moderate to high | *Low to moderate* | Low | High |
| Duration of existence | High | Low to moderate | *Low to moderate* | High | High |
| Stability of membership | High | Low to moderate | *Low to moderate* | High | High |
| Diversity of members in functional backgrounds | Low | High | *High* | Low | High |

---

### BOX 6-3
### TEAM MEMBERS NEED TO GIVE EQUAL ATTENTION TO:

1. What they are doing (goal or the task they are trying to achieve),
2. How they (are going to) do it, and
3. Ensuring that all group members feel valued, included, and well treated, and that no one member dominates the other group members or uses the group for their own purposes (self-oriented behavior).

---

difficulties that arise will not be effective in moderating self-oriented behavior. Consequently, they will not perform as effectively as groups that are able to do this. While this may sound complicated on paper, it just means that to be able to effectively work together, team members need to give equal attention to all three issues identified in Box 6.3.

It is therefore important to understand how emotional issues can affect group behavior, acknowledge the legitimacy of others' feelings, and recognize how emotions may drive self-oriented behavior. If any group member becomes emotionally triggered by the group, it is important to discuss their feelings with the group. If team members cannot speak honestly when something is bothering them and deal with their feelings constructively, they may well behave in ways that are counterproductive (e.g., with anger, negativity, resentment, or withdrawal).

It is important that all group members participate in the group and work toward achieving inclusivity. This means more vocal group members should take care not to dominate discussions but ensure that quieter members get their say. Quieter members also have a responsibility to be more courageous and not just leave group problem solving to others. This also extends to group members contributing to keeping the group on track and highlighting issues that may be hindering the group's progress.

## STAGES OF TEAM DEVELOPMENT

Tuckman (1965) identified four basic stages that work groups go through while developing into teams.

1. **Forming**—In this stage, members focus on accepting each other and learning more about the group and its purpose. This is a period of uncertainty, self-consciousness, and superficiality. Effective group leaders help orient members, clarify the group's purpose, and work on establishing trusting relationships. By the end of this stage, members feel like they belong to the group.

2. **Storming**—Members must give up some individuality to belong to any group. This is quite difficult for many people, and tension, criticism, and confrontation are typical of this stage. The group becomes polarized, subdivides into cliques, and challenges the leader and other members. Effective leadership involves helping the group focus on a common vision, modeling constructive conflict management, and legitimizing expressions of individuality that do not hinder productivity. Skilled leaders ensure that the group is a safe place for all members. They also reassure members that storming is a normal stage in a group's development that paves the way for later.

3. **Norming**—Members develop shared expectations about group roles and norms. This stage is characterized by collaboration, commitment, increased cohesion, and identification with the group. Effective leaders continue to help set norms, provide positive feedback on the group's progress, and prevent groupthink, which is the tendency for members of a cohesive group to seek consensus so strongly that they fail to explore alternative courses of action.

4. **Performing**—At this stage, the group focuses its energy on achieving its goals and being productive. There is increased cohesion, acceptance of individual differences, and mutual support. Skilled leaders help the group lead itself at this point, foster the development of group traditions, and encourage the group to evaluate its effectiveness.

In 1977 Tuckman added a fifth stage to his model.

5. **Adjourning**—Temporary groups disband and focus less on performance and more on closure. In this stage, members struggle with holding on (nostalgia) and letting go (looking ahead

to the future). Effective leaders encourage the group to reflect on and celebrate its achievements (Tuckman & Jensen, 1977). These stages are illustrated in Fig. 6-1. What is notable is that group productivity remains relatively low for quite some time in the early stages of development. This can be a difficult situation for leaders to handle as it requires both acceptance that productivity will be limited for a time and patience to work through the forming, storming, and norming stages.

## SUMMARY POINTS

- There is general agreement in research literature that teamworking can lead to superior outcomes.
- Calling a work group a team does not make it one.
- It takes a lot of time and effort to develop a group into a team and then maintain effective teamworking.
- Teams operate in different contexts with different team members. This means the leadership demands may vary considerably in different teams.

- In health and social care settings, work groups are increasingly made up of a wide range of different professionals and members with other essential skills. This places unique demands on leaders in interdisciplinary teams.

## LEADERSHIP AND TEAMS

The relationship between the concepts of leadership and teamwork represents somewhat of a paradox. According to Alimo-Metcalfe and Alban-Metcalfe (2003) traditional theories of leadership are largely focused on a "heroic" model. Their focus is on individuals who, through traits or behavioral skills, can transform poorly performing organizations and extract the maximum commitment and effort from followers. The paradox is that, at the same time, teamworking, which includes dispersing management responsibility to groups that operate through collective effort (and often shared leadership), is seen by many as the key to high performance organizations.

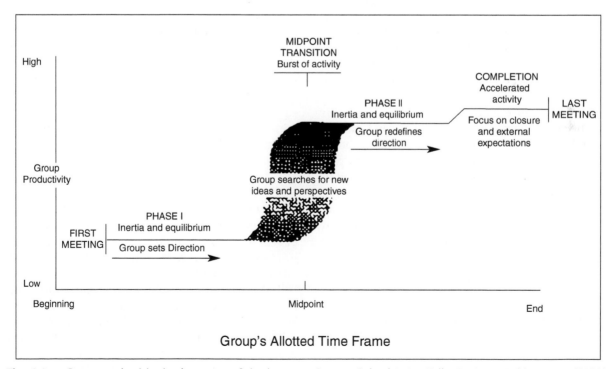

**Fig. 6-1** ■ Group productivity in the stages of development. Source: Osland J. A., Kolb, D. A., & Rubin, I. M. (2000). *Organizational behaviour: An experiential approach* (7th Ed.). Pearson.

Unsurprisingly then, some literature focuses on the issue of whether teams need a leader or at least to what extent teams can or should be self-managed (Hayes, 2002). Pivotal to this strand of literature is Meindl (1990), who asserts that good performance in organizations or teams is often over-attributed to leaders. Bennis and Biederman (1997) point out that very little writing attributes fantastic accomplishments to the talented workgroups/teams that produced them. Manz (1992) finds that what organizations often labeled as self-managed teams were far from self-managed. However, he advocates that organizations could go much further and work groups could and should be given almost complete autonomy (Manz & Sims, 2001). Hackman (2002) asserts that there is a propensity to assign team successes and failures to individuals. He calls this natural tendency to find individual heroes or scapegoats "leader attribution error" (Hackman, 2002, p. 200). He argues that individual leaders do not shape team performance. Rather, performance is more a combined effect (Box 6-4).

When these design elements are successfully put in place, team performance processes are maximized. The team leader's role is to provide the elements necessary for high performance, and the main mechanism for achieving this within a team is expert coaching. However, the day-to-day leadership within the team should be shared by the team members, who, if membership is diverse, each have strengths and weakness that are complementary.

There is evidence, however, that self-managed teams often become directionless, unproductive, and stuck in minor conflicts (Laiken, 1994). Group autonomy should therefore be an endpoint, not a beginning, and the process of achieving it requires a significant investment in time and skilled leadership (Munro & Laiken, 2003). Significantly, Hackman (2002) also asserts that the performance research for self-managed teams over-attributes performance gains to teams.

---

**BOX 6-4**

Compelling direction
Enabling team structure
A supportive organizational context

---

Hackman, J. R. (2002). *Leading teams: Setting the stage for great performance*. Harvard Business School Press.

---

## THE KEY ELEMENTS OF EFFECTIVE LEADERSHIP IN TEAMS

While the authors of the above critiques attack the mainstream discourses about both teamworking and leadership, they, together with virtually every writer on the subject of teams, acknowledge that effective leadership is important for teams to work successfully.

Staniforth and West (1995) point toward a dearth of research that specifically focuses on team leadership. However, there is more research on teamworking, which includes the findings on the key elements of team leadership and proposes outline models (Hackman, 1990, 2002; Hayes, 2002; Katzenbach & Smith, 2015; Lafasto & Larssen, 2002; Larssen & Lafasto, 1989; Shackleton, 1995; Staniforth & West, 1995; Stoker, 2008). This body of research proposes the following elements of team leadership, summarized in Box 6-5.

### Empowerment

The concept of empowerment is central to teamworking (Hayes, 2002) and differs markedly from delegating (Shackleton, 1995). There are six aspects of empowerment, as shown in Box 6-6.

An effective leader achieves empowerment through expert coaching (Hackman, 2002), active listening, encouragement, building self-confidence and capabilities, and ensuring small successes. Appropriate structure and support are provided to both the team and individuals, contingent upon circumstances, their relative expertise, and confidence levels.

### Focus on the Team's Goals, Performance, and Approach

The team leader helps the team understand its purpose and key role (Staniforth & West, 1995), clarifies its aims and values (Katzenbach & Smith, 2015), and takes responsibility for providing direction and compelling vision (Hayes, 2002). In creating favorable performance conditions (Hackman, 1990), team leaders steer their team rather than control and drive it like hierarchical leaders do (Katzenbach & Smith, 2015).

## BOX 6-5
## GENERIC TEAM LEADERSHIP FRAMEWORK

### PERSON-FOCUSED LEADERSHIP— TRANSFORMATIONAL LEADERSHIP

*Focus on the team's goals, performance, and approach*

Help the team understand its purpose and key role (Staniforth & West, 1995).

Clarify aims and values (Katzenbach & Smith, 2015).

Take responsibility for direction and compelling vision (Hayes, 2002).

Create favorable performance conditions (Hackman, 1990).

Steer team progress, rather than control and drive it (Katzenbach & Smith, 2015).

*Empowerment*

Provide expert coaching (Hayes, 2002).

Show respect and belief in staff.

Display confidence in self and others.

Establish training opportunities to develop team skills.

Establish clear boundaries for autonomy and empowerment.

Ensure that the team has the information and resources for the job.

Ensure rate of progress to meet organizational schedules (Shackleton, 1995).

*Ensure a Collaborative Climate*

Create a safe climate for team members to discuss any issue related to team success (Larssen & Lafasto, 1989).

Balance group autonomy and the leader's role power (Hackman, 2002).

Judge when to use power and when to empower (i.e., create group autonomy).

Observe and analyze patterns of interaction and performance processes within the team

Intervene when required (Hackman, 2002; Staniforth & West, 1995).

*Building Confidence and Commitment (Motivation)*

Highlight successes and positives (Katzenbach & Smith, 2005)

Acknowledge the contributions of team members (Larssen & Lafasto, 1989)

Show appreciation for initiative.

Encourage the team to value each other's skills and talents (Katzenbach & Smith, 2005).

### TASK-FOCUSED LEADERSHIP

*Initiating Structure*

Manage Performance

Create an enabling team structure (Hackman, 2002).

Balance rate of work to meet organizational schedules.

Confront and resolve issues around inadequate performance (Larssen & Lafasto, 1989).

Ensure that everyone, including themselves, does equal amounts of work.

Do not delegate difficult or nasty tasks to others (Katzenbach & Smith, 2015).

Use mistakes as opportunities for team learning.

Encourage team responsibility for failures as well as successes.

Foster constructive, collaborative problem-solving (Katzenbach & Smith, 2015).

Match responsibilities and support to individual experience/expertise (Stoker, 2008).

*Set Priorities for the Team*

Clarify the parameters of the team's responsibilities (Hackman, 1990; Hackman, 2002).

Set team priorities (Lafasto & Larssen, 2002; Larssen & Lafasto, 1989).

Give contingent rewards.

*Manage Relationships with Outsiders (Boundary Spanning)*

Represent the team to the rest of the organization (Hayes, 2002; Katzenbach & Smith, 2015).

Communicate its values and aims (Katzenbach & Smith, 2015).

Remove obstacles from the team's path.

Obtain necessary resources, support (Hackman, 2002), and information (Shackleton, 1995)

Arrange education and training (Hackman, 2002).

Work to create a supportive organizational context (Hackman, 2002).

*Ensure the Correct Mix and Level of Skills in the Team*

Ensure that the team is the right size and has an appropriate skill mix (Hackman, 1990).

Recruit staff with appropriate technical skills and experiences to undertake team tasks.

Establish opportunities for training, learning, and development (Shackleton, 1995).

Develop teamworking and leadership skills in the team (Staniforth & West, 1995).

Create opportunities for team members to develop.

Share opportunities that arise in the organization with the team.

Ensure team members are credited for their achievements (Katzenbach & Smith, 2015).

*Demonstrate Expertise*

Demonstrate high levels of expertise and technical know-how.

Do real work (Katzenbach & Smith, 2015; Larssen & Lafasto, 1989).

Understand the technical issues in achieving the team's goals (Adair, 2005)

---

**BOX 6-6**
## SIX ASPECTS OF EMPOWERMENT

1. **Respect and belief**. Leaders need to respect their staff and show belief that they are capable of high performance.
2. **Confidence**. Leaders need to be confident in their own abilities, both in terms of technical expertise and their ability to lead. Those who lack confidence may feel that the only way to show their competence is by controlling and directing people, so empowering followers is a potential threat.
3. **Training**. Leaders must strike the correct balance between respecting the team's abilities and establishing training opportunities to develop necessary skills.
4. **Boundaries**. There need to be clear boundaries regarding areas of empowerment. The team cannot decide absolutely everything about what it does and when.
5. **Information**. The team specifies what information it needs to do the job, when they need it, and from whom. A key job of the leader is to get them the information they need to work effectively.
6. **Rate of progress**. There needs to be a balance between allowing the team to decide its own rate and pushing it to ensure that organizational schedules are met.

---

## Set Priorities for the Team

Setting priorities and clarifying the parameters/boundaries of the team's responsibilities (Hackman, 1990; Hackman, 2002) are an important part of the leader's role.

## Manage Relationships with Outsiders

A supportive organizational context is vital to any team's success, and its creation is part of the team leader's job (Hackman, 2002). This includes representing the team to the rest of the organization to communicate its values and aims (Hayes, 2002; Katzenbach & Smith, 2015), removing obstacles from the team's path, and winning resources and support (Hackman, 2002). Included is obtaining the information the team needs (Shackleton, 1995) and arranging the education and training required for it to effectively complete its tasks (Hackman, 2002).

## Build Confidence and Commitment

The team leader achieves this by highlighting successes and positives (Katzenbach & Smith, 2015) acknowledging the contributions of team members (Larssen & Lafasto, 1989), showing appreciation for members' initiative, and encouraging the team to value each other's skills and talents (Katzenbach & Smith, 2015).

## Ensure a Collaborative Climate

The team leader creates a safe climate for team members to openly and supportively discuss any issue related to the team's success (Larssen & Lafasto, 1989) and empowers the team to take joint responsibility for achieving its goal (Hayes, 2002). However, empowerment does not involve leaving the team to their own devices (Staniforth & West, 1995) but rather balancing group autonomy and the leader's role authority (Hackman, 2002). The balance is delicate and requires skilled judgement to decide when to empower (i.e., create group autonomy) or when it is right for the leader to exercise role power. It requires sensitivity and awareness to observe and analyze team interaction patterns and work processes and make timely interventions when required (Hackman, 2002; Staniforth & West, 1995). Some leaders can mask their lack of confidence by becoming overly autocratic and authoritarian (Hayes, 2002).

## Manage Performance

While the team leader empowers the team—giving it high levels of autonomy to manage its own work—this does have boundaries; the team leader must strike a balance between allowing the team to decide its own rate of work and setting the rate required to meet organizational schedules (Shackleton, 1995). To achieve this, members must ensure that everyone on the team, including themselves, does roughly equal amounts of work and does not delegate difficult or unpleasant tasks to others (Katzenbach & Smith, 2015; Staniforth & West, 1995). They must also be willing to confront and resolve issues associated with inadequate performance by team members (Larssen & Lafasto, 1989). When issues do arise or mistakes occur, it is important for the team leader not to blame team members but solve the problem without placing undue pressure on the people involved. Mistakes are best considered an opportunity for team learning or for developing new levels of understanding. Having said this, shortfalls in team performance should always be acknowledged and efforts made to sort out problems. By taking responsibility for failures as well as successes, the team leader enhances the feeling of teamwork and fosters constructive, collaborative problem-solving (Katzenbach & Smith, 2015).

However, with reference to the central debates on democratic versus autocratic styles and generic versus situational leadership, it is notable that the levels of expertise and confidence of individual team members need to be taken into consideration. Stoker's (2008) empirical study reports on the effects of team tenure and leadership in self managing teams. See Box 6-7.

## Demonstrate Expertise by Doing Real Work

It is important to understand that a team leader's role differs from that of a team manager. A team leader is located within the team and works alongside other team members to achieve team goals, while a team manager is generally located outside the team. Team managers may manage several teams, and their role is to ensure that the team achieves the overall organizational goals that are set for it and has the resources and support it requires (Hayes, 2002). Because the team leader works as part of the team, it is important that they demonstrate high levels of expertise and technical know-how so they can fully appreciate the technical issues that must be faced to achieve the team's goals.

In professional organizations, this technical expertise is extremely important. Without it, leaders of teams of professionals find it difficult to command the respect of other team members, and their position can quickly become untenable (Adair, 2005).

## Ensure the Correct Mix and Level of Skills in the Team

An essential team leadership function is ensuring that the team's characteristics are appropriate for its role and the tasks it must achieve. The team leader therefore has to ensure that the team is the right size and has an appropriate skill mix (Hackman, 1990). When recruiting team members with the essential technical skills and experiences to undertake team tasks, it is important not to assume that the individuals are already equipped to be team players. Teamworking and team leadership skills are not naturally bountiful and generally need to be developed (Staniforth & West, 1995). Again, there is an important balancing act between respecting the team's abilities and establishing opportunities for training, learning, and development (Shackleton, 1995). An important mechanism is to create opportunities for team members to develop, share opportunities that arise in the organization, and ensure that team members are credited for their achievements, rather than the team leader alone. This both develops member skills and builds commitment to the team (Katzenbach & Smith, 2015).

## LEADING INTERDISCIPLINARY HEALTH AND SOCIAL CARE TEAMS

There is growing literature on teamwork in health and social care teams. Again, as with the wider organizational literature on teamworking, few studies focus directly on leadership. The following leadership variables are therefore derived from studies of teamworking in health and social care.

## Facilitate Shared Leadership

For interdisciplinary teams to work effectively, each team member must accept responsibility as a member-leader to step in and out of the leadership role when their professional expertise or particular

---

### BOX 6-7
### FINDINGS OF AN EMPIRICAL STUDY

- New team members reported high levels of individual performance when their team leader demonstrated directive behavior.
- They reported lower levels of individual performance and greater emotional exhaustion when their team leader adopted more coaching behavioral styles.
- Finally, individual performance was greater and emotional exhaustion less for team members with relatively long team tenure when their team leader exhibited a behavioral coaching style.

Stoker, J. I. (2008). Effects of team tenure and leadership in self-managing teams. *Personnel Review, 37*(5), 564–582.

knowledge of a client or situation comes to the fore. This process requires a formal leader who has overall responsibility for the team's performance, but consciously shares the leadership function, facilitating joint decision-making, and delegates leadership roles (McCallin, 2003; Mickan & Rodger, 2000; Smith et al, 2018; West et al., 2003). The key mechanism for achieving this is empowerment (McCray, 2003). Interdisciplinary team leaders (IdTLs) actively work to develop/maintain non-hierarchical, democratic structures (Ovretveit, 1997). They coach team members (Maister, 1993) to develop the skills required (McCallin, 2003), share their ideas, work to create agreement, and supply the information the team requires (Mickan & Rodger, 2000).

## Leadership Clarity

Teams with a specific team leader have higher levels of staff satisfaction than teams where the leadership role is split (Nancarrow et al., 2009). Leadership clarity is associated with clear team objectives, high levels of participation, commitment to excellence, and support for innovation (West et al., 2003). Primary health care team members rated their effectiveness more highly when they had both strong leadership and high team member involvement (Rosen & Callaly, 2005).

## Transformation and Change

Transformational leadership is important (Irizarry et al., 1993; McCray, 2003). The IdTL acts as a role model, consistent with their espoused values (Pollard, Miers, & Gilchrist, 2005; West et al, 2014), to create a climate in which staff are inspired, challenged, supported, motivated, and rewarded (Irizarry et al., 1993); respond to change in a flexible way (Suter et al., 2007); and facilitate or act as a catalyst for practice change (Willumsen, 2006).

## Personal Qualities

The IdTL must act as a role model, displaying a strong, confident manner and high work standards (Smith et al., 2018). Through their enthusiasm and dedication, they inspire commitment (Abreu, 1997; Pollard, Miers, & Gilchrist, 2005), the ability to empathize (McCray, 2003), and knowledge of people (Suter et al., 2007).

## Aligning Goals with the Organization

The IdTL works to influence the group's direction and climate to ensure alignment with the organization's goals and productivity (Cook & Leathard, 2004). They do this by ensuring that the team has articulated a clear and inspiring vision of its work, creating regular times when it can review its performance (Lyubovnikova et al., 2015), and providing feedback to highlight important issues (Cook & Leathard, 2004; Mickan & Rodger, 2000).

## Creativity and Innovation—Developing the Service

A productive balance of harmony and debate is vital to ensure creativity (Cook & Leathard, 2004), innovation, and the development of new practice models (Smith et al, 2018; Suter et al., 2007). To achieve this, it is essential to provide feedback on important issues (Mickan & Rodger, 2000).

## Communication

A team leader must facilitate interaction processes that develop/sustain clear communication channels within the team (Blewett et al., 2010; Ovretveit, 1997; Suter et al., 2007; Willumsen, 2006). They can do this by initiating constructive discussion; modeling good practices (Lyubovnikova et al., 2015; Mickan & Rodger, 2000); and supporting, actively listening to, and trusting team members (Cook & Leathard, 2004; Mickan & Rodger, 2000). A leader must also manage conflicts that arise, ensuring a productive balance between harmony and healthy debate (McCray, 2003; Mickan & Rodger, 2000).

## Team Building

Teamwork is not a naturally occurring phenomenon (Lyubovnikova et al., 2015). A team leader must therefore invest time in team building, setting expectations for working together (Smith et al., 2018; Suter et al., 2007) and creating a climate of mutual respect (Cook & Leathard, 2004; Ovretveit, 1997). They work to ensure cohesion (Willumsen, 2006), developing the team's interpersonal skills (Ovretveit, 1997; West & Slater, 1996), promoting interdisciplinary collaboration through group reflection on practice (Branowicki et al., 2001; McCallin, 1999), and ensuring socialization of new or inexperienced team members (McCray, 2003).

Collaboration is promoted by allowing enough time for discussion and reflection on practice and encouraging staff to interact with those outside their profession (Branowicki et al., 2001; McCallin, 2003; Suter et al., 2007). To effectively build a team, the IdTL needs to have a good understanding of group dynamics and must also manage members' well-being (Smith et al., 2018).

### Setting Direction

The leader ensures that the team retains a focus on its priorities and goals and that individual team members maintain the correct focus (Mickan & Rodger, 2000). They work to manage team processes (Maister, 1993), including setting clear tasks (Ross et al., 2000), coordinating work (Mickan & Rodger, 2000), and ensuring equitable allocation (Pollard, Miers, & Gilchrist, 2005). Within this framework, it is also important to match tasks to individual expertise (Stoker, 2008).

### External Liaison

A team leader must take external responsibility for the team (Irizarry et al., 1993), ensuring that it is represented and gains the resources it requires (Maister, 1993). This requires entrepreneurial skills to promote the team's work (Smith et al., 2018), the ability to develop networks and linkages (Pollard, Miers, & Gilchrist, 2005), demonstrations of effectiveness through data collection and evaluation (Irizarry et al., 1993), and ensuring the team understands its clients (Willumsen, 2006).

### Skill Mix and Diversity

The IdTL needs to ensure that the team has the right skill mix and diversity to achieve its goals and tasks. This involves both external recruitment and internal development (Ross et al., 2000) with regular supervision, annual performance/development reviews, and providing access to relevant training (Burton et al., 2009; Smith et al, 2018).

### Clinical and Contextual Expertise

Professionals will only be accepted into IdTL roles if they prove their professional expertise (Branowicki et al., 2001; Maister, 1993; Smith et al., 2018). Knowledge of the professional roles of others is also a key competency (MacDonald et al., 2010). Within this, it is important that the team leader balances focus between the needs of the patient, the organization, and the team. Understanding the organization's mission, structure, economics, politics (Branowicki et al., 2001), and current development programs (West et al., 2014), combined with a sound historical perspective, are also important for facilitating an understanding of the context and ensuring that all perspectives are considered (Abreu, 1997) (Box 6-8).

## CONCLUSION

There is good evidence overall that teams can produce superior performance in a variety of work settings, including health and social care. However, achieving the potential performance gains is not easy. Continual efforts to develop teams are required for any performance gains to be achieved. Just labelling a work group a team is unlikely to have any real effect.

In health and social care, teams generally comprise a range of staff from different professions and disciplines. Within these interdisciplinary teams, effective leadership is complex. For interdisciplinary teams to work effectively, each member must accept that they have respoithnsibilities as a member-leader (McCallin, 1999). This entails team members stepping in and out of the leadership role when their (professional/disciplinary) expertise or contextual knowledge of a particular client or situation is needed. The shifting dynamics of shared leadership in interdisciplinary teams depends on the problem at hand and requires that all team members equally participate and take responsibility for both informal and formal leadership responsibilities, according to the continually changing situation. For this process to work, however, it must be facilitated by an overall team leader who is a respected professional, understands the roles of other team members, and is prepared to step in and take formal authority when there is a high level of risk in the team's work. This leads to a somewhat paradoxical conclusion that effective teams need a clear team leader, whose primary job is to facilitate shared leadership (Smith et al., 2018).

## BOX 6-8
## INTERDISCIPLINARY HEALTH AND SOCIAL CARE TEAM LEADERSHIP FRAMEWORK

### FACILITATE SHARED LEADERSHIP

Consciously involve team members in decision-making and delegate responsibilities appropriately (NHS Leadership Academy, 2011; McCallin, 1999; Mickan & Rodger, 2000; Ovretveit, 1997; Smith, Fowler-Davis, Nancarrow, Ariss, & Enderby, 2018; West et al., 2003).

Empower team members (McCray, 2003).

Develop and maintain non-hierarchical structures (Ovretveit, 1997).

Work to create agreement (Mickan & Rodger, 2000).

Coach colleagues in shared leadership (Maister, 1993; McCallin, 2003).

### LEADERSHIP CLARITY

Ensure clarity of leadership (Nancarrow et al., 2009; West et al., 2003).

Combine strong leadership and high involvement (Rosen & Callaly, 2005).

### TRANSFORMATION AND CHANGE (Irizarry et al., 1993; McCray, 2003)

Create a climate where staff are challenged, supported, motivated, and rewarded (West et al., 2003).

Respond to change flexibly (Suter et al., 2007).

Facilitate or act as a catalyst for practice change (Willumsen, 2006).

Act as a role model (Pollard, Ross, & Means, 2005; West et al., 2014).

Inspire other team members (West et al., 2003).

### PERSONAL QUALITIES

High standards (Smith et al., 2018).

Enthusiasm.

Commitment (Abreu, 1997).

Empathy (McCray, 2003).

Knowledge of people (Suter et al., 2007).

### GOAL ALIGNMENT

Ensure the team has articulated a clear and inspiring vision of its work (Lyubovnikova et al., 2015).

Assure productivity and goals are in line with those of the organization (Cook & Leathard, 2004).

Create regular time for the team to review its performance (Lyubovnikova et al., 2015).

Provide feedback about important issues (Cook & Leathard, 2004; Mickan & Rodger, 2000).

### CREATIVITY & INNOVATION

Establish a productive balance of harmony and debate to ensure creativity (Cook & Leathard, 2004).

Develop innovations and new practice models (Smith et al., 2018; Suter et al., 2007).

Ensure effective leadership and team work processes (West et al., 2003).

### COMMUNICATION

Maintain clear communication channels and facilitate interaction processes (Blewett et al., 2010; Ovretveit, 1997; Suter et al., 2007; Willumsen, 2006).

Listen to, support, and trust team members (Cook & Leathard, 2004; Mickan & Rodger, 2000).

Initiate constructive debates and share their own ideas (Lyubovnikova et al., 2015; Mickan & Rodger, 2000).

Manage conflict and maintain a productive balance between harmony and healthy debate (McCray, 2003; Mickan & Rodger, 2000).

### TEAM BUILDING

Set expectations for working together (Smith et al., 2018 Suter et al., 2007).

Create a climate of mutual respect (Cook & Leathard, 2004; Ovretveit, 1997).

Ensure cohesion (Willumsen, 2006).

Develop the team's interpersonal skills (Ovretveit, 1997).

Ensure the contextual socialization of new/inexperienced team members (McCray, 2003).

Promote interprofessional collaboration (Branowicki et al., 2001; McCallin, 2003; Suter et al., 2007).

Facilitate group reflection on practice (Branowicki et al., 2001; McCallin, 1999).

### SETTING DIRECTION

Coordinate tasks (Mickan & Rodger, 2000).

Manage processes (Maister, 1993).

Ensure work is allocated equally (Pollard, Ross et al., 2005).

Set clear tasks (Ross et al., 2000).

### EXTERNAL LIAISON

Represent the team externally (Irizarry et al., 1993).

Ensure necessary resources are made available (Maister, 1993).

Develop entrepreneurial skills to promote the team (Smith et al., 2018).

Develop strategies for promoting the team's work (Irizarry et al., 1993).

Demonstrate effectiveness through data collection and evaluation (Irizarry et al., 1993).

Ensure the team understands its customers and can exploit new opportunities (Willumsen, 2006).

Develop networks and linkages (Pollard, Ross et al., 2005).

*(continued)*

**BOX 6-8**
## INTERDISCIPLINARY HEALTH AND SOCIAL CARE TEAM LEADERSHIP FRAMEWORK— CONT'D

### SKILL MIX AND DIVERSITY

Recruit externally and develop internally (Ross et al., 2000).

Ensure regular supervision and personal development review (Burton et al., 2009).

Assure access to relevant training (Burton et al., 2009; Smith et al., 2018).

### CLINICAL AND CONTEXTUAL EXPERTISE

High levels of professional expertise (Branowicki et al., 2001; Irizarry et al., 1993; Maister, 1993; Smith et al., 2018).

Demonstrate in-depth understanding of the organization (Branowicki et al., 2001) and current development programs (West et al., 2014).

Balance focus among the needs of the patient, organization, and team (Branowicki et al., 2001).

Facilitate understanding of context and ensure all perspectives are considered (Abreu, 1997).

Knowledge of the professional roles of others (MacDonald et al., 2010).

## REFERENCES

Abreu, B. (1997). Interdisciplinary leadership: The future is now. *OD. Practitioner, 2*(3), 20–25.

Adair, J. (2005). *The action-centred leader.* Jaico Publishing.

Alimo-Metcalfe, B., & Alban-Metcalfe, J. (2003). Leadership. Stamp of greatness. *Health Service Journal, 113*(5861), 28–32.

Bennis, W., & Biederman, P. W. (1997). *Organising genius: The secrets of creative collaboration.* Addison-Wesley Publishing.

Blewett, L. A., Johnson, K., McCarthy, T., Lackner, T., & Brandt, B. (2010). Improving geriatric transitional care through inter-professional care teams. *Journal of Evaluation in Clinical Practice, 16*(1), 57–63. https://doi.org/10.1111/j.1365-2753.2008.01114.x.

Branowicki, P. A., Shermont, H., Rogers, J., & Melchiono, M. (2001). Improving systems related to clinical practice: An interdisciplinary team approach. *Seminars for Nurse Managers, 9*(2), 110–114.

Burton, C. R., Fisher, A., & Green, T. L. (2009). The organisational context of nursing care in stroke units: a case study approach. *International Journal of Nursing Studies, 46*(1), 85–94. https://doi.org/10.1016/j.ijnurstu.2008.08.001. Epub 2008 Sep 17. PMID: 18801481.

Cohen, S. G., & Bailey, D. E. (1997). What makes teams work: Group effectiveness work from the shop floor. *Journal of Management, 23*, 239–290.

Cook, M. J., & Leathard, H. L. (2004). Learning for clinical leadership. *Journal of Nursing Management, 12*(6), 436–444.

Currie, V. L., & Harvey, G. (2000). The use of care pathways as tools to support the implementation of evidence-based practice. *Journal of Interdisciplinary Care, 14*, 311–324.

Department of Health. (2002a). *The NHS Plan: A plan for investment, a plan for reform.* HMSO.

Department of Health. (2002b). *Shifting the balance of power: The next steps.* HMSO.

Department of Health. (2008). *NHS next stage review: A high-quality workforce.* HMSO.

Freidson, E. (1970). *The profession of medicine: A study of the sociology of applied knowledge.* Harper & Row.

Hackman, J. R. (2002). *Leading teams: Setting the stage for great performance.* Harvard Business School Press.

Hackman, J. R. (Ed.), (1990). *Groups that work (and those that don't): Conditions for effective teamwork.* Jossey-Bass.

Hayes, N. (2002). *Managing teams: A strategy for success.* Cengage Learning EMEA.

Irizarry, C., Garneau, B., & Walter, R. (1993). Social work leadership development through international exchange. *Social Work in Health Care, 18*(3–4), 35–46.

Katzenbach, J. R., & Smith, D. K. (2015). *The wisdom of teams: Creating the high-performance organisation.* Harvard Business Review.

Lafasto, F. M. J., & Larssen, C. E. (2002). *When teams work best: 6,000 team members tell what it takes to succeed.* Sage Publications.

Laiken, M. (1994). Conflict in teams: Problem or opportunity?: *Lectures in Health Promotion Series 4.* Centre for Health Promotion, University of Toronto.

Larssen, C. E., & Lafasto, F. M. J. (1989). *Teamwork: What must go right, what can go wrong.* Sage Publications.

Leathard, A. (2003). *Interdisciplinary collaboration: From policy to practice in health and social care.* Brunner-Routledge.

Lyubovnikova, J., West, M. A., Dawson, J. F., & Carter, M. R. (2015). 24-Karat or fool's gold? Consequences of real team and co-acting group membership in healthcare organizations. *European Journal of Work and Organizational Psychology, 24*(6), 929–950. https://doi.org/10.1080/1359432X.2014.992421.

MacDonald, M., Bally, J., Ferguson, L., Murray, B., Fowler-Kerry, S., & Anonson, J. (2010). Knowledge of the professional role of others: A key interprofessional competency. *Nurse Education in Practice, 10*(4), 238–242.

Maister, D. H. (1993). *Managing the professional service firm.* Free Press.

Manz, C. C. (1992). Self-leading work teams: Moving beyond self-management myths. *Human Relations, 45*(11), 1119–1140.

Manz, C. C., & Sims, H. P. (2001). *The new superleadership: Leading others to lead themselves.* Berrett-Koehler.

McCallin, A. (1999). Revolution in healthcare: Altering systems, changing behaviour: *Ph.D.* Gaithersburg: Changing Behaviour. https://scholar.google.com/scholar_lookup?title=Revolution%20in%20Healthcare%3A%20Altering%20Systems&publication_year=1999&author=McCallin%2CA.

McCallin, A. (2003). Interdisciplinary team leadership: a revisionist approach for an old problem? *Journal of Nursing Management, 11*(6), 364–370. https://doi.org/10.1046/j.1365-2834.2003.00425.x.

McCray, J. (2003). Leading interprofessional practice: A conceptual framework to support practitioners in the field of learning disability. *Journal of Nursing Management, 11*(6), 387–395.

Meindl, J. R. (1990). On leadership: An alternative to the conventional wisdom. *Research in Organisational Behaviour, 12*, 329–341.

Mickan, S. M., & Rodger, S. A. (2000). Characteristics of effective teams: A literature review. *Australian Health Review, 23*(3), 201–208.

Moran, A. M. (2008). A study to examine the contribution of support workers to the delivery and outcomes of community rehabilitation and intermediate care services in England: *PhD.* University of Sheffield.

Munro, C. R., & Laiken, M. (2003). Developing & sustaining high performance teams. *OD Practitioner, 35*(4), 63.

Nancarrow, S., Enderby, P., Ariss, A., Smith, T., Booth, A., & Campbell, M. (2012). *Enhancing the effectiveness of interdisciplinary working: costs and outcomes.* NIHR Service Delivery and Organisation Programme.

Nancarrow, S., Moran, A. M., Enderby, P., Parker, S., Dixon, S., Mitchell, C., … Buchan, J. (2009). *The impact of workforce flexibility on the costs and outcomes of older peoples' services.* National Co-Ordinating Centre for NHS Service Delivery and Organisation.

Osland, J. A., Kolb, D. A., & Rubin, I. M. (2000). *Organizational behaviour: An experiential approach* (7th Ed.). Pearson.

Ovretveit, J. (1997). How to describe interprofessional working. In J. Ovretveit, P. Mathias, & T. Thompson (Eds.), *Interprofessional working for health and social care* (pp. 9–33). Palgrave.

Pollard, K. C., Miers, M. E., & Gilchrist, M. (2005). Collaborative learning for collaborative working? Initial findings from a longitudinal study of health and social care students. *Health and Social Care in the Community, 12*(4), 346–358.

Pollard, K. C., Ross, K., & Means, R. (2005). Nurse leadership, interprofessionalism and the modernization agenda. *British Journal of Nursing, 14*(6), 339–344. https://doi.org/10.12968/bjon.2005.14.6.17805.

Reeves, S., Macmillan, K., & Van Soeren, M. (2010). Leadership of interprofessional health and social care teams: A socio-historical analysis. *Journal of Nursing Management, 18*(3), 258–264.

Rosen, A., & Callaly, T. (2005). Interprofessional teamwork and leadership: Issues for psychiatrists. *Australasian Psychiatry, 3*, 234–240.

Ross, F., Rink, E., & Furne, A. (2000). Integration or pragmatic coalition? An evaluation of nursing teams in primary care. *Journal of Interprofessional Care, 14*(3), 259–267.

Schein, E. H. (2016). *Organizational culture and leadership* (5th Ed.). John Wiley & Sons.

Sennett, R. (1998). *The corrosion of character: The personal consequences of work in the new capitalism.* W. W. Norton.

Shackleton, V. J. (1995). *Business leadership.* Routledge.

Smith, T., Fowler-Davis, S., Nancarrow, S., Ariss, S., & Enderby, P. (2018). Leadership in interprofessional health and social care teams: A literature review. *Leadership in Health Services, 31*(4), 452–467. https://doi.org/10.1108/LHS-06-2016-0026.

Staniforth, D., & West, M. A. (1995). Leading and managing teams. *Team Performance Management, 1*(2), 28–33.

Stoker, J. I. (2008). Effects of team tenure and leadership in self-managing teams. *Personnel Review, 37*(5), 564–582.

Suter, E., Arndt, J., Lait, J., Jackson, K., Kipp, J., Taylor, E., & Arthur, N. (2007). How can frontline managers demonstrate leadership in enabling interprofessional practice? *Healthcare Management Forum, 20*(4), 38–43.

Tuckman, B. W. (1965). Developmental sequence in small groups. *Psychological Bulletin, 63*(6), 384–399. https://doi.org/10.1037/H0022100.

Tuckman, B. W., & Jensen, M. A. C. (1977). Stages of small-group development revisited. *Group and Organization Studies, 2*(4), 419–427.

West, M. A., & Slater, J. (1996). *The effectiveness of teamworking in primary health care.* The Health Education Authority.

West, M. A., Borrill, C. S., Dawson, J. F., Brodbeck, F., Shapiro, D. A., & Haward, B. (2003). Leadership clarity and team innovation in health care. *The Leadership Quarterly, 14*(4–5), 393–410.

West, M. A., Lyubovnikova, J., Eckert, R., & Denis, J. (2014). Collective leadership for cultures of high quality health care. *Journal of Organizational Effectiveness: People and Performance, 1*(3), 240–260.

Willumsen, E. (2006). Leadership in interprofessional collaboration – The case of childcare in Norway. *Journal of Interprofessional Care, 20*(4), 403–413.

Xyrichis, A., & Lowton, K. (2008). What fosters or prevents interprofessional teamworking in primary or community care? A literature review. *International Journal of Nursing Studies, 45*(1), 140–153.

Yukl, G. (2019). *Leadership in organisations* (9th Ed.). Pearson Education Ltd.

NHS Leadership Academy (2011). Leadership Framework, Institute for Innovation and Improvement. https://www.leadershipacademy.nhs.uk/wp-content/uploads/2012/11/NHSLeadership-Framework-LeadershipFramework.pdf

## REFLECTIVE QUESTIONS

- What are the most important skills for health and social care leaders to develop?
- What are the benefits of teamworking in health and social care workplaces?
- From your experience of team leadership, is it better to have a single leader or should leadership be shared?
- What are the main demands placed upon the leaders of interdisciplinary teams?
- In your opinion, why might a leader take back control of the shared leadership at particular times?
- What are the skills that you feel are necessary for a leader to embody in an interdisciplinary health and social care team?

# 7

# RESILIENCE: MANAGING SELF AND MANAGING RISK

CAROL J. CLARK

■ ■ ■ ■ ■ ■ ■ ■ ■ ■ ■ ■ ■ ■ ■ ■ ■ ■ ■ ■ ■

## OBJECTIVES

*After reading this chapter, you should be able to:*

■ Identify and reflect on factors you believe may have contributed to your own resilience and how you might use this knowledge to continue to build this strength in your leadership.

■ Analyze the factors that are contributing to psychosocial risk and the resilience of your department/institution/ organization.

■ Critically discuss factors that you currently use to identify and manage risk and consider what advice you might provide to colleagues to ensure risk is limited and managed as far as is practical.

■ Broadly consider how you might build your own resilience and that of the staff in your organization throughout their careers.

## INTRODUCTION

Chapter 7 broadly considers leadership, resilience, and managing risk for individuals and organizations by providing examples from health and social care in the United Kingdom, while also drawing on examples of practices from other industries. The importance of leadership and resilience in health and social care cannot be underestimated, as the National Health Service (NHS) and Social Care employ 1.4 million and 1.6 million people, respectively (NHS Information Centre, 2013; Skills for Care, 2010). These large influential organizations provide valuable lessons related to institutional resilience and risk across the spectrum of good and poor practices. Consideration is given to exploring what can be done to build individual resilience, manage psychosocial issues that might undermine

resilience, and the life experiences that help people "bounce back" and grow. Building resilient organizations is a prerequisite for ensuring stable health and social care workforces and for the health and well-being of the individuals within them. Adverse events are normal in all organizations, and regulators, policy makers, and leaders need to address these with openness and transparency, learning as much from the aspects that succeed as from those that fail. Ultimately, resilient organizations with a shared vision that manage risk can become "go to" organizations.

## BUILDING INDIVIDUAL RESILIENCE

Individual resilience may be considered a way of facing and understanding the world; it may be innate and therefore embedded in everything we do. It is a philosophy that we may not be aware of until we begin to deconstruct its meaning. We might only understand the term in the context of our own world view, as resilience lies on a spectrum and is influenced by a bricolage of worldly experiences (Pietrzak & Southwick, 2011). Resilience is summarized as the ability to adapt in a time of difficulty, for example, following a catastrophe, traumatic event, or significant periods of stress caused by personal, health, social, employment, or financial issues (Palmiter et al., 2012).

All adult learners will have had life experiences that contribute to their level of resilience. Higher education and work place institutions should be supported in their efforts to ensure health and social care students understand how they might build their resilience and what factors might mitigate risk to resilience. As already alluded to, a traumatic experience can affect a person's resilience (Southwick et al., 2014). It is not a trait that belongs to some and not others; rather, it is one that evolves through learning and developing thoughts, behaviors, and actions in which anyone can participate.

Building resilience requires engaging with some important steps, including facing reality, taking responsibility, understanding reality, and improvising solutions (Coutu, 2002). Resilience has four core components: connection, wellness, healthy thinking, and meaning. These components are embedded within each person and ultimately impact what we think and do as individuals and as leaders (Palmiter et al., 2012). Building resilience requires understanding and reflecting on how to connect with taking responsibility, facing reality, and working on solutions that ensure the health and well-being of individuals and organizations.

Increased resilience correlates with the ability to manage stress and recognizing that stress is a risk factor for conditions such as anxiety and depression. It impacts the workforce in terms of health and well-being, productivity, and recruitment and retention. Work-related stress is a person's reaction to undue pressures and demands placed on them at work (HSE, 2019). This definition is limited, as it does not consider the broader stressors placed on employees outside the work environment that may also contribute. In the United Kingdom, the size of the problem can be understood by reviewing the NHS data for January 2020, which shows overall workforce sickness at 4.8% for that month; the most common reasons cited were anxiety/stress/depression, with these conditions accounting for nearly one-fourth of all sickness (NHS, 2020).

In 2018, 602,000 workers across the United Kingdom (excluding Northern Ireland) suffered from work-related stress, leading to 12.8 million lost workdays, with an average of 21.2 days per person. This makes up about half of all self-reported work-related illnesses. Workplace stress was greater in large public sector organizations such as education and health and social care and was correlated with increased workload stress. The major causes of work-related stress (including depression and/or anxiety) are workload pressures (tight deadlines, high workload), too much responsibility, and a lack of support. In combination with organizational change and conflict (violence, bullying, and threats), these constituted 80% of all work stresses (HSE, 2019). These data highlight the need not only for

resilient individuals but also for resilient organizations within which employees feel supported.

## Generational Response to Stress

In 2019, NHS England published its Long-Term Plan (LTP) (NHS, 2019), presenting an overall vision for the development of the NHS over the next 10 years. This plan recognizes the key role of staff, existing pressures, ways of working, and how these might impact retention and recruitment. With more than 1.4 million staff spanning five generations, it is important to explore how work-related stress is responded to across the generations.

The five generations are described by the year of birth, as follows: Traditionalists, born before 1945; Baby Boomers (BB) 1945–1960; Generation X (Gen X) 1961–1980; Generation Y (Gen Y) 1981–1995; and Generation Z (Gen Z), born after 1995. Each generation has different work priorities and training requirements, which will affect policies around issues such as recruitment and retention. A survey that compared the views of Gen Z with those of BB found that 55% of Gen Z had taken time off as a result of work-related stress compared with 17% of BB (CIPD, 2008). Moreover, the cost of mental health per employee as a proportion of their earnings is much higher (8.3%) in 18–29 year-olds compared with that of all other age groups (5.8%) (Deloitte, 2020). Therefore, possible solutions to reduce stress in the BB generation aimed at staff retention and/or preparation for retirement might be different from the solutions for Gen Z in relation to initial recruitment and retention. However, there is evidence of similarities across the generations within staff in the NHS around factors that reduce stress and support retention, including support, flexibility, and being appreciated (NHS HEE, 2019).

In 2018, the NHS workforce comprised 13% BB, 51% Gen X, 33% Gen Y, and 3% Gen Z. This is in the context of reports that there were 100,000 vacancies across NHS Trusts, with 20% of staff leaving their roles in community trusts in 2017–18 (NHS HEE, 2019). Key issues for recruitment and retention are interlinked, as inadequate staff numbers can contribute to increased workload stress and anxiety levels; these in turn lead to psychosocial risk factors that undermine the resilience of both individuals and organizations and generate subsequent costs. Work-related stress is showing a rising trend, with a reported increase of 1.3% from 2016 to 2017. In addition, the costs of stress-related illness are significant, averaging £1794–2174 per recorded illness in 2014 (NHS HEE, 2019).

Undergraduate or pre-registration health and social care students represent the future workforce, and their health and well-being need to be considered. There is recognition that educational attrition rates could be high in some health professional groups, for example, with up to 30% of nursing students leaving some programs in the United Kingdom (Crombie et al., 2013), some of whom opt to defer their studies due to emotional health issues. Enhancing resilience is likely to be an important element in the tool kit of health and social care professionals across generations who work in complex, stressful, and emotionally challenging environments (Sanderson & Brewer, 2017). There is no reason this tool kit cannot be part of the undergraduate curricula.

## RISK MANAGEMENT

Work-related and psychosocial stress are now widely recognized as major challenges to occupational health in workplaces worldwide and can be summarized as the stress experienced when job demands exceed an individual's ability to cope with or control a situation (European Foundation, 2007). Health and social care environments are well recognized as emotionally challenging and stressful. Health and social care professions have raised concerns with key bodies, including the Medical Research Council and the Economic and Social Research Council, acknowledging the size of the problem (Windle et al., 2011). Factors that are considered to contribute to stress in the workplace are the interactions between job content and the management, organization, and environmental conditions, and an employee's competencies and requirements. Many people spend the majority of their waking hours in their working environment. Providing the "right" environment and "risk managing" that environment may help mitigate psychosocial stress, leading to a healthier and more productive workforce. Conversely, if these elements are not considered, there may be a rise in absenteeism, presenteeism (working more hours than required or working when unwell—in both cases being less productive), and/or people opting to take early retirement.

Leaders and managers play a key role in recognizing, understanding, and managing psychosocial risk factors. In the first instance, they may need training to recognize the risk factors in their particular setting. This training and organizational support will only be available in institutions that foster an environment where the need to manage risk factors is recognized and understood. At an individual level, the job content should match the employee's competencies and ambitions. With the right support, employees may "grow" into their jobs and blossom in their careers. Elements that might facilitate such a trajectory include regular meetings with a leader to review workload and content, discussions about career plans (appraisals), opportunities for meaningful training, and a supportive environment when things go wrong. This approach takes time and effort on the part of leaders and managers, which is often unrecognized in their workload. Chapter 13 explores and broadens the discussion of these issues.

Cox (1993) first discussed psychosocial hazards, a term later adopted by the European Framework for Psychosocial Risk Management (PRIMA-EF, 2008). The framework presents a holistic set of guidelines to support the recognition and management of psychosocial risk in the workplace. These can be broadly divided into three main themes, with a fourth theme that influences the three main themes. The first theme encompasses job content, workload, pace, and schedule and the interaction with meaningful work and a career trajectory. The second theme relates to the organization and includes the physical, social, and cultural environment and a person's role and function within this environment. The third theme is the home–work interface; this can be an area of significant conflict as families juggle dual careers and caring responsibilities. The fourth theme, which influences all the other themes, relates to "control." Employers and employees need to recognize the aspects of these three themes that are within their control and those that are not, so there can be a focus on managing elements that may become stressors (Cox, 1993).

It is important to recognize that stressors are individual and change over time. There are also some broader strategies that can be used as part of a risk management strategy aimed at improving the general work environment. In the scientific literature, three main types of work-related stress prevention strategies have been identified and are broadly described under the terms primary, secondary, and tertiary (PRIMA-EF, 2008).

## Primary Prevention

Primary prevention requires considering how aspects of work are organized and managed. This might include designing an organizational structure that ensures employees have a line manager and appraiser who have time to meaningfully engage in line management and appraisal processes. To improve staff retention, these conversations should be career developing as opposed to career limiting. In the health and social care sector, this may involve providing opportunities for colleagues to take on post-graduate education to enhance leadership or advanced clinical/social care practice. Enhanced skills increase productivity, improve retention, and ultimately benefit the organization.

## Secondary Prevention

Secondary prevention requires considering approaches that an organization can use to combat work-related stress. This might involve staff being offered time management training and flexible working arrangements. With the advent of virtual meetings, staff who work across sites can be encouraged to attend meetings virtually, thereby spending less time travelling. Additional measures for health and social care staff might include providing childcare and flexible working during school holidays. This is particularly relevant to a workforce that includes many women, who often carry the bulk of childcare responsibilities. For example, 80% of both the nonmedical NHS workforce and the adult social care workforce are women (NHS Information Centre, 2008; Skills for Care, 2010).

## Tertiary Prevention

Tertiary prevention approaches are those that aim to reduce the impact of work-related stress on an individual's health. This might involve working with a colleague after their return to work to identify an appropriate phased return. This includes working with the individual's team/work colleagues to make sure others are not overloaded. The case study in Box 7-1 is one example.

> **BOX 7.1**
> **CASE STUDY #1**
>
> Janet was an Allied Health Professional who returned to work following six months off work for a stress-related illness and back pain. A three-month phased return interspersed with annual leave was initially put in place to support her return, with a follow up scheduled after the initial two weeks. It soon became apparent that the planned phased return was too ambitious. Within two weeks, Janet recognized that she could not work at the pace she had anticipated. This caused immense stress, as she felt she was letting her colleagues and patients/clients down. It also produced emotional stress for her colleagues as they tried to encourage and support her but felt unable to do so.
>
> **Reflect**: As a manager/leader, consider what psychosocial hazards may be contributing to Janet's stress and what prevention approaches might mitigate future absences caused by stress.

## CORPORATE AND INDIVIDUAL RESPONSIBILITY

There is an ethical requirement for organizations to demonstrate corporate social responsibility that goes beyond the organization and considers global challenges. Global challenges include achieving a sustainable future across nations and relate to poverty, inequality, climate change, environmental degradation, peace, and justice. Strategies that are aimed at economic growth also need to address health and social needs, education, and job opportunities while protecting the planet (United Nations, 2015). Institutions and corporations are responsible to their internal environment and employees and to the external environment. The focus of this next section is on exploring corporate responsibility for the internal environment.

There may be competing priorities within an organization, but one of the most strategically important priorities is looking after the workforce to achieve a sustainable future and ensure a resilient organization. Promoting well-being in the workplace and addressing physical and psychosocial issues fall within the scope of corporate social responsibility. This involves recognizing psychosocial issues at the heart of an organization in strategies, plans, and processes. Doing so ensures that psychosocial issues are recognized, understood, and managed throughout the organization and that the organization works with stakeholders to ensure their voices are heard (PRIMA-EF, 2008).

Integrating psychosocial issues into strategies, plans, and processes requires clear demonstration of the organization's vision, how the vision will be achieved, and how psychosocial issues have been considered. This firstly requires the whole organization to "buy" the vision, as well as transparency of work processes and the working environment, to ensure a supportive environment is maintained that will mitigate psychosocial issues. The second issue highlights the need for psychosocial issues to be recognized and managed. This requires ensuring that leaders have the tools, such as training and fostering innovation, to address the risks. Ultimately, this will enhance the staff experience, which will benefit recruitment and retention. The third consideration is to ensure a balance between implementing systems, internalizing values, and organizational learning; it can be easy for an organization to focus on implementing systems and lose sight of what is happening within the organization.

The events that led to the Francis Report (Francis, 2013) illustrate this point. The Trust board was focused on implementing systems and, in particular, achieving "Foundation Trust status" to gain greater autonomy. This focus resulted in a series of collective failures across the organization, leading to patient suffering. Interestingly, the Trust and its many stakeholders did not recognize or acknowledge the failures in a timely manner (Francis, 2013). This brings the discussion to the fourth action for addressing psychosocial risk, which is maintaining meaningful engagement with stakeholders. The greater the involvement of key stakeholders, the more likely it is that psychosocial elements will continue to be highlighted. Stakeholders can include but are not limited to patients/clients, health and social care institutions, employment agencies, unions, professional and statutory bodies, and higher education institutions. This gives importance to having systems in place so that all of these collective voices can be heard.

Finally, even in health and social care institutions, the health of employees is unlikely to feature as a primary business interest. There is likely to be concern about how ill health affects the delivery of services, but less interest in the idea that the delivery of services might be contributing to ill health. The costs of ill health cannot be ignored; in 2017, 38% of NHS staff reported feeling unwell as a result of work-related stress (NHS Survey Coordination Centre, 2018), and mental ill health among employees cost UK employers £42–£45 billion each year (Deloitte, 2020). Since 2017, more businesses have been providing training for managers to help them support staff with mental health problems, and there is evidence that each £1 spent results in a £5 return (Deloitte, 2020). Supporting the workforce and caring about their welfare in turn contribute to staff retention and a more productive and resilient organization.

## RESILIENCE WITHIN AN ORGANIZATION

Elements that enable resilience within an organization can be observed in an organization that faces reality, holds on to reality, and improvises solutions that are continually adapted to meet the ever-changing needs of the internal and external environments (Coutu, 2002). Nurturing the right culture to ensure resilience in an organization requires valuing relationships based on trust with all staff and key stakeholders. One example of how this might be achieved was modeled by Virgin Atlantic, who situated senior members of the organization in a place that was regularly accessible by all (i.e., the corner of an open plan office). The organization provided an environment in which staff as stakeholders had a voice that could be heard. This simple innovation led to employees building a relationship of trust and understanding within the organization.

### Resilience and Leadership During a Crisis

In 2020, our understanding and experience of resilience has been influenced by the COVID-19 global pandemic. This pandemic has led to unprecedented changes across all our lives, with a major impact in the health and social care sector.

As "lockdown" was initiated in the United Kingdom, health and social care organizations were bracing themselves to manage the pandemic. Change occurred quickly and required leaders to work with colleagues to manage new work environments and swiftly navigate and embrace new norms (work and home) at a time of high stress and anxiety. Individuals' perceptions and how these changes affected them will have differed. In other situations, people with negative coping behaviors who report high levels of perceived stress are less resilient (Rahimi et al., 2014). Conversely, the ability to cope, reflect, and take ownership are features that correlate with resilience (Sanderson & Brewer, 2017).

Quick judgements had to be made with limited time to explore risks. Those with backgrounds in health and social care may be viewed as better able to manage in times of crisis; they are well versed in exercising professional judgement and managing risk because they have learned to integrate their explicit and tacit knowledge (Holroyd, 2015). While this may be the case for some, it will not have been the case for all, partly because the crisis was not only happening at work, it was also occurring in people's home lives. One major feature was that schools and nurseries closed and grandparents were requested to isolate, making childcare and home schooling a significant consideration for employees with school-age children.

Returning to the notion of explicit and tacit knowledge, explicit knowledge relates to the objective skills of understanding facts, data, research, and policies, while tacit knowledge can be described as softer, innate skills, including intuition, insight, and pragmatism. In the early stages of the pandemic in the United Kingdom, there was limited explicit knowledge, which required leaders to use their tacit knowledge with compassion, empathy, and reassurance to support the resilience of their teams. As people emerge from a crisis, they can grow their own resilience by reflecting on their experiences and sharing stories with others, including problem solving and strategies for managing their own health and well-being, as suggested by Sanderson and Brewer (2017).

## Building Individual Resilience

Building resilience involves the interaction of biological, psychological, social, and cultural factors along a continuum. It may involve actively seeking a way forward that has the capacity to be dynamic and therefore allows an individual to adapt successfully (Southwick et al., 2014). An individual's resilience is the ability to "bounce back" after a "crisis;" it is what helps us recover and remain robust (Francke, 2016). We do not know what makes some people more resilient than others or what helps people "bounce back." It is suggested that it might be in our biology but influenced by our experiences and environment (for example,

our support systems). It is likely to be adaptive and embedded in close relationships and emotional security (Southwick et al., 2014). Most leaders and managers who have dealt with "significant issues" at work will have had their confidence dented, been affected emotionally, and generally acknowledge that it has impacted their personal and work lives (Skoberne et al., 2016). One of the pivotal tools that supports the ability to "bounce back" is being able to learn from what has gone wrong and to move on and focus on future success (Redmond & Crisafulli, 2010).

From a cultural perspective, the word "hope" and the ability to think about and believe in a meaningful future are considered important elements for building resilience (Panter-Brick & Eggerman, 2012). This might be achieved through storytelling and collaborating with others to gain a sense of meaning (a concept also discussed in Chapter 11). Another element could be providing individuals with resources that facilitate their ability to construct a better future that is realistic and meaningful. It is important to build and nurture resilience early, for example, in children, and provide individuals with agency, flexibility, motivation, and a sense of belonging with meaningful occupation through life (Masten, 2014; Southwick et al., 2014).

Nurses reported that attending a training program provided them with an opportunity to learn from the program and peers and to affirm and strengthen their current practice in resilience (Foster et al., 2018). Resilience may be enhanced by training individuals to (a) read the situation or context sensitivity, (b) have a repertoire of behaviors, and c) have the ability to regroup using constructive feedback (Bonanno & Burton, 2013), which in some cases may be facilitated by cognitive behavioral therapy (Foster et al., 2018). It has also been proposed that there should be a cultural expectation early in life that individuals will need to deal with adversity, thereby preparing them and ensuring adversity is perceived as a norm rather than something unusual (Southwick et al., 2014).

## Training to Increase Resilience

Most health and social care undergraduate programs use reflective practice as a method for engaging students in lifelong learning. Reflective practice is also a requirement for continuing professional development and maintaining professional registration; it is one of the six themes identified by Low et al. (2019) in a recent scoping review aimed at exploring educational strategies for teaching resilience. The other five themes were storytelling; practicing mindfulness and meditation; enhancing self-knowledge and personal competencies; mentoring and professional support; and mentoring and peer support (Low et al., 2019) (Box 7-2).

Career-long educational programs can provide reinforcement to staff that there are many things they can do for themselves that can help them manage their situation. These might include better communication, empathizing with patients/clients, building trusting relationships, using skills gained through mindfulness practice, and reflective practice. However, individual resilience can be eroded if the external stressors that an individual has little control over are not managed. These might include, for example, a high workload, insufficient resources, and high staff turnover. In addition to educational programs that enhance an individual's confidence and resilience, there also needs to be a structure and organization that enables resilience (Foster et al., 2018). There is a requirement for all individuals to have confidence in their leaders and know that someone is "watching their back."

## Building Resilient Teams

Across health and social care, teams will be made up of many professionals working together (see Chapter 6 for a further discussion). The most productive and resilient teams will be those who have good interprofessional working relationships built on trust and understanding. The activities of building an understanding of the different professional groups and working in teams needs to start in undergraduate programs with interprofessional learning and can also be part of continuing professional development. In health and social care, we rarely work in isolation and our individual resilience is influenced by how our teams function (it is also recognized that we may be a member of many teams). Resilient teams have four things in common: trusting one another and feeling safe with colleagues, an ability to improvise, a belief in the team's ability to deliver a task, and a shared understanding of how the team works (Kirkman et al., 2019).

Feeling safe with a team means having the confidence to raise new ideas and know they will not be ridiculed; it also enables the team to improvise new solutions. Social interactions with shared stories can help team members feel a sense of belonging and build trust. If everyone understands the team's purpose and how it works, and has a shared vision, the chances of delivering the task and being successful will be improved. The shared journey to achievement is one way to build resilience (Box 7-3 and Box 7-4).

---

**BOX 7.2**
**STRATEGIES FOR BUILDING RESILIENCE***

- Legitimizing failure and empowering people to learn and move on—most people learn from their mistakes.
- Understanding the importance of a supportive culture: inclusion, not exclusion.
- Recognizing and identifying psychosocial risk factors.
- Exploring how risk factors can be mitigated/managed.
- Identifying key stakeholders and working with them to ensure their voices can be heard.
- Enabling individuals to face reality (with a balanced mindset), to keep reviewing the environment, and remain focused on the vision and values.
- Recognizing the benefits of mentoring and/or coaching—including sharing experiences of failure and success.
- Recognizing the importance of support networks at home and at work.

Coutu (2002); Redmond & Crisafulli (2010); Skoberne et al. (2016); Amalberti & Vincent (2020).
*This is not an exhaustive list.

---

**BOX 7.3**
**CASE STUDY #2**

A successful community nursing team of four had received accolades for their service, which was very much in demand. One year later they had been unable to recruit to fill a vacancy when a member of the team retired. To mitigate the lack of resources, the team restructured and reprioritized to manage service requirements. In the last month, one member of the team had been promoted and another member of the team with significant caring responsibilities had taken temporary sick leave due to stress.

**Reflect** As the team lead, consider the factors that are threatening this team's resilience and what measures might be put in place.

## Building Resilient Organizations

Finding meaning in one's environment is an important aspect of building resilient organizations (Coutu, 2002); the term "finding meaning" might be interpreted as values. These values can be used as a scaffold to build an organization and create a resilient culture. The values are core to an organization and can help it frame its strategies, policies, and decisions.

The six values of the NHS are referred to in the NHS constitution (Department of Health and Social Care, 2015). The importance of these values should not be underestimated, as Coutu (2002) suggests that an organization's values contribute more to its resilience than does the resilience of the individuals in the workforce. It is argued that if the entire workforce is following the same values, then they will all be pulling together in the same direction. However, if all employees are resilient but interpret the values differently, it may lead to conflict of decisions and actions. The first step in building resilience in an organization such as the NHS is to ensure the vision and values are simple, relatable, and embedded throughout the organization. They will only be memorable if they have meaning for employees. Ensuring transparency and embedding the values of the NHS and a Trust organization were part of the recommendations in the King's Fund Report (2013). I have focused on employees, but the values also need to be memorable for other NHS stakeholders (i.e., patients/clients/service users, senior civil servants, and politicians).

Another facet that can influence resilience is "facing down reality" (Coutu, 2002). This relates to an organization having a clear sense of reality (risks are defined and considered) and includes ensuring that the vision's focus and values are not lost or interpreted too optimistically. In the Mid Staffordshire enquiry (Francis, 2013), it appears that "reality" was lost for a number of reasons, one of which was the multiple reorganizations that led to a loss of institutional memory (of previous risks). A second reason was the loss of understanding regarding the Trust's core business. The focus for the trust board was on the systems and processes required to build a Trust and meet financial targets, which was at odds with the core business of delivering health and social care. When an organization addresses the reality of its environment, it prepares to act in a way that ensures endurance and survival. This includes listening to colleagues and ensuring that everyone knows and is constantly reassessing the reality (risks) and working together toward the same values.

The third cornerstone of organizational resilience is "ritualized ingenuity;" this is described as the ability to improvise solutions to problems (Coutu, 2002) and "'making do" in challenging times. There are many excellent examples of how colleagues in the NHS have used ingenuity, innovation, and creativity to manage significant risks and crises. Emergency departments in the NHS are particularly adept at improvising on a regular basis, and, in spite of challenges, have continued to deliver high quality care. However, of note is the suggestion that dependence on individual leaders is one of the limiting factors in an organization's ability to manage resilience and improvise (Amalberti & Vincent, 2020) (Box 7-5).

## CONCLUSION

This chapter has defined and introduced the term "resilience," providing us with a broad context of a term that explains how we face and understand the world. It may be seen by others as adapting well to adversity. Resilience correlates with the ability to manage stress, and although it is normal to experience stress through life, there are times when this can adversely affect a person's health and well-being and lead to conditions such as anxiety and depression. Work-related stress is a significant burden on the workforce, and within the large health and social care sector, the importance of recognizing factors that may reduce resilience need due consideration. Case studies stimulate thinking

## BOX 7.5
## CASE STUDY #3

Alex is a mid-career social worker with a young family and recently achieved promotion, moving to a job in a different part of the country. The job had a demanding caseload, including managing several teams with numerous stakeholders. Two months after starting, her line manager had to take extended time off work following an accident and Alex was expected to deputize. Shortly after this, there was a serious complaint about the conduct and professionalism of a staff member, and Alex was assigned to lead the investigation.

Work pressure began to mount as she tried to maintain focus on her normal work activities, manage the additional responsibilities of her line manager, and progress the investigation. There was conflicting and confusing input from the next level manager and human resources department, and she felt she was receiving insufficient understanding and support. She spent increasing hours at work, compromising the attention she was able to give to her family, and she began to sleep badly, feel unwell, and was unable to function.

**Reflect**: As Alex's line manager returning from sick leave to this situation, how would you address it and what features might a more resilient organization have in place to mitigate the impact?

about psychosocial factors in a workplace that may increase the risk of stress-related illness and how these might be mitigated to improve health and well-being as well as workforce productivity.

This chapter considered building resilience in the workforce across teams and organizations. It incorporated references to learning from a variety of organizations. Consideration of the tools that might be useful in training programs has also been addressed as encouragers and enablers of resilient behaviors. Organizations with a shared vision that includes addressing psychosocial risk factors form the basis of a resilient organization. Resilient organizations attract employees, enabling successful recruitment and retention and the health and well-being of the workforce, ultimately improving productivity. As leaders, if we are to support the resilience of individuals and teams, educating the workforce is only part of the solution; the other major aspect is the social responsibility of organizations to openly risk manage the work environment. Workforces need to be offered a clear vision of an organization's values and behaviors; individuals then feel trusted and supported to perform.

## REFERENCES

Amalberti, R., & Vincent, C. (2020). Managing risk in hazardous conditions: Improvisation is not enough. *BMJ Quality & Safety*, 29(1), 60–63. https://doi.org/10.1136/bmjqs-2019-009443.

Bonanno, G. A., & Burton, C. L. (2013). Regulatory flexibility: An individual differences perspective on coping and emotion regulation. *Perspectives on Psychological Science*, 8(6), 591–612.

Chartered Institute of Personnel Development (CIPD). (2008). *Gen Up: How the four generations work*. <https://www.criticaleye.com/inspiring/insights-servfile.cfm?id=2183>

Coutu, D. L. (2002). How resilience works. *Harvard Business Review* <http://factoroh.com/wp-content/uploads/How-resilience-works.pdf>

Cox, T. (1993). *Stress research and stress management: Putting theory to work*. HSE Books.

Crombie, A., Brindley, J., Harris, D., Marks-Maran, D., & Thompson, T. M. (2013). Factors that enhance rates of completion: What makes students stay? *Nurse Education Today*, 33(11), 1282–1287. https://doi.org/10.1016/j.nedt.2013.03.020.

Deloitte. (2020). *Mental health and employers: Refreshing the case for investment*. <https://www2.deloitte.com/content/dam/Deloitte/uk/Documents/consultancy/deloitte-uk-mental-health-and-employers.pdf>

Department of Health and Social Care. (2015). *The NHS constitution for England*. <https://www.gov.uk/government/publications/the-nhs-constitution-for-england/the-nhs-constitution-for-england>

European Foundation for the Improvement of Living and Working Conditions. (European Foundation). (2007). *Fourth European working conditions survey*. Office for Official Publications of the European communities. <http://www.eurofound.europa.eu/ewco/surveys/index.htm>

Foster, K., Cuzzillo, C., & Furness, T. (2018). Strengthening mental health nurses' resilience through a workplace resilience programme: A qualitative inquiry. *Journal of Psychiatric & Mental Health Nursing*, 25(5–6), 338–348. <https://onlinelibrary.wiley.com/doi/10.1111/jpm.12467>

Francis, R. (2013). Report of the Mid Staffordshire NHS Foundation trust public enquiry. *TSO London* <https://assets.publishing.service.gov.uk/government/uploads/system/uploads/attachment_data/file/279124/0947.pdf>

Francke, A. (2016). Foreword. In K. Skoberne, L. Plas, S. Ghezelayagh, & P. Woodman (Eds.), *Bouncing back. Leadership lessons in resilience* (pp. 3). Chartered Management Institute. <https://www.managers.org.uk/~/media/Files/PDF/BouncingBackLeadershipLessonsinResilienceFullreportJune20.pdf>

Health and Safety Executive (HSE). (2019). *Work-related stress, anxiety or depression statistics in Great Britain* (pp. 1–9). <https://www.hse.gov.uk/statistics/causdis/stress.pdf>

Holroyd, J. (2015). *Self-leadership and personal resilience in health and social care*. SAGE. ISBN: 978-1-4739-1624-1.

King's Fund Report. (2013). *Patient-centred leadership. Re-discovering our purpose*. <https://www.kingsfund.org.uk/sites/default/files/field/field_publication_file/patient-centred-leadership-rediscovering-our-purpose-may13.pdf>

Kirkman, B., Stoverink, A. C., Mistry, S., & Rosen, B. M. (2019). The four things resilient teams do. *Harvard Business Review* https://hbr.org/2019/07/the-4-things-resilient-teams-do>

Low, R., King, S., & Foster-Boucher, C. (2019). Learning to bounce back: A scoping review about resiliency education. *The Journal of Nursing Education*, 58(6), 321–329. https://doi.org/10.3928/01484834-20190521-02.

Masten, A. S. (2014). Global perspectives on resilience in children and youth. *Child Development*, 85(1), 6–20. <https://eds-a-ebscohost-com.libezproxy.bournemouth.ac.uk/eds/pdfviewer/pdfviewer?vid=15&sid=e86bf447-a67c-41a4-a02e-fb19142bbdfb%40sessionmgr4007>

NHS. (2019). *The long-term plan*. <https://www.longtermplan.nhs.uk/wp-content/uploads/2019/08/nhs-long-term-plan-version-1.2.pdf>

NHS. (2020). *Statistics*. <https://digital.nhs.uk/data-and-information/publications/statistical/nhs-sickness-absence-rates/january-2020-provisional-statistics>

NHS Health Education England. (NHS HEE). (2019). *Research evidence of the impact of generational differences on the NHS workforce*. <http://allcatsrgrey.org.uk/wp/download/management/human_resources/Generational-Differences-Deep-Dive.pdf>

NHS Information Centre. (2008). *Report NHS Staff 1997–2007* (non-medical).

NHS Information Centre. (2013). *Report NHS Workforce: Summary of staff in the NHS: Results from September 2012 census*. <https://digital.nhs.uk/data-and-information/publications/statistical/nhs-workforce-statistics-overview/nhs-workforce-summary-of-staff-in-the-nhs-results-from-september-2012-census>

NHS Survey Coordination Centre. (2018). *NHS staff survey 2017*. <http://www.nhsstaffsurveys.com/Caches/Files/P3088_ST17_National%20briefing_v5.0.pdf>

Palmiter, D., Alvord, M., Dorlen, R., Comas-Diaz, L., Luthar, S. S., Maddi, S. R., … Tedeschi, R. G. (2012). *Building your resilience. American Psychological Association*. <https://www.apa.org/topics/resilience#:~:text=Psychologists%20define%20resilience%20as%20the,or%20workplace%20and%20financial%20stressors>

Panter-Brick, C., & Eggerman, M. (2012). Understanding culture, resilience and mental health: The production of hope. In M. Ungar (Ed.), *The social ecology of resilience: A handbook of theory and practice* (pp. 369–386). Springer. e-ISBN: 978-1-4614-0586-3.

Pietrzak, R. H., & Southwick, S. M. (2011). Psychological resilience in OEF-OIF veterans: Application of a novel classification approach and examination of demographic and psychosocial correlates. *Journal of Affective Disorders*, 133(3), 560–568. <https://www-sciencedirect-com.libezproxy.bournemouth.ac.uk/science/article/pii/S0165032711001959?via%3Dihub>

PRIMA-EF. (2008). Guidance on the European framework for psychosocial risk management. A resource for employers and worker representatives. In S. Leka, & T. Cox (Eds.), *Approaches to work-related stress prevention and management*. <https://www.who.int/occupational_health/publications/PRIMA-EF%20Guidance_9.pdf?ua=1>

Rahimi, B., Baetz, M., Bowen, R., & Balbuena, L. (2014). Resilience, stress, and coping among Canadian medical students. *Canadian Medical Education Journal*, 5(1) <https://journalhosting.ucalgary.ca/index.php/cmej/article/view/36689/29550>

Redmond, A., & Crisafulli, P. (2010). *Comebacks: Powerful lessons from leaders who endured setbacks and recaptured success on their terms*. Josey-Bass. ISBN: 978-0-470-58375-3.

Sanderson, B., & Brewer, M. (2017). What do we know about student resilience in health professional education? A scoping review of the literature. *Nurse Education Today*, 58, 65–71. <https://www.sciencedirect.com/science/article/abs/pii/S0260691717301806?via%3Dihub>

Skills for Care. (2010). Report: The state of the adult social care workforce in England.

Skoberne, K., Plas, L., Ghezelayagh, S., & Woodman, P. (2016). *Bouncing back: Leadership lessons in resilience*. Chartered Management Institute. <https://www.managers.org.uk/~/media/Files/PDF/BouncingBackLeadershipLessonsinResilienceFullreportJune20.pdf>

Southwick, S. M., Bonanno, G. A., Masten, A. S., Panter-Brick, C., & Yehuda, R. (2014). Resilience definitions, theory and challenges: Interdisciplinary. *perspectives. European Journal of Psychotraumatology*, 5(1) <https://eds-a-ebsco-host-com.libezproxy.bournemouth.ac.uk/eds/pdfviewer/pdfviewer?vid=20&sid=e86bf447-a67c-41a4-a02e-fb19142bbdfb%40sessionmgr4007>

United Nations. (2015). *Transforming our world: The 2030 agenda for sustainable development*. General Assembly Resolution 70/1. <https://www.un.org/ga/search/view_doc.asp?symbol=A/RES/70/1&Lang=E>

Windle, G., Bennett, K. M., & Noyes, J. (2011). A methodological review of resilience measurement scales. *Health & Quality of Life Outcomes*, 9(1), 8. https://doi.org/10.1186/1477-7525-9-8.

## REFLECTIVE QUESTIONS

- From your own perspective, deconstruct your own resilience. How good are you at facing reality, taking responsibility, understanding reality, and improvising solutions?
- From your own experience, think of an employee and consider what factors in the workplace might be risk factors for their resilience.
- What measures could you put in place to mitigate risk factor(s) identified for an employee?
- Within your own organization, consider if policies and plans for supporting psychosocial well-being in the workplace are transparent and easy to access.
- What strategies would you like to implement in the workplace to build your own resilience and that of your workforce?

# 8

# THE IMPORTANCE OF COMMUNICATION IN LEADERSHIP AND MANAGEMENT IN HEALTH AND SOCIAL CARE

CLARE FELICITY JANE PRICE-DOWD

## OBJECTIVES

*After reading this chapter, you should be able to:*

- Define five levels of communication.
- Identify types, styles, and purposes of communication.
- Critically analyze how approaches to communication are changing with the growing use of technology in health care.
- Identify how to adapt different communication approaches to changing health and care contexts.
- Apply communication tools to maximize impact in your practice.

## INTRODUCTION

In the context of leading and managing in health and social care, there is a recognized need for effective and impactful communication. Communication is essential for achieving the outcomes and outputs desired in workplaces, either through direction and process as managers or relationships and behaviors as leaders. Any exploration into the subject of communication, therefore, needs to address with equal importance both message content and how it is relayed. Effective communication supports rapid and accurate exchanges of information, bridges gaps between those giving and receiving care, and creates a shared sense of purpose in improving population health while supporting sustainable public services.

Better communication for improved outcomes continues to be a focus in health and social care policy in England. The NHS Long-Term Plan (NHS England, 2019) identifies the possibility for greater shared decision-making between professionals and patients through enhanced communication. In addition, it commits to a new contract that sets out the leadership behaviors that are expected. The document, "We are the NHS: People Plan for 2020/2021—action for us all" (NHS England, 2020) develops this further, citing many new ways of working that have only been made possible by normalizing conversations that have not been part of routine practice to date. Communication is one of the Chief Nursing Officer's 6Cs of Nursing (NHS England, 2012), in addition to featuring in every part of the NHS Constitution (Department of Health and Social Care, 2015); yet, year-on-year, communication is cited as either the cause or a contributory factor in numerous complaints within the UK National Health Service (NHS). It is often how the message is relayed—insincerity, jargon, poor attention—rather than the content that leads to discontent. The report, "Learning from Deaths" (NHS England, 2018), states that communication needed to be compassionate, but also clear and honest. At the most basic level, failing to communicate effectively risks being misunderstood; at an extreme level, it could and has led to catastrophic harm. From individual cases detailed by the UK Parliamentary and Health Service Ombudsman (2020) to the Public Inquiry into Mid Staffordshire NHS Foundation Trust in England (Francis, 2013), poor communication between staff and from staff to patients as well as externally with other organizations has been a key feature in downward spirals resulting in multiple preventable injuries and deaths.

Probably the most famous social movement involving health care staff in recent years was the result of poor communication. While undergoing cancer treatment, the late Dr Kate Grainger, a geriatrician in England, noted the number of fellow professionals who failed to introduce themselves as they treated her. The result—a simple, standard introduction, "Hello my name is….," at the beginning of every health and care interaction—has now become routine worldwide. Additional research by McDonald (2016) for Marie Curie Cancer Care estimates that the NHS wastes over £1 bn each year that is attributable to poor communication, which directly leads to poor adherence to treatment, unnecessary appointments, and litigation.

While these two examples show the results of poor communication, research in both the United States and the United Kingdom also shows that effective communication is instrumental in building positive relationships between staff and between staff and patients while increasing compliance and trust (Allinson & Chaar, 2016; Step et al., 2009). Quite simply, effective communication is within everyone's ability to achieve.

This chapter considers communication from a range of perspectives. First, the levels, style, types, and purposes of communication are explored. This is followed by an examination of how technology has changed the way we communicate forever. Finally, there is consideration of how to improve the practice of communication by both understanding the barriers and being able to adapt to changing contexts, which leads to greater effectiveness in the workplace.

## WAYS TO UNDERSTAND COMMUNICATION

Optimizing communication requires an appreciation of what "good" looks like. This can be achieved by examining the **levels**, **styles**, **types**, and **purposes** of communication.

### Levels of Communication

Think for a moment about learning to drive a car or ride a bike. Initially, it is wobbly, the gears are clunky, and every moment is spent in intense concentration trying to avoid accidents or falling off. Communication

is the very opposite. Despite being fundamental to everything we do, generally little or no attention is paid to how we communicate. Simmonds (2019) describes communication using five levels ranging from unconscious to fully conscious (Box 8-1).

## Communication Types, Styles, and Purposes

In addition to the five levels in Box 8-1, there are a number of other ways that we can examine communication: by type, style, and purpose.

### Type of Communication
#### Verbal
Verbal communication refers to human interaction using words and usually refers to speech or oral communication. However, written communications and sometimes sign language can also be encompassed in the term. It is distinguished from nonverbal communication whilst recognising that they complement each other (Reference, 2021).

**ORAL.** Can be face-to-face or electronic, such as telephone, Skype, TV, and radio. It is influenced by "para-language" accents, speed, clarity, volume, choice, complexity of words, humor, and the cultures of the speaker and recipient. It can range from one-to-one to one-to-millions. The advantages are the speed of exchange, personalization, and, if the exchange is face-to-face, the opportunity for clarification. Disadvantages include lack of proof that the communication took place if not recorded or witnessed and its unsuitability for lengthy messages due to the inability of listeners to retain information.

**WRITTEN.** Includes words, signs, symbols, and uses mediums like letters, reports, case notes, email, post-it notes, Apps, Text SMS, Instagram, and Facebook. Written communication is influenced by the words chosen, grammar and flow, writing style, and clarity of message. The advantages are that the written imprint can be retained if the message is long; disadvantages include the risk of breaches in confidentiality and the need for a level of literacy that may not be present.

#### Non-verbal
Often referred to as "body language," non-verbal communication is often a supplement to verbal communication and comes in many forms:

## BOX 8.1
### FIVE LEVELS OF COMMUNICATION FROM SUBCONSCIOUS TO FULLY CONSCIOUS

**Level 1** Communication is subconscious, habitual, and shows no self-awareness. Information about the integration is by "telling." The operational impact of change may be included, but there is little or no checking of understanding or concern for emotional impact on the receivers. Misunderstanding and alienation are possible.

**Level 2** Communication is also largely subconscious, with suboptimal listening skills shown. There may be superficial attempts to rectify misunderstanding on major points such as changes to role or base, but conversations are fleeting. Few exchanges are present with no desire to move to anything beyond shallow. Questioning is often closed and there is little attempt to build trust or gain depth of understanding between parties. Opportunity for questions may be time-limited with little enthusiasm for further exploration, leading to ambiguity and confusion.

**Level 3** Effective exchanges can take place by applying some communication skills. Leaders and managers demonstrate willingness to listen and are mindful of language and the non-verbal cues they demonstrate. They show the ability to respond and react appropriately to others. Here, the detail and implications might be segmented for different staff groups, such as clinical and non-clinical staff.

**Level 4** Communication shows the application of a variety of skills. At this level, we see leaders and managers building rapport and showing genuine concern for how their message is received by staff. The language and style used are adjusted to match the situation, and shared understanding is achieved by imparting detail. Stakeholders can debate and negotiate without becoming defensive.

**Level 5** Communication occurs in a way that demonstrates full consciousness in all aspects of the interactions. Unconscious bias is consciously acknowledged and sufficient time is given; rather than imparting lots of information, the opening may be short to elicit a response and the interaction is one of equals. There is clarity of thinking and a desire for collaboration; while the tone can be passionate, it does not tip into anger. They know how to "disagree well" without a resulting breakdown in trust or the relationship.

Simmonds, N. (2019). Five levels of communication. www.consciouscommunication.co.uk

**KINESICS.** Includes gesturing; facial expressions of happiness, anger, sadness, and so on; eye contact; and posture. In the COVID-19 pandemic, the wearing of personal protective equipment by health and social care staff and especially the face coverings generally worn have greatly impacted the ability to read kinesics.

This can be especially challenging for those who rely on non-verbal cues, such as those who are hearing impaired.

**ATTITUDE.** For example, not doing what we say or not turning up for meetings can communicate a lack of respect.

**ARTEFACTS.** For example, a uniform, accessories, and appearance are used to convey a message.

**HAPTICS.** Touch, which can be equally supportive and threatening.

**PROXEMICS.** Space distancing, which can be either "intimate" (very close), "personal" (still close but not immediate), "social," or "public." Proxemics are situational; a patient who is distressed may welcome communicating in an intimate space, which may also include touch; the same proximity is not universally acceptable (Hall, 1966). Proximity that is too close can inhibit communication; think about how everyone stops talking in an elevator. Communication can close down when personal space is diminished.

**CHRONEMICS.** The time of messaging. A call at 3 a.m. or on a nonworking day might indicate a need for urgent action; whatever the message, the "timing" itself is a communication.

**SIGNS AS LANGUAGE.** This includes gesturing, but also symbols such as warnings against hazards; think of the messages these signs portray.

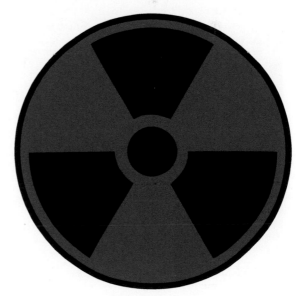

Radiation hazard

## Styles of Communication

Research in the United States by Killingsworth and Gilbert (2010) and Kane et al., (2007, 2017) finds that almost half of our working time is spent on "automatic pilot," being totally unconscious of how we feel, act,

Safety hazard

or speak to others. While each person's communication style has unique nuances, there are a number of models that attempt to define the different types of subconscious default styles. Two examples are Jackson and Smith (2013) and Bourne (1995). Jackson and Smith offer four styles: **Assertive**—bold and direct; **Animated**—energetic and fun; **Attentive**—caring and listening; and **Accurate**—precise and detailed. Bourne (1995) identifies five styles: **Assertive, Aggressive, Passive-aggressive, Submissive**, and **Manipulative**.

South African Psychologist Claire Newton effectively summarizes Bourne's (1995) five styles in the illustrations below.

1. **Assertive style** is found in those with high levels of self-worth, but not so high as to tip into arrogance and disregard of others (Fig. 8-1). This is considered the healthiest form of communication because it welcomes the opinions of others, knowing that they can hold their

| Behavioral characteristics | Non-verbal behavior |
|---|---|
| Achieving goals without hurting others | Voice – Medium pitch, speed, and volume |
| Protective of own rights and respectful of others' rights | Posture – Open posture, symmetrical balance, tall, relaxed, no fidgeting |
| Socially and emotionally expressive | Gestures – Even, rounded, expansive |
| Making your own choices and taking responsibility for them | Facial expression – Good eye contact |
| Asking directly for needs to be met, while accepting the possibility of rejection | Spatial position – In control, respectful of others |
| Accepting compliments | |

### Assertive Style

| Language | People on the receiving end feel: |
|---|---|
| "Please would you turn the volume down? I am really struggling to concentrate on my studies." | • They can take the person at their word |
| "I am so sorry, but I won't be able to help you with your project this afternoon, as I have a dentist appointment." | • They know where they stand with the person |
| | • The person can cope with justified criticism and accept compliments |
| | • The person can look after themselves |
| | • Respect for the person |

Fig. 8-1 ■ The assertive style of communication. Reproduced with permission from Newton (2011), based on Bourne (1995).

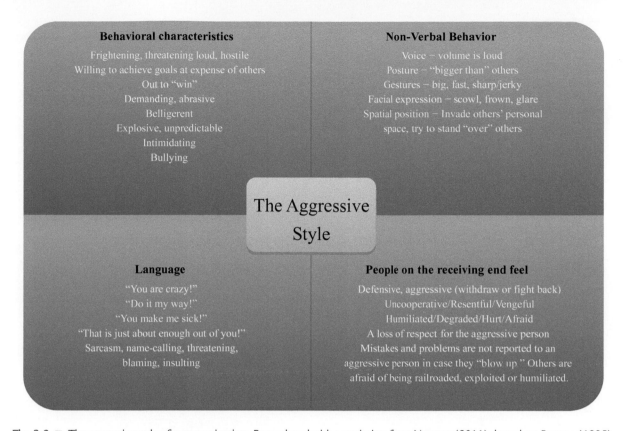

**Behavioral characteristics**

Frightening, threatening loud, hostile
Willing to achieve goals at expense of others
Out to "win"
Demanding, abrasive
Belligerent
Explosive, unpredictable
Intimidating
Bullying

**Non-Verbal Behavior**

Voice – volume is loud
Posture – "bigger than" others
Gestures – big, fast, sharp/jerky
Facial expression – scowl, frown, glare
Spatial position – Invade others' personal
space, try to stand "over" others

The Aggressive
Style

**Language**

"You are crazy!"
"Do it my way!"
"You make me sick!"
"That is just about enough out of you!"
Sarcasm, name-calling, threatening,
blaming, insulting

**People on the receiving end feel**

Defensive, aggressive (withdraw or fight back)
Uncooperative/Resentful/Vengeful
Humiliated/Degraded/Hurt/Afraid
A loss of respect for the aggressive person
Mistakes and problems are not reported to an
aggressive person in case they "blow up." Others are
afraid of being railroaded, exploited or humiliated.

**Fig. 8-2** ■ The aggressive style of communication. Reproduced with permission from Newton (2011), based on Bourne (1995).

opinion with confidence and avoiding manipulation. However, despite being the most effective style, it is the least used.

2. **Aggressive style** is about being the "winner" in any exchange (Fig. 8-2). The wants or needs of others are not relevant; one's own viewpoint is considered right and superior. Aggressive communicators, despite their self-belief, are ineffective because their message gets lost due to the negative effect their style has on recipients.

3. **Passive-Aggressive** communicators often appear amiable on the surface but underneath are thinking and acting in a totally different way (Fig. 8-3). Passive aggression stems from feelings of being out of control and having no power in a situation. The result is undermining, lack of cooperation, or failing to follow through on promises. The feeling of powerlessness prevents them from showing their resentment openly, so the behavior seen is to undermine remotely.

4. **Submissive** style is used by "people pleasers;" they hate conflict and will do anything to keep the work and team harmonious (Fig. 8-4). They believe everyone has more important needs than their own and often go out of their way to make sure everyone is happy.

5. **Manipulative** style is seen in people labeled as scheming and calculating. They can be described as "playing games" and are not easily trusted (Fig. 8-5). Manipulative communicators are skilled at influencing or controlling for their own advantage while concealing underlying messages.

### Purposes of Communication

A third way to examine communication is by considering the purpose. The purpose is determined by the direction of the communication (one-way or two-way), whether the communication is cooperative or competitive, and whether the goal can be achieved by talking "at" someone or if it needs their reciprocal input. Below

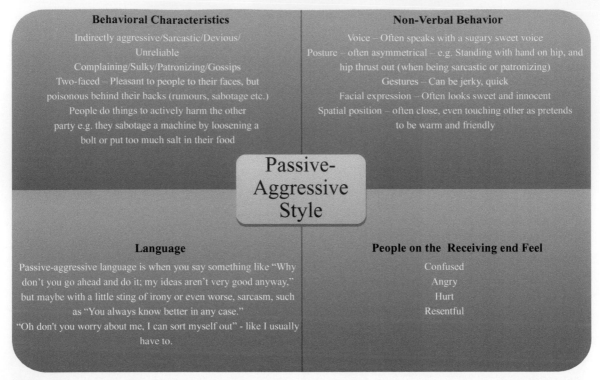

**Behavioral Characteristics**

Indirectly aggressive/Sarcastic/Devious/
Unreliable
Complaining/Sulky/Patronizing/Gossips
Two-faced – Pleasant to people to their faces, but
poisonous behind their backs (rumours, sabotage etc.)
People do things to actively harm the other
party e.g. they sabotage a machine by loosening a
bolt or put too much salt in their food

**Non-Verbal Behavior**

Voice – Often speaks with a sugary sweet voice
Posture – often asymmetrical – e.g. Standing with hand on hip, and
hip thrust out (when being sarcastic or patronizing)
Gestures – Can be jerky, quick
Facial expression – Often looks sweet and innocent
Spatial position – often close, even touching other as pretends
to be warm and friendly

**Passive-Aggressive Style**

**Language**

Passive-aggressive language is when you say something like "Why
don't you go ahead and do it; my ideas aren't very good anyway,"
but maybe with a little sting of irony or even worse, sarcasm, such
as "You always know better in any case."
"Oh don't you worry about me, I can sort myself out" - like I usually
have to.

**People on the Receiving end Feel**

Confused
Angry
Hurt
Resentful

Fig. 8-3 ■ The passive-aggressive style of communication. Reproduced with permission from Newton (2011), based on Bourne (1995).

are five different communication purposes and how leaders and managers might apply them (Box 8-2).

The role for leaders and managers is encouraging healthy dialogue, where the emphasis is on creating understanding, which ultimately reduces the level of workplace conflict. Dialogue is essential for building collaboration and teamworking, based on creating respect for the views of others.

## SUMMARY POINTS

- To communicate effectively, leaders and managers must use different approaches and pay equal attention to content and method.
- Much of the time, we communicate without paying any attention to how we do this, which impacts the quality and outcome of the interaction.
- There are a number of ways to consider communication; here, we have considered the levels, types, styles, and purposes of communication.

## THE ROLE OF TECHNOLOGY IN COMMUNICATION

Much of what has been considered to this point may already be familiar. This section considers the role of technology and its influence on how we interact. Communication technology has enabled rapid, safer, and more effective delivery within health and social care and can be the difference between dependence and independence. The terms "digital communication" or "technology-assisted communication" are often used. This relates to how we communicate optimally using electronic channels—email, intranets, social media, telemedicine, Skype, video conferencing, instant messaging, and often via mobile phones—and not the hardware used.

Chokshi's (2019) principles, referred to in Chapter 1, describe the commonalities that affect health care worldwide and the four principles that guide common solutions. Chokshi's principle three refers to delivering

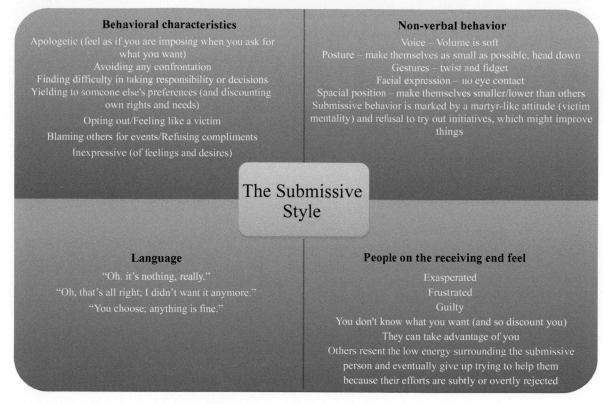

**Behavioral characteristics**

Apologetic (feel as if you are imposing when you ask for what you want)
Avoiding any confrontation
Finding difficulty in taking responsibility or decisions
Yielding to someone else's preferences (and discounting own rights and needs)
Opting out/Feeling like a victim
Blaming others for events/Refusing compliments
Inexpressive (of feelings and desires)

**Non-verbal behavior**

Voice – Volume is soft
Posture – make themselves as small as possible, head down
Gestures – twist and fidget
Facial expression – no eye contact
Spacial position – make themselves smaller/lower than others
Submissive behavior is marked by a martyr-like attitude (victim mentality) and refusal to try out initiatives, which might improve things

The Submissive Style

**Language**

"Oh. it's nothing, really."
"Oh, that's all right; I didn't want it anymore."
"You choose; anything is fine."

**People on the receiving end feel**

Exasperated
Frustrated
Guilty
You don't know what you want (and so discount you)
They can take advantage of you
Others resent the low energy surrounding the submissive person and eventually give up trying to help them because their efforts are subtly or overtly rejected

**Fig. 8-4** ■ The submissive style of communication. Reproduced with permission from Newton (2011), based on Bourne (1995).

care close to the patient, integrating their physical, emotional, and social care with the additional use of digital technology, while principle four relates to using data to guide care delivery, drive improvement, and identify gaps in data. These principles not only relate to care delivery using digital methods; they also include all aspects of the interaction, such as communication between colleagues, the multi-disciplinary team, families, and patients.

Today, we take for granted technology that would have seemed impossible only a generation ago. As long ago as 1995, Bill Gates, co-founder of the US firm Microsoft, imagined the "Wallet PC;" we now have everything he imagined and more within a smart phone (Gates et al., 1995). A proportion of the health and care workforce will have never known a world without home computers or mobile phones. Electronic

communication is so integral to life now, it is easy to overlook how it impacts the way we communicate.

The UK Government' Digital Strategy emphasized "Digital by default" for how we receive and consume information (Department of Health, 2012). Initially, there were platforms that made electronic communication possible, followed by the explosion of channels for the narrative—YouTube, Facebook, Twitter, Instagram, personal emails, and now tens of thousands of Apps that support health care. In 2019, the NHS Long-Term Plan described "a digital NHS 'front door' through [which] the NHS App will provide advice, check symptoms and connect people with health care professionals—including through telephone and video consultations" (Section 1.43, p. 26). There is no more waiting for the professional: the professional is now personally on-call for us at any time, in any loca-

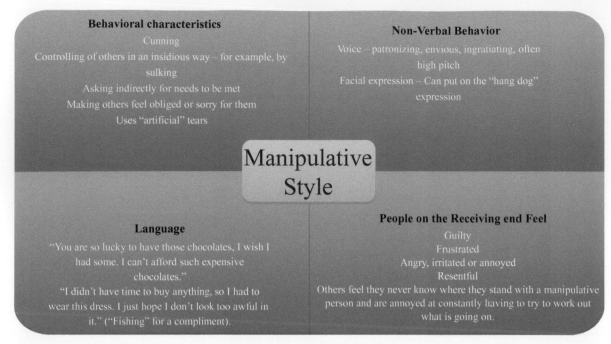

**Fig. 8-5** ■ The manipulative style of communication. Reproduced with permission from Newton (2011), based on Bourne (1995).

tion. The COVID-19 pandemic saw this become a reality at great speed, with over a half million video consultations being conducted in primary and secondary care, and 2.3 million online consultations taking place in primary care in the month of June 2020 (NHS England, 2020).

It is doubtful that many health professionals would want to go back to paper-based systems. For example, in the past, contacting a colleague who was "on call" involved telephoning a "switchboard" for a message to be sent to their pager and then being required to wait for a call back. We can now instantly message people using Facetime and send status reports and imaging with the click of a mouse. The ubiquity of the Internet has brought the latest evidence into our pockets, enabling everyone to access information as never before and share it instantly with others. According to Matei (2019), the average person in the United States is now either sending or receiving communication electronically, on average, for 3 hours and 15 minutes per day, which equates to a total of 35 days per year.

Despite innovations and subsequent improvements in technology, the one constant remains: the need to create meaningful narrative and connections that inform and engage.

Technology is liberating, but the true purpose remains the need to enhance human-to-human relationships. Technology is a means, not an end, if meaningful communication is still going to take place.

## Synchronous and Asynchronous Communication

Communication can be synchronous or asynchronous in terms of both time and place, as shown in Table 8.1, with the number of channels available to facilitate this growing rapidly.

The flexibility of text, email, and voicemail has reduced the frustration of missed calls and slow postal methods, while asynchronous communication enables "sending" and "receiving" content at any time and in any location, to be consumed when convenient. Additionally, asynchronous communication

## BOX 8-2
### FIVE DIFFERENT PURPOSES FOR COMMUNICATION WITH APPLICATION FOR LEADERS AND MANAGERS

1. **Debate**—two-way and competitive, with the purpose of winning an argument either directly with another or to win over a group of observers. Example: when a manager and team members disagree over introducing a new process with increased paperwork or data burden.
2. **Discussion**—also two-way and can be competitive or cooperative. Sometimes considered as debate but without hostility; the purpose is still to get across a particular view while challenging those of others.
3. **Dialogue**—two-way cooperative for the exchange of ideas or information. There is no desire to win; the goal here is listening, understanding, and building a shared sense of purpose. Example: how a team might approach a project and team goals or how a clinician and patient might achieve consensus on treatment options.
4. **Discourse**—one-way cooperative with the aim of delivering information but not inviting or making response possible. Example: in a cardiac arrest situation, the senior clinician directs the team knowing they will cooperate in the best interests of saving the patient.
5. **Diatribe**—one-way competitive with the aim of getting across views that are forceful and attacking. Example: the need to implement an unpopular policy where negotiation is not an option.

### TABLE 8.1
#### Synchronous and Asynchronous Communication

|  | Time | Place |
|---|---|---|
| Synchronous communication | Face-to-face, Telephone, Facetime via smartphone, Skype, Webcam, Video conferencing, | Face-to-face |
| Asynchronous communication | Email, Voicemail, Text, MSN, WhatsApp, etc. | Email, Telephone Text/MSN, Skype, Webcam, Video conferencing, Chat-bots |

gives those who prefer to reflect or have a preference for introversion the space to process information before communicating responses.

### Challenges of Synchronous and Asynchronous Communication

Technology is not a panacea for communication opportunities. Research in the United States by Misra et al. (2014) finds that while technology freed us from the need to synchronize with those we are relaying information to, a disconnect leads to diminished ability to connect on a human level at other times. This in turn can have a negative effect on how we build relationships, collaborate, and solve problems, all of which are essential leadership and management functions.

### Knowing How you "Sound"

Unconsciously, emotional states can be evident in messages that are sent. In his seminal work on emotional intelligence, US psychologist Goleman (1995) advocates knowing one's internal states, preferences, resources, and intuitions through emotional intelligence to understand how emotions impact everyday interactions. It can be tempting to use the fact that a conversation is not face-to-face as an excuse for a diatribe or difficult message, but it is poor practice to hide behind the "send" button. Emotions such as urgency, irritation, and anger can manifest in the use of **Bold**, CAPITAL LETTERS, underlined text, and excessive use of!!! or worse, **ALL FOUR!!!** This betrays the emotion at the time of writing. On the surface, a sender may not find communications inappropriate for a mass joke—"a bit of fun"—but the message received could be one of racism, sexism, or homophobia. Once you hit send, it is out of your control. Thus, quite simply, do not communicate anything asynchronously that you would not say face-to-face.

Left unchecked or handled badly, how you unconsciously portray your emotions risks damaging team relations; loss of performance and respect; and ultimately, loss of staff. Asynchronous in time and place does not make it any less "you" that sent the message, and all electronic messages leave an imprint. Even after you think they have been deleted, your words can live on forever in a screenshot.

---

**BOX 8-3**
## STOP, THINK, LISTEN, COMMUNICATE

**Stop**—A response in haste may escalate an already poor situation. Removing heated emotions allows for organizing thoughts so what comes next has impact and flows well.

**Think**—What do you want to achieve? a) Change the other person's opinion; b) change the situation, change yourself. Make sure you know the purpose.

**Listen**—Don't jump into formulating a response straight away; listen to what is being said, paying attention to both verbal and non-verbal content.

**Communicate**—When you finally embark on the communication, you will have greater clarity of purpose.

Cahn, D., & Abigail, R. (2007). *Managing conflict through communication*. Pearson

---

However tempting it may be to let off steam in an email, imagine how you would feel as the receiver. Write it—then send it to yourself. Chances are you will change it.

Cahn and Abigail (2007) developed the S-TLC [Stop – Think, Listen, Communicate] tool, which can be used effectively in this situation. It is effective because it considers the behaviors of both sides of the communication and helps each engage effectively in the interaction (Box 8-3).

## Boundaries 1—Personal and Private Time

Digital communication has revolutionized flexible working but has also blurred the professional boundaries that exist between leaders, managers, and their teams, which has implications for their duty of care. The COVID-19 pandemic "lockdown" saw a huge shift to home working with the provision of work-owned laptops, tablets, and phones to maintain business continuity. The move has been from "working at home" to "living at work." Even before this global situation, the obligation for 24/7 availability was creating a "new nightshift," where employees "log back on" or "never log off." The need to be constantly connected leads to conflict in work–life balance and emotional and psychological trauma (Boswell et al., 2016; Shoukat, 2019) with devices being considered as addictive as some narcotics (Alavi et al., 2012).

What would previously be considered "teleworking" or home based during office hours is being replaced by around-the-clock availability with distortion between necessity, extended availability during peaks of activity, and perpetual presence. A good practice tip is to add an email signature that includes phrases such as "I work flexibly and may send emails outside of usual working hours. I do not expect you to respond outside of your working hours."

## Boundaries 2—Work and Non-Work Persona

Social media communicates our non-work persona to the professional world. Add to this non-verbal communication in the form of gestures or artefacts like clothing and this takes on extra significance. In the extreme, the case of English nurse Rebecca Leighton saw personal Facebook posts used in the media to create a false impression of her life. While the allegation was wholly untrue, the media portrayal persisted of a party-loving "Angel of Death" who murdered her patients (BBC, 2011). In a survey of 1000 private sector human resource managers by The Harris Poll on behalf of CareerBuilder, 70% checked the social media presence of prospective employees; 57% said it stopped them from offering positions; half looked at how current employees present themselves online, and over one-third have reprimanded or fired current staff as a result of what is posted (CareerBuilder, 2018). Reasons included discriminatory comments related to race, gender, or religion (37%); poor communication skills (27%); inappropriate comments about past organizations or colleagues (25%); and sharing confidential information. To avoid problems, people are advised to use privacy settings on social media to protect the private from becoming public.

## Clarity

Using email and text may feel like a conversation—but it is not. Think about this simple sentence "*I didn't tell the Dr you were worried.*" Consider all the ways this could be interpreted if you received it—just like this, with no emphasis or punctuation—as a text or an email and at a time when you could not seek clarity. As the recipient, you could interpret the sentence in any of the following ways:

*I* didn't tell the Dr you were worried.
I ***didn't*** tell the Dr you were worried.
I didn't ***tell*** the Dr you were worried.
I didn't tell the ***Dr*** you were worried.
I didn't tell the Dr ***you*** were worried.
I didn't tell the Dr you ***were*** worried.
I didn't tell the Dr you were ***worried***.

In the first, the sender is suggesting someone else told the Dr; in the second, they are denying something was said, while in the third, they are disputing the method by which the communication was transmitted—was it written? Who knows? In the fourth, the recipient is in question; in the fifth, the person who is worried is in question. In the sixth, it is the timing of the worry, and in the seventh, the "worry" is the focus—what was the Dr told about you? One message, with seven possible interpretations, demonstrates why clarity is especially important, as you may not be there at the time the communication is read.

### The "Safety Net"

A cautionary note—asynchronous communication may require a safety net. Clicking "send" is no guarantee; just because an email, text, or voice mail has gone, it does not mean that the intended recipient has received or understood it. In synchronous communication, there are opportunities to add clarity and ensure understanding through two-way dialogue; the same care needs to be paid to asynchronous communication. Safety netting ensures that messages are received and understood. Consider the potential consequences for you as a leader or manager if you failed to safety net in the following situations:

- You ask a colleague to "tell others when you see them" to prepare something for a meeting tomorrow.
- You email your team to change the time and place of an event.
- You leave a voicemail urgently requesting a patient to contact a health care professional.

The result might be a minor annoyance, embarrassment at lack of preparedness, a wasted journey or frustration, but it could also be harmful if treatment is delayed.

If you think you will forget a safety net, set a reminder in your work calendar for when you would have expected a response but not so far into the future that the delay might cause a risk to well-being.

### SUMMARY POINTS

- Technology has changed how we communicate forever. It can be synchronous or asynchronous, increasing the freedom of how and when we interact.
- Leaders and managers in health and social care need to be mindful of the changing boundaries that communicating using technology brings and that sender and recipient may have different expectations.
- Being removed from the people we communicate with requires attention to clarity of message and follow up to ensure the message has been received and understood.

## DEVELOPING EFFECTIVE COMMUNICATION IN YOUR PRACTICE

Communication can be ineffective purely because there is failure to mitigate barriers, adapt style to changing contexts, or have difficult conversations in a way that enables positive change. The final section considers those elements and the techniques that are useful for facilitating successful outcomes.

### "Difficult" Conversations

The nature of health and social care means no leader or manager can avoid the circumstances from which difficult conversations will arise. They are uncomfortable, and there may be the temptation to hope the situation just goes away. However, having challenging conversations might be the only way for things to improve. People can avoid difficult conversations due to fear of being undermined, long-lasting damage to relationships, or not being liked/respected. Often, people can inadvertently be partly to blame for a situation, perhaps by not being clear enough in setting the objectives or failing to set parameters. It can be tempting to minimize a situation when what is needed is direct, yet skillful action. In any difficult conversation, think three Cs: confident, clear, and controlled.

## Preparation is Key

It will prevent a communication from becoming derailed. Have all the information—facts, not hearsay—and intervene at the right time. Too soon and there could be accusations of not allowing the person sufficient opportunity to perform well; too late and the situation may be irretrievable. Ensure sufficient time is set aside and clearly articulate the meeting purpose in advance: "We need a conversation about the department" is very different from "I have received a number of complaints about the department. We need to meet in the next week to discuss why this is happening so that we can improve."

By initiating a conversation, the person with the authority owns that there is a problem. The goal is to get acceptance from the other person that the problem is real and that they also need to take responsibility. This is the point that action moves from "managing" the situation to "leading."

Table 8.2 helps with preparation for a difficult conversation. By identifying what you want to avoid, it is easier to plan how you want it to progress.

## Addressing Barriers

Often, effective communication can be enabled simply by identifying and removing controllable barriers to prevent situations from arising. Consider the following barriers (Box 8-4):

## Adapting Communication to the Situation

Goleman (2000) describes leadership as being like an expert golfer who ensures success by instinctively choosing the right club for each shot. The same premise can be applied to communication. By adapting "what" and "how" we communicate, it is possible to increase understanding in addition to enhancing the message's impact. A global study of 550 human resource senior managers performed by Burin (2019) for Sage People reveals that any workplace may now routinely contain three, four, or even five generations with Traditionalists, Baby Boomers, Generation X, Millennials (Generation Y), and those born after 1997 (Generation Z) Fuhl (2020). Coupled with the ever-changing work environment, this exemplifies why leaders and managers must be able to seamlessly adapt

| TABLE 8.2 | |
|---|---|
| **Planning for a Difficult Conversation** | |
| **Plan to Avoid:** | **Plan to Promote:** |
| Opportunistic and haphazard | Showing you value the person through time and preparation |
| Negative criticism | Constructive challenge |
| Personal attack and blame | Concern and positive regard |
| Hearsay and gossip | Facts and evidence |
| Issues other than the one you are addressing now "You always fail at..." | A focus on the issue to be addressed; if other things arise, note and plan to deal with when appropriate |
| Dominating and authoritarian | Approachable, open demeanor. Listen and respond; there may be a backstory you know nothing about |
| Anger and aggression | Calm and professional; the person may not react how you expect, instead attacking, submissive, or tearful |
| Inflexible approach | Knowing when to persist but knowing when to quit |
| Punishment | Developmental opportunities "I can see you are currently struggling with...let's look at how can we support..." |

to the presenting situation and not communicate on autopilot.

It can be helpful to think about the audience being communicated to, choose the channel, understand the context, and use practical models.

### Audience

It does not matter if you are speaking in a one-to-one situation or to thousands of people, the issue is the same: understand the audience you are communicating with. Factors such as professional background, level of understanding, seniority, formal/casual, and tone all matter, so do not guess. For example, it is tempting to think that busy senior managers only have time for brief facts; they are the very people that may need all the detail. The implications for getting this wrong are logistical—you need time to repeat the communication to give the required detail—and reputational—you risk loss of credibility.

---

**BOX 8-4**
## BARRIERS TO COMMUNICATION

**Language**—Twelve percent of the total health and social care workforce in the United Kingdom is made up of overseas nationals who may not be conversing in a primary language (Baker, 2019). Consider the impact that jargon, abbreviations, local colloquialisms, and accents can have on understanding meaning. For example, think of the implications of not understanding the phrase "grab me when you are free."

**Physical**—Consider hearing or speech impairment, pain that inhibits attentive listening, or lack of sight resulting in the inability to notice non-verbal cues. Open plan environments, noise, heat, cold, marked territories, open or closed doors, and the manager's proximity to the team can all serve as physical barriers to communication.

**Psychological**—Fear or intimidation removes the psychological safety needed to have truly open and honest exchanges without reprisal.

**Cultural**—Stereotyping based on gender, age, or perceptions of background, status, or social class.

**Systemic**—Access to communication technology being restricted by "grade" or limiting who can send and receive emails or have access to work communication accounts.

**Digital literacy** may be poor where not expected. Research done in 2020 in the United Kingdom by the telecommunications regulator Ofcom (2020) finds that it is no longer possible to accurately categorize those who might have poor digital literacy or be considered disadvantaged by electronic methods. There is no correlation between disability, age, or geography and digital literacy, and while socioeconomic class might influence the amount spent on a device, accessibility is greater than ever before.

---

### Choose the Channel

Match the audience to the methods people engage with most but remember that company culture is not static. Have a couple of options, one synchronous and one asynchronous, to maximize engagement.

### Understand the Context

The COVID-19 pandemic is a once-in-a-career situation. The pressures of such a crisis situation dictate how communication needs to happen, which may be at odds with usual practices. Team members may not be used to being given commands and will remember how it makes them feel when told what to do rather than consulted and included in decision-making. However, in situations of extreme stress, calm, clear,

and confident communication reduces uncertainty, chaos, friction, ambiguity, and fear. Clearly articulating purpose and intent—<u>what</u> needs to be done rather than <u>how</u>—nurtures trust and respect. It can be tempting to believe others need much more information than they actually do. Long narratives and giving the full picture can lead to confusion by overexplaining. The listener does not need every bit of information to understand the situation.

### Practical Models

It takes practice to become a leader like the intuitive golfer that Goleman (2000) described. Fortunately, there are some simple models to support effective communication, such as when integrating health and social care services across a given locality.

### Feel-Felt-Found

This model was developed for customer care and sales and is a well-used technique in that sphere. However, it can be a good model for framing communication with people who are worried or undecided about an issue, offering reassurance and helping them think more positively. It acknowledges concern, gives an example of how others in similar circumstances have felt, and finally shows the benefits that people in similar circumstances found from supporting the change.

It might sound like this…

> *"I understand that change is difficult and that you are <u>feeling</u> anxious about the integration and what it might mean for your role in the team. Change can be very unsettling and lots of your colleagues <u>felt</u> the same when I spoke to them; I did myself when it was first suggested. I have spoken to another department that has done this, and they <u>found</u> that once they got going, patients liked the new services much better and the staff found much less duplication across all areas of work."*

### The 5-point Assertive Conversation

This can be helpful if a particular person or group is exhibiting a behavior or attitude you want to address. In this case, it could be undermining progress toward the agreed way forward. It praises the person for what they are good at (1), calls out the negative behavior directly (2), states what you want to happen (3), states what will happen if they positively change (4), and what will happen if they do not (5).

> *"(Name), you are an excellent manager; everyone really values the way you have supported the team since the integration of services was announced (1). I've noticed lately that while you are keeping your own team updated, you are refusing to meet with new colleagues and have been very negative about the proposal (2). What I would really like you to do is plan joint meetings with new colleagues so everyone can be clear on responsibilities (3). If you do, we will build relationships quickly and we can get our joint services advertised to patients (4). If you do not, it means that there will be confusion between teams, and patients risk not getting the care they need (5).*

### SBAR (Situation, Background, Actions, Recommendation)

SBAR was originally designed for relaying information in emergency situations in the US military, then adapted for health care by Kaiser Permanente. The SBAR tool is now applied worldwide across health and social care. In situations like the COVID-19 pandemic, health and social care staff across the United Kingdom have found themselves working in new, rapidly created teams and unfamiliar settings. SBAR enables information to be transferred accurately using four sections with standardized prompt questions. The structure reduces the likelihood of errors and need for repetition. It ensures just the right level of detail is given, while the receiver knows what to expect. SBAR is particularly effective when the giver and receiver may be of different professional backgrounds or have different levels of understanding, but it can be used in any context (NHS Improvement, 2014).

**S—situation**—Identify self, where you are, reason for the call, your concern

**B—background**—Reason for call, significant context, or patient history

**A—assessment**—"I think the problem is…" or "I don't know what the problem is, but the following is happening," vital signs, etc.

**R—recommendation**—What you would like to happen… "I need you to come and see the patient now/within the next half hour," being very explicit by adding clarification: "Is there anything I need to do until you get here?"

## SUMMARY POINTS

- Difficult conversations are not easy but are sometimes necessary, and there are ways to help them be effective.
- Communication can be impeded by a range of barriers. Many are within the manager or leader's control to address.
- Your default style of conversation will not be appropriate in all settings. Adapting can ensure you meet both your needs and those of the recipient.
- Structured communication models can help develop clear, concise interactions and keep people on track, especially in situations of stress or when a consistent message is needed.

## CONCLUSION

What enhances and impedes good communication is ever changing. This chapter has considered the positive effect that improved communication can have on the practice of leadership and management within health and social care. While the underlying theories of communication are well established, the context in which they are practiced and the channels through which people communicate are far from static. Technology has afforded greater freedom by removing the need to physically be with others in both time and place. However, this disconnect brings new challenges, which include the need to ensure that the messages we relay are received and understood as intended, regardless of the medium.

The importance of communication in leadership and management in health and social care cannot be overemphasized. Not all communication is going to be positive or go as planned. However, the models suggested can help leaders and managers be prepared for the unexpected. The key to all effective and impactful communication starts with self-awareness. Knowing that everyone has a default autopilot style is crucial as a starting point. An awareness of how to adapt that style to fit the presenting need is an essential skill and one that can be developed over time. This can enhance the effectiveness of practice and teams and ultimately improve the partnerships and services for those requiring care.

## REFERENCES

Alavi, S. S., Ferdosi, M., Jannatifard, F., Eslami, M., Alaghemandan, H., & Setare, M. (2012). Behavioural addiction versus substance addiction: Correspondence of psychiatric and psychological views. *International Journal of Preventive Medicine, 3*(4), 290–294.

Allinson, M., & Chaar, B. (2016). How to build and maintain trust with patients. *Pharmaceutical Journal, 297*(7895), 993.

Baker, C. (2019). *NHS Staff from Overseas – Statistics. Briefing Paper 7783.* Commons Library Briefing. <https://commonslibrary.parliament.uk/research-briefings/cbp-7783/>

BBC (2011). Stepping Hill Hospital: Nurse arrested in murder probe. https://www.bbc.com/news/uk-england-14214375.

Boswell, W. R., Olson-Buchanan, J. B., Butts, M. M., & Becker, W. J. (2016). Managing 'after hours' electronic work communication. *Organizational Dynamics, 45*(4), 291–297. https://doi.org/10.1016/j.orgdyn.2016.10.004.

Bourne, E. J. (1995). *The anxiety and phobia workbook (2nd Ed.).* New Harbinger Publications, Inc.

Burin, P. (2019). 17 to 70: Managing a multi-generational workforce. Meeting the challenges and opportunities of today's new multigenerational workforce. Sage People. <https://www.sagepeople.com/17-70/multigen-research>

Cahn, D., & Abigail, R. (2007). *Managing conflict through communication.* Pearson.

CareerBuilder. (2018). More than half of employers have found content on social media that caused them NOT to hire a candidate. <http://press.careerbuilder.com/2018-08-09-More-Than-Half-of-Employers-Have-Found-Content-on-Social-Media-That-Caused-Them-NOT-to-Hire-a-Candidate-According-to-Recent-Career-Builder-Survey>

Chokshi, D. A. (2019, October 22). Four principles for improving health care around the world. *Harvard Business Review* <https://hbr.org/2019/10/4-principles-for-improving-health-care-around-the-world>

Department of Health. (2012). Digital strategy. Crown Copyright. <https://assets.publishing.service.gov.uk/government/uploads/system/uploads/attachment_data/file/213222/final-report1.pdf>

Department of Health and Social Care. (2015). The NHS constitution for England. <https://www.gov.uk/government/publications/the-nhs-constitution-for-england/the-nhs-constitution-for-england>

Francis, R. (2013). Report of the Mid Staffordshire NHS Foundation Trust public inquiry. <https://assets.publishing.service.gov.uk/government/uploads/system/uploads/attachment_data/file/279124/0947.pdf>

Fuhl, J. (2020). 5 ways to successfully manage a mulit-generational workforce. <https://www.sage.com/en-gb/blog/five-ways-manage-multi-generational-workforce/>

Gates, B., Myhrvold, N., & Rinearson, P. (1995). *The road ahead.* Viking Books.

Goleman, D. (1995). *Emotional intelligence: Why it can matter more than IQ.* Bantam Books.

Goleman, D. (2000). Leadership that gets results. *Harvard Business Review, 78,* 78–90.

Hall, E. T. (1966). *The hidden dimension.* Anchor Books.

Jackson, J., & Smith, L. B. (2013). *Leveraging your communication style: Enhance relationships, build bridges and reduce conflict* (pp. 1458). Jessup Press. e Book ISBN: 978-0-9884306-00.

Kane, M. J., Brown, L. H., McVay, J. C., Silvia, P. J., Myin-Germeys, I., & Kwapil, T. R. (2007). For whom the mind wanders, and when: An experience sampling study of working memory and executive control in daily life. *Psychological Science, 18*(7), 614–621.

Kane, M. J., Gross, G. M., Chun, C. A., Smeekens, B. A., Meier, M. E., Silvia, P. J., & Kwapil, T. R. (2017). For whom the mind wanders, and when, varies across laboratory and daily life settings. *Psychological Science, 28*(9), 1271–1289.

Killingsworth, M. A., & Gilbert, D. T. (2010). A wandering mind is an unhappy mind. *Science, 330,* 932.

Matei, A. (2019, August 29). Shock! Horror! Do you know how much time you spend on your phone? *Guardian Newspaper.* <https://www.theguardian.com/lifeandstyle/2019/aug/21/cell-phone-screen-time-average-habits!>

McDonald, A. (2016). *The long and winding road – Improving communication with patients in the NHS.* Marie Curie Cancer Care. <https://www.mariecurie.org.uk/globalassets/media/documents/policy/campaigns/the-long-and-winding-road.pdf>

Misra, S., Cheng, L., Genevie, J., & Yuan, M. (2014). The iPhone effect: The quality of in-person social inter- actions in the presence of mobile device. *Environment and Behavior,* 1–24.

Newton, C. (2011). *Five communication styles.* <http://www.claire-newton.co.za/my-articles/the-five-communication-styles.html>

NHS England. (2012). *Compassion in practice.* Department of Health. <https://www.england.nhs.uk/wp-content/uploads/2012/12/compassion-in-practice.pdf>

NHS England. (2018). Learning from deaths: A guide for NHS Trusts on working with bereaved families and carers. <https://www.england.nhs.uk/publication/learning-from-deaths-guidance-for-nhs-trusts-on-working-with-bereaved-families-and-carers/>

NHS England. (2019). The long-term plan. <https://www.longtermplan.nhs.uk>

NHS England. (2020). We are the NHS: People plan 2020/1 – Action for us all.

NHS Improvement. (2014). *SBAR communication tool – Situation, background, assessment, recommendation.* Online library of Quality, Service Improvement and Redesign tools. <https://improvement.nhs.uk/documents/2162/sbar-communication-tool.pdf>

Ofcom. (2020). Adults media use and attitudes at: <https://www.ofcom.org.uk/__data/assets/pdf_file/0031/196375/adults-media-use-and-attitudes-2020-report.pdf>

Reference, Oxford (2021). A Dictionary of Media and Communication. Oxford University Press. https://www.oxfordreference.com/view/10.1093/oi/authority.20110803115457102.

Shoukat, S. (2019). Cell phone addiction and psychological and physiological health in adolescents. *EXCLI Journal, 18,* 47–50. <https://www.ncbi.nlm.nih.gov/pmc/articles/PMC6449671/>

Simmonds, N. (2019). Five levels of communication. <http://www.consciouscommunication.co.uk>

Step, M. M., Rose, J. H., Albert, J. M., Cheruvu, V. K., & Siminoff, L. A. (2009). Modelling patient-centered communication: Oncologist relational communication and patient communication involvement in breast cancer adjuvant therapy decision-making. *Patient Education and Counselling Journal, 77*(3), 369–378.

UK Parliamentary and Health Service Ombudsman. (2020). *The ombudsman's casework report 2019*. Parliamentary and Health Service Ombudsman (PHSO). <https://www.ombudsman.org.uk/publications/ombudsmans-casework-report-2019-0>

## REFLECTIVE QUESTIONS

- Consider how you communicate when on "autopilot;" how does this change when you are busy or under stress? What could you do to be more mindful of the impact that this has on others?

- Consider all the channels you use to communicate. When you communicate asynchronously using technology, do you change your tone or manner? What effect might this have on those receiving your communication?

- Reflect on a difficult conversation you have had. Think about what you have learned in this chapter and how you might apply it to the next difficult conversation you have.

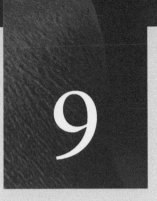

# 9

# MAKING DATA MATTER FOR STRATEGIC LEADERSHIP

SARAH SCOBIE

## OBJECTIVES

*After reading this chapter, you should be able to:*

- Understand the scope for using data to improve health and social care management.
- Develop a broad understanding of how data and information can enhance decision-making at different levels.
- Understand the impact of digital technology on the availability and use of data, including both challenges and opportunities.
- Recognize the importance of leadership for analytics and the role of all leaders in making effective use of data.

## INTRODUCTION

Effective use of data is critical to the decision-making process and, as such, is an essential tool for health and social care leaders.

In the United Kingdom (UK), which is the focus of this chapter, there is a long history of using data for management; indeed, Florence Nightingale pioneered the collection and analysis of data to reduce hospital infections. More recently, during the 1970s, a major shift occurred in resource allocation for health services: data on population health, service use, and the cost of providing services began to be used to enable the UK National Health Service (NHS) to move closer to its founding principle of providing services based on need.

This chapter analyzes how examining data is crucial for strategic leadership. First, the health and social care data context in the UK is set by outlining the main organizations involved in collecting and using data and how this is governed. Five applications of data analysis are then discussed to illustrate how data are used in practice across health and social care organizations and systems. This is followed by a discussion of the challenges and opportunities in using data at a time when digital delivery and consumption of health care are increasingly the norm. The chapter concludes with a discussion of leadership for analysis in health and social care.

However, this chapter focuses primarily on health rather than social care, with the recognition that the concepts will fit both disciplines. Many of the same principles and lessons apply, but there are currently fewer examples of using data from social care.

## CONTEXT: POLICY AND GOVERNANCE RELATING TO DATA FOR HEALTH AND SOCIAL CARE

The responsibility for collecting, managing, analyzing, and publishing data on health and social care straddles a large number of local and national organizations (Government Statistical Service, 2021). This results in a complicated landscape for data use, which can make it difficult to know what data are available and how to access and interpret the data. While individual organizations may have access to detailed information about their own patients or clients, they may lack the relevant information to compare their services with others.

Organizations may also find it challenging to share data across organizational boundaries, for example, health and social care providers working in the same geographic area (National Audit Office, 2020).

Complex governance arrangements and infrastructure have been established that seek to support the best use of data, while balancing its risks and benefits. This is an area of rapid development, and there is considerable debate about whether the checks and balances that currently exist are right. This section briefly introduces the main sources of health and social care data, considers how collection and management of these data are regulated, and describes particular issues relating to social care data.

## HOW ARE HEALTH AND SOCIAL CARE DATA COLLECTED?

Most health and social care data originate from care providers. This routine data, as it is called, can be collected directly during the process of care, for example, dates of appointments or admission to a hospital. Data may also be derived from the patients' clinical notes, such as details of diagnoses and procedures, which are coded after discharge. Routine data are used within organizations to manage services and also submitted to national bodies for distribution and analysis. For example, in England, hospital activity data are submitted by hospitals to NHS Digital (2020), who then makes the data available in pseudo-anonymized form to commissioners, central bodies, and for research.

A massive amount of detailed analysis can be undertaken using routine datasets, but there are important limitations in the data's scope and quality (Deeny & Steventon, 2015). One significant limitation of much routine data is that the data lack information on health outcomes. For this reason alone, it is important to also draw on additional sources, which include clinical audits, patient and staff surveys, vital statistics, and data from research studies. The opportunities emerging by using data from digital sources, including directly from patient-held devices, are discussed further below.

## HOW ARE COLLECTION AND USE OF DATA REGULATED?

Collection and use of data are regulated through a range of mechanisms along the data journey. Professional regulation of clinical notes predates the digital collection and analysis of data, and these requirements are an important part of the framework for data collection. Although guidance has been updated to reflect changes in data capture methods over time, moving from analog to digital data collection raises a number of important clinical and legal issues about the responsibility for data in clinical records.

Once data are extracted from patients' records and collated for analysis, the NHS data dictionary defines individual data items. For data submitted nationally, additional data standards may apply, and regulation of data flows in the NHS results in multiple requirements, which may sometimes conflict (Parkin & Loft, 2020). There are legal requirements for managing privacy, which are set out in the General Data Protection Regulation (GDPR), the NHS Caldicott principles for the use of data, requirements of regulators including the Care Quality Commission (CQC) and professional bodies, reporting requirements between commissioners and providers of services, and data required by national bodies for managing the NHS as a whole (NHS Digital, 2019).

There is growing concern that regulation is not keeping pace with the rapid growth in data sources and analysis methods. This could cause harm, either directly such as through breach of confidentiality, or indirectly through analysis resulting in decisions that disadvantage some groups and exacerbate health inequalities. A framework for regulating artificial intelligence (AI) aims to address these issues (Gould, 2020).

## SOCIAL CARE DATA

While routine health data undoubtedly have limitations, there are national standards for data collection and management and established flows of data for analysis purposes. The same infrastructure does not exist for social care, with minimal standards for data collection and mandatory data collection limited to infrequent, usually aggregated data (Steventon et al., 2020).

The organization of social care introduces additional challenges. For example, a large proportion of social care is self-funded. Local authorities, the statutory bodies responsible for social care, do not have a comprehensive picture of social care use within their area because many people arrange care directly with providers. Data sources for social care are distributed across local authority funders; the regulator for social care, CQC; and other national bodies (Office for National Statistics, 2020). While a number of developments are in the pipeline, given the current starting point, there are likely to be significant gaps for some time to come.

## SUMMARY POINTS

- The use of data, from collection, storage, and analysis through to publication and release is a resource-intensive activity and has significant ethical and legal dimensions.
- Routine data, generated from delivering care, are extremely valuable, despite limitations that include the lack of health outcome measures.
- Standards for data and data sharing are critical for effective use of data but need to keep pace with data sources and analysis methods.
- In the UK, the infrastructure for social care data is less developed than that for health care data.

## DATA AND ANALYTICS IN PRACTICE

This section discusses five applications of data analysis to illustrate how this underpins delivering and managing safe care in a sustainable way. While not exhaustive, the examples span direct patient care to national decision-making and introduce a range of analytical approaches.

### Predictive Analytics for Direct Care and Population Health

Predictive analytics use large data sets covering previous use of health care or clinical conditions to predict future health needs or a patient's prognosis. This can enable clinicians to identify escalating problems, intervene more quickly, and improve understanding of the needs of populations to enable provision of more targeted services.

Frailty scores, which are used in both hospitals and primary care, are one example. These can be used to improve the care of individual patients (Lansbury et al., 2017) and to shape service delivery and working across health and community organizations (Devereux et al., 2019).

Predictive tools usually include demographic data about patients, such as age, gender, and measures of deprivation, linked with data on clinical risk factors and outcomes. The tools are developed by analyzing historic data using statistical methods such as multiple regression to develop a model. This is then validated on a separate dataset to ensure the findings are accurate. With the rapid growth in detailed clinical and other data, new methods are being adopted, such as AI and machine learning (Academy of Medical Royal Colleges, 2019).

There are a number of challenges when using predictive tools. Predictive tools are only as good as the data available to develop the model. For example, models predicting who is likely to be admitted to a hospital are generally limited to demographic and clinical data; important social factors, such as whether the patient lives alone, has recently been bereaved, or has significant social needs, are not routinely collected (Lewis et al., 2017). Further, the data used to develop the model need to be representative of the population for which future care needs are being predicted and are limited to predicting future needs based on past access to services. If access to services was not equitable, using historic data can reinforce this bias by estimating future needs for health care that are also inequitable (Obermeyer et al., 2019).

A second type of problem with predictive analytics is how to effectively use the results. The usefulness of risk tools depends to a large extent on there being an effective intervention for high-risk patients. Predictive tools to identify high-risk patients in primary care have been difficult to use in practice because they are limited to effective interventions, and primary care teams have found it difficult to respond proactively while also dealing with high levels of demand (Salisbury et al., 2018).

With the huge growth in clinical data and the growth in predictive tools across all aspects of life, predictive tools are here to stay in health and social care. Key questions to consider when using predictive tools include (Box 9-1):

### Quality Improvement

Quality improvement can take place at the individual team level, across an organization, or even at a system level.

A core component of quality improvement is using data to understand what problems or issues exist and monitoring the impact of changes in practice or pathways to improve services (Box 9-2). There are many examples of using data and analytics for quality improvement, but there are also examples of challenges.

One of the biggest challenges is defining and measuring the quality of care. Outcomes data are sparse within routinely collected data, so bespoke data collections can be needed; maintaining this and scaling up data collection are difficult. Initiatives to support better outcomes data collection for local improvement work at a team level risk becoming performance measures; for example, the NHS patient safety thermometer was designed for local use and is not appropriate for comparison across organizations (Armstrong et al., 2018). However, the process of developing measures can be important in itself, as it requires agreement on what it is that matters.

A second major challenge is that quality improvement projects may not be resourced to undertake robust evaluations or get independent advice on how to

measure impact. Improvements that are thought to be effective by their originators may on further evaluation be found to be ineffective or any benefits obtained may not be maintained over time (Dixon-Woods, 2019).

Developing analytical support for quality improvement work can address some of these challenges by drawing on wider data sources, comparative analysis, and external expertise.

### Performance Management

Health and social care services collect and analyze data for performance management at all levels—from team through to organization, local system, and nationally. There are several frameworks nationally that shape what is measured and how data are used, including the NHS constitution, the NHS outcomes framework, strategic plans, and annual planning documents. This results in a complex set of interrelated performance requirements, which can sometimes be contradictory, but which all generate the need for analysis of data across multiple organizations and teams.

In the UK, performance of waiting times for treatment illustrates how data can be used for performance management and the challenges encountered. Targets for waiting time for treatment are enshrined in the NHS constitution, and these are operationalized each year in annual planning guidance. Since 2004, there has been a standard for patients to be treated within 18 weeks from referral by a general practitioner (GP). Currently, the target is for 92% of patients to meet this standard, although this has not been met since 2016 (The King's Fund, 2019).

Data used for monitoring times are collected along the patient pathway: at referral, when appointments or tests are booked, on the date of the appointment, and at discharge following completion of treatment. Waiting times are monitored by tracking the activity and number of people waiting over time (NHS Improvement, 2018). This could also include sub-group analysis, for example, for different groups of patients, clinical specialties, or geographic areas. Modeling expected future waiting times is also valuable, using data on throughput, numbers of new referrals, and number of people leaving (either because their treatment has ended or for another reason).

Challenges with analyzing waiting times are numerous. First, the data set for waiting times is dynamic;

patients are being added or removed continuously, based on actions taken by clinical teams or by patients themselves. Validating data can be problematic, especially if organizations have multiple data sources, such as at the individual clinic level or across a hospital (NHS Improvement, 2017). As with any modeling (see below), the assumptions used for planning future capacity are critical.

There are also wider challenges with performance targets to consider (Bevan & Hood, 2006). Emphasis on targets can distort clinical priorities, for example, leading to patients with less urgent issues being treated to avoid breaching the target, while more serious cases wait longer. How data are recorded can also be influenced, and organizations can spend a disproportionate amount of time correcting data rather than fixing underlying data collection or service issues.

Performance management in the NHS has undoubtedly been effective in driving service changes, particularly when the historic improvements over the last 20 years are considered. However, they can do this most effectively when data are used to understand why the target is not being met and engage clinical teams in identifying how to improve the patient pathway.

## PLANNING AND SERVICE TRANSFORMATION

Analysis for strategic planning and service transformation can be used at an organization or system level to understand the impact or requirements for changing services. Examples could be physical service changes, such as relocating a GP practice or hospital, or changes to patient pathways, such as streamlining the referral process or introducing new criteria for accessing services.

A first step in this situation will be to undertake a baseline analysis to understand how services are currently being used. This could include using activity data in addition to feedback from patients and staff, data on health outcomes, and information on resources and workforce. Ideally, the baseline analysis will consider trends over time so historic patterns of service use and the direction of change can be considered, along with analysis of variation between patient groups and benchmarking with other areas or services. This will enable the service change to consider strengths and weaknesses of the current service delivery and how equitable the service is.

Once a baseline for the current service has been developed, the next step will usually be to model alternative future scenarios (ACT Academy, 2020). A key part of this is developing a range of plausible assumptions for future services. Involving a wide range of stakeholders is critical here, and the range should ideally include patients, the public, and a spectrum of staff involved in delivering the service. The process of developing assumptions is critical because it makes the parameters for the decision clearer and more transparent.

The results of modeling can be used to develop an expected plan for what the future service will deliver once implemented. This can be used as the basis for monitoring the implementation and could also inform a contract for the service. Monitoring over time should consider tracking whether the assumptions on which the model was based have held up (for example, progress in recruiting staff or referring patients to a service) as well as metrics for the service delivered (for example, number of appointments) and the outcomes.

The challenges with strategic planning analysis of this kind include both technical and relational. On the technical side, it can be difficult to find the data needed to properly understand how the current service is working, particularly in relation to quality and outcomes, and to identify data relevant for future alternative service models. For example, there have been attempts to develop contracts for health services that move away from activity to outcomes for the population served. These are challenging to implement in practice because inadequate data are available to properly define the population and service needs (National Audit Office, 2016).

However good the data and modeling technique are, the model will only be as good as the assumptions that are used. It can be challenging to get buy-in from relevant stakeholders, including clinicians, patients, and public partnerships. Without this, decisions made based on the model are likely to be challenged.

Modeling methods are likely to become increasingly complex as the data available to feed them grows. This can address some of the challenges of models that over-simplify reality. However, for models to be useful, the assumptions and sources of data used for them need to be transparent so that patients and the public, in addition to clinical and managerial decision-makers, can engage with the results.

## EVALUATING INNOVATION IN HEALTH AND SOCIAL CARE

There is a growing focus within health and social care to innovate, but also an expanding body of research that demonstrates why innovations may not be adopted or may not yield the benefits expected (Greenhalgh et al., 2017). Clinical interventions that are demonstrated to be effective in clinical trials may not produce the same benefits when rolled out; factors such as staff training and capacity, how well the new intervention fits with existing pathways, and acceptability to patients and staff are all important. Furthermore, clinical trial data, which is the standard for drug treatment, may not be available for other types of service changes or digital innovations, such as apps to support self-management, algorithms to identify high risk patients, or digital diagnostic tools.

Evaluating innovations is recognized as a core part of enabling health and social care services to innovate by providing the evidence about what does or does not work, as well as why it works and in what context. This can support scaling up and adoption of innovations.

Routine data play a crucial role in evaluations because they reduce the data collection required; their use can also mean that the impact of the evaluation can be compared against a counterfactual drawn from a control group among a similar population. Questions that routine data can be used to answer might include whether patients who receive the intervention go on to use other services more or less and potentially shed light on health outcomes.

However, routine data alone are unlikely to be sufficient. Information will be needed about the roll-out of the intervention, including recruitment and uptake. Qualitative information from patients and staff enables evaluators to understand the context in which the intervention was rolled out and why it did or did not work. This is crucial for assessing what aspects of innovation are scalable and what conditions could enable it to be adopted more widely.

Evaluations of complex interventions are complex projects in themselves. Interest is growing in undertaking rapid evaluations because of resource constraints and to ensure learning from the innovation can be quickly fed into service improvements. Potential practical challenges to consider earlier on in the process involve access to data, including how to link data about the intervention with routine data, how to access data about control groups, and how information will be collected from patients and staff and analyzed, because qualitative data collection and analysis is resource intensive. While all these practical issues are important, even more crucial are early discussions with commissioners about what the results will be used for and how negative findings will be used. Evaluations may not show the results that commissioners were hoping for and considering this in advance can help improve both interventions and the evaluation process (Kumpunen et al., 2019).

Looking forward, the ability to monitor service changes using routine data will support evaluations of innovations, and there is considerable interest in how the NHS can become a Learning Health System (discussed later).

### SUMMARY POINTS

- Data and analysis inform all aspects of managing health care and are critical to bringing about quality improvements and enabling services to adapt and meet new requirements.
- The technical aspects of analysis—such as having the right data and using appropriate methods—are necessary but not sufficient; effective data analysis needs the right stakeholders to be involved from the start so the objectives are clear and underlying assumptions are transparent.

## OPPORTUNITIES AND CHALLENGES USING DATA IN THE DIGITAL AGE

Policymakers are depending on digital innovation driven by better use of data concerning current health service performance to enable service transformation and a more sustainable health system. Across health and social care, rapid advances are being made in the use of digital technology. These range from automating administrative functions to using AI to interpret diagnostic tests to enabling patient appointments to be handled remotely.

All of these activities leave a digital footprint. There is a growing volume of data being generated that are not being used to their full effect. Opportunities to use these data more effectively, the challenges that restrain this, and how these might be addressed is the next topic.

## Digital Data Opportunities

Digitizing transactional activities in the NHS, such as booking appointments, managing stock, or processing repeat prescriptions, can provide a huge volume of additional data. For example, enabling patients to select their own appointment times provides data on which appointments are most convenient for which groups of patients, which could in turn be used to schedule clinics more productively. Routine operational data, such as bed numbers or staffing in hospitals, are usually very dispersed and not consistently recorded. Transactional data from electronic health records about which staff logged in to use the system could provide useful data on staffing in different parts of an organization. Electronic prescribing in primary care, where information on a patient's prescription is transferred electronically to community pharmacies, has generated huge savings in time and improved safety for patients, practices, and pharmacies. In addition, it provides richer data on prescribed medicines; analysis of these data enables practices to know which patients have actually collected their medicine and allows trends in prescribing patterns to be monitored, considering the health condition for which the medicine was prescribed.

Digitizing health care will bring richer clinical data into the hands of clinicians in real-time. This provides the opportunity for data to be used directly for patient care. Electronic health records offer the ability to develop much more sensitive measures of risks and harms, considerably extending the measures that can be developed from retrospective analysis of routine data. This could also provide the opportunity for real-time surveillance and feedback to improve care. One example is the use of the National Early Warning Score (NEWS) to spot patients whose conditions are deteriorating and trigger an effective response (Inada-Kim & Nsutebu, 2018). In primary care, the PINCER initiative uses data to identify prescribing risks and harms, enabling pharmacists to work with GP practices to resolve issues and prevent recurrence (Avery et al., 2012).

Further, health and social care record systems are being developed that connect data from different care settings, both for direct care and for analysis (Local Government Association, 2018). The development of linked datasets opens the door to developing measures of safety at the interface between services: for example, to identify gaps in care and safety issues arising from poor coordination of care between settings. Linked datasets covering the local population that use primary care data also provide the opportunity to develop measures of quality relevant to particular cohorts of patients, for example, people with multiple long-term conditions and complex needs (Hays et al., 2017).

Increasingly, health data may also come directly from patients themselves through wearables and apps (Cresswell et al., 2019). This could provide the opportunity to understand safety and risk in a much wider range of care settings, including at home, where the majority of patient time is spent and where there is currently a gap in our knowledge.

## Risks and Obstacles to Making Better Use of Data

However, there are obstacles to making better use of data from either digital solutions or more conventional data sources. Significantly, making better use of data requires developing skills and capacity in the clinical and non-clinical workforce. Making sense of potentially huge quantities of clinical data requires analytical, systems, and clinical knowledge. Individuals with this combination of skills are in short supply: analytical resources in the NHS have focused on performance and regulation rather than quality improvement and service transformation (Goldacre et al., 2020). There is a need to build a better combined understanding among analysts, clinicians, and others about how to use data effectively at different levels—from direct care, at ward or team level, through to the whole organization or population level.

Allied to this, there are currently few protocols or consistent approaches published for analyzing many of the data sources that are becoming available from digital systems. For example, despite NEWS being rolled out for clinical use across the NHS, there is no standardized way of analyzing NEWS data. Developing and sharing methods and standards for analyzing similar electronic health record data need to be a priority.

Underlying these challenges, planning for how data will be analyzed and used needs to start at the outset of digital developments. Thinking about how the data will be managed and used is too often left until after implementation, by which time opportunities to capture data in a way that will support analysis are lost. This can lead to a loss of faith between front-line clinicians who want to access their data and analytics teams who do not have the means or capacity to extract and make use of the data.

Patients and the public are rightly concerned about who has access to their health data (Understanding Patient Data, 2020). While patient identifiable data can be shared for direct patient care, information for analysis should be anonymized. As data become more critical to delivering care, the boundary between direct care and secondary analysis is less clear. It also becomes more challenging to fully anonymize data: the rich linked data that is most useful for improv-ing health services is also more likely to allow identi-fication of individuals.

## A POTENTIAL WAY FORWARD: LEARNING HEALTH SYSTEMS IN THE UNITED KINGDOM

Learning health systems (LHS) aim to address the chal-lenge of ensuring that the huge growth in digital health and social care data can be used to improve care, shorten the timeframe of improvement projects, and ensure these are based on real world data (Nwaru et al., 2017). Briefly, the learning health system cycle captures current care and outcomes by analyzing data from clinical encoun-ters, combines local knowledge with evidence from else-where to understand quality of care and how it could be improved, and turns this knowledge into action, which is undertaken by the learning community (Fig. 9-1).

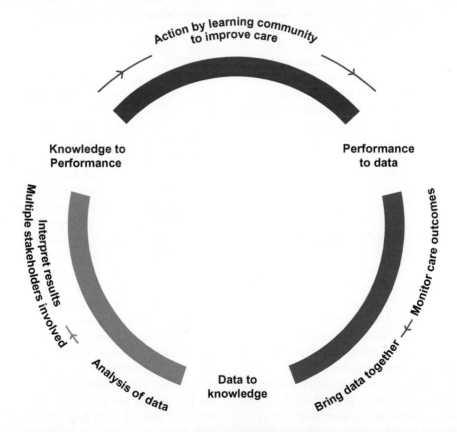

**Fig. 9-1** ■ Learning health system cycle Source: Scobie, S., & Castle-Clarke, S. (2019). *What can the NHS learn from Learning Health Systems?* Nuffield Trust. https://www.nuffieldtrust.org.uk/research/what-can-the-nhs-learn-from-learning-health-systems

A key feature of LHS, which differentiates them from research, is that for each improvement project, there is a learning health community that takes on the responsibility for acting on the learning, not just creating new evidence. Proponents of LHS have identified key characteristics of learning health communities, which need to be all inclusive, involving both the whole health care team and the patient; trusted; decentralized; and reciprocal, such that participants who create data also receive access to that data and the tools to analyze it. The experiences of organizations and health systems that have adopted this approach are that collaboration is an essential ingredient for a learning community to be effective in improving care (Seid et al., 2014).

In addition to the cultural factors that provide motivation and enable learning, several building blocks contribute to effective LHSs that can operate at scale. The NHS is already investing in some of these building blocks, but there are some gaps and also significant challenges to achieving the current aspirations.

A key question for the UK NHS and likely other health systems is whether the right incentives are in place to enable better use of health data for improvement at scale, both in terms of driving the right culture and developing the infrastructure. Currently there are too few external incentives for clinicians to engage in quality improvement, given the absence of outcomes measurement and the lower status of implementation compared to original research. Currently, NHS analytics functions are more focused on regulation and performance than on quality improvement and transformation.

## SUMMARY POINTS

- Digital technology increasingly supports the delivery and consumption of health care, leaving a detailed digital footprint.
- The resulting data can be used to improve how services are organized, enhance clinical decision-making, understand gaps in care between service providers and allow patients to be more engaged in their care.
- These new opportunities bring challenges, including developing the workforce able to use and understand the data, improving methods, and addressing privacy and data sharing concerns.

- A learning health systems approach is a potential model for maximizing the use of data in the digital age.

## CONCLUSION

The context within which data and analysis are used in health and social care has been outlined and some of the benefits and challenges have been explored within the background of developing greater use of digital technology in health and social care. Now, the question of leadership for analytics is addressed.

The starting point for the chapter was that use of data and analysis is critical to making good decisions. Analysis can help frame questions for decision-makers so that the issues are clear and allow making explicit assumptions in the absence of evidence and the values implicit in the decision-making process. For example, by asking questions about the impact of a decision on different population groups or asking about the impact on patient experience as well as costs, analysis can broaden the frame of reference for managers. Ultimately, analysis should reduce uncertainty for decision-makers about the potential impact of different decisions.

However, how well do leaders and decision-makers use data? Although health care prides itself on taking an evidence-based approach, very different standards of evidence can apply to policy and management decisions compared to those used in clinical care. There is often a separation between decision-makers and analysts, which can limit how well analysis is used (Goldacre et al., 2020). Further, the limited analytical workforce in the NHS is often primarily addressing performance reporting rather than transformation or improvement objectives. Analysis can also sometimes be requested after a decision is made. There has rightly been a focus on relationships within and across health and social care organizations, but this can lead to over-reliance on management decisions based on intuitive prior assumptions and not being engaged with evidence from data analysis being deemed acceptable for managers.

Leaders have clear responsibilities for the ethical use of data and analysis. Examples discussed here have included where the choice and scope of analysis will impact the conclusions reached. This will have very real impacts on individuals and populations, for example, regarding how resources are deployed and who has access to care. Analysis of variation between different patient groups is a vital tool for reducing inequality and improving outcomes. Leaders also need to consider diversity issues within their analysis by engaging with communities impacted by their work and considering diversity within their own teams.

As digital technology and data come to play an increasingly large part in health and social care, it must be the case that organizations that are not making good use of data are not high performing. Leaders of organizations and health systems need to consider what strategies they have to improve the use of data analytics and build capability and capacity across the workforce, both of analytical staff and users of data and analysis. Regulatory scrutiny has a part to play in ensuring that organizations are using their data assets effectively.

During the Pandemic, the COVID-19 response has demonstrated that the health and social care system in the UK can make huge strides in using data by taking a more collaborative approach. The common goal of responding to COVID-19 largely dissolved barriers that previously prevented analytical teams from sharing resources, such as data, access to models and methodologies, code and report formats, and specialist skills and expertise. Networks were set up to enable analysts to work more effectively and yielded tangible results that will be important to maintain. Critical to this will be support from managers within organizations; NHS management teams have often taken a proprietorial approach to analytical outputs rather than agreeing to work from a shared evidence base.

The starting point for good use of data and analysis is communication and dialogue between managers and analysts to shape the questions being asked. This will drive both better analysis and also improved transparency about the level of evidence available, the uncertainty of conclusions, and the values underpinning decisions.

## REFERENCES

Academy of Medical Royal Colleges. (2019). *Artificial intelligence in healthcare*. <https://www.aomrc.org.uk/wp-content/uploads/2019/01/Artificial_intelligence_in_healthcare_0119.pdf>

ACT Academy. (2020). *Modelling and simulation. Online library of quality, service improvement and redesign tools*. NHS Improvement. <https://improvement.nhs.uk/documents/2136/modelling-simulation.pdf>

Armstrong, N., Brewster, L., Tarrant, C., Dixon, R., Willars, J., Power, M., & Dixon-Woods, M. (2018). Taking the heat or taking the temperature? A qualitative study of a large-scale exercise in seeking to measure for improvement, not blame. *Social Science & Medicine, 198*, 157–164. https://doi.org/10.1016/j.socscimed.2017.12.033.

Avery, A. J., Rodgers, S., Cantrill, J. A., Armstrong, S., Cresswell, K., Eden, M., … Prescott, R. J. (2012). A pharmacist-led information technology intervention for medication errors (PINCER): A multicentre, cluster randomised, controlled trial and cost-effectiveness analysis. *The Lancet, 379*(9823), 1310–1319.

Bevan, G., & Hood, C. (2006). Have targets improved performance in the English NHS? *BMJ, 332*, 419–422.

Cresswell, K., McKinstry, B., Wolters, M., Shah, A., & Sheikh, A. (2019). Five key strategic priorities of integrating patient generated health data into United Kingdom electronic health records. *Journal of Innovation in Health Informatics, 25*, 254–259. https://doi.org/10.14236/jhi.v25i4.1068.

Deeny, S. R., & Steventon, A. (2015). Making sense of the shadows: Priorities for creating a learning healthcare system based on routinely collected data. *BMJ Quality & Safety, 24*, 505–515. https://doi.org/10.1136/bmjqs-2015-004278.

Devereux, N., Ellis, G., Dobie, L., Baughan, P., & Monaghan, T. (2019). Testing a proactive approach to frailty identification: The electronic frailty index. *BMJ Open Quality, 8*, e000682. https://doi.org/10.1136/bmjoq-2019-000682.

Dixon-Woods, M. (2019). How to improve healthcare improvement – An essay by Mary Dixon-Woods. *BMJ, 367*, l5514. https://doi.org/10.1136/bmj.l5514.

Goldacre, B., Bardsley, M., Benson, T., Cheema, K., Chinn, R., Coughlan, E., … Morley, J. (2020). Bringing NHS data analysis into the 21st century. *Journal of the Royal Society of Medicine, 113*(10), 383–388. https://doi.org/10.1177/0141076820930666.

Gould, M. (2020). *Regulating AI in health and care*. NHS Digital. <https://digital.nhs.uk/blog/transformation-blog/2020/regulating-ai-in-health-and-care>

Government Statistical Service. (2021). <https://gss.civilservice.gov.uk/user-facing-pages/health-and-care-statistics/hc-statistics-landscape/>

Greenhalgh, T., Wherton, J., Papoutsi, C., Lynch, J., Hughes, G., A'Court, C., … Shaw, S. (2017). Beyond adoption: A new framework for theorizing and evaluating nonadoption, abandonment, and challenges to the scale-up, spread, and sustainability of health and care technologies. *Journal of Medical Internet Research, 19*, e367. https://doi.org/10.2196/jmir.8775.

Hays, R., Daker-White, G., Esmail, A., Barlow, W., Minor, B., Brown, B., … Bower, P. (2017). Threats to patient safety in primary care reported by older people with multimorbidity: Baseline findings from a longitudinal qualitative study and implications for intervention. *BMC Health Services Research, 17*, 754. https://doi.org/10.1186/s12913-017-2727-9.

Inada-Kim, M., & Nsutebu, E. (2018). NEWS 2: An opportunity to standardise the management of deterioration and sepsis. *BMJ* <https://blogs.bmj.com/bmj/2018/02/08/news-2-an-opportunity-to-standardise-the-management-of-deterioration-and-sepsis/>

Kumpunen, S., Edwards, N., Georghiou, T., & Hughes, G. (2019). *Evaluating integrated care: Why are evaluations not producing the results we expect?*. Briefing: Nuffield Trust. <https://www.nuffieldtrust.org.uk/resource/evaluating-integrated-care-why-are-evaluations-not-producing-the-results-we-expect>

Lansbury, L. N., Roberts, H. C., Clift, E., Herklots, A., Robinson, N., & Sayer, A. A. (2017). Use of the electronic Frailty Index to identify vulnerable patients: A pilot study in primary care. *British Journal of General Practice, 67*, e751–e756. https://doi.org/10.3399/bjgp17X693089.

Lewis, G., Curry, N., & Bardsley, M. (2017). *Choosing a predictive risk model: A guide for commissioners in England*. The Nuffield Trust. <https://www.nuffieldtrust.org.uk/resource/choosing-a-predictive-risk-model-a-guide-for-commissioners-in-england>

Local Government Association, NHS England. (Local Government Association). (2018). *Local health and care record exemplars*. <https://www.england.nhs.uk/wp-content/uploads/2018/05/local-health-and-care-record-exemplars-summary.pdf>

National Audit Office. (2016). Investigation into the collapse of the UnitingCare Partnership contract in Cambridgeshire and Peterborough. HC 512 SESSION 2016-17. https://www.nao.org.uk/press-release/investigation-into-the-collapse-of-the-unitingcare-partnership-contract-in-cambridgeshire-and-peterborough/.

National Audit Office. (2020). *Digital transformation in the NHS*. <https://www.nao.org.uk/wp-content/uploads/2019/05/Digital-transformation-in-the-NHS.pdf>

NHS Digital. (2019). *Data security and information governance*. <https://digital.nhs.uk/data-and-information/looking-after-information/data-security-and-information-governance>

NHS Digital. (2020). *About NHS Digital*. <https://digital.nhs.uk/about-nhs-digitalhttps://digital. At: http://nhs.uk/about-nhs-digital>. Digital.

NHS Improvement. (2017). *Referral to treatment pathways: A guide to managing efficient elective care, third edition*. Elective care guide. NHS Improvement. <https://improvement.nhs.uk/documents/986/Elective_care_guide_third_edition_-_May_2017.pdf>

NHS Improvement. (2018). *Making data count*. <https://improvement.nhs.uk/resources/making-data-count/>

Nwaru, B. I., Friedman, C., Halamka, J., & Sheikh, A. (2017). Can learning health systems help organisations deliver personalised care?

*BMC Medicine, 15*, 177. https://doi.org/10.1186/s12916-017-0935-0.

Obermeyer, Z., Powers, B., Vogeli, C., & Mullainathan, S. (2019). Dissecting racial bias in an algorithm used to manage the health of populations. *Science, 366*, 447–453. https://doi.org/10.1126/science.aax2342.

Office for National Statistics. (2020). UK adult social care statistics landscape. <https://www.ons.gov.uk/releases/ukadultsocialcarestatisticslandscape>

Parkin, E., & Loft, P. (2020). *Patient health records: Access, sharing and confidentiality (Briefing Paper No. Number 07103)*. House of Commons Library.

Salisbury, C., Man, M. S., Bower, P., Guthrie, B., Chaplin, K., Gaunt, D. M., … Mercer, S. W. (2018). Management of multimorbidity using a patient-centred care model: A pragmatic cluster-randomised trial of the 3D approach. *The Lancet, 392*, 41–50. https://doi.org/10.1016/S0140-6736(18)31308-4.

Scobie, S., & Castle-Clarke, S. (2019). *What can the NHS learn from learning health systems?*. The Nuffield Trust. <https://www.nuffieldtrust.org.uk/research/what-can-the-nhs-learn-from-learning-health-systems>

Seid, M., Margolis, P. A., & Opipari-Arrigan, L. (2014). Engagement, peer production, and the learning healthcare system. *JAMA Pediatrics, 168*, 201–202. https://doi.org/10.1001/jamapediatrics.2013.5063.

Steventon, A., Deeny, S., & Coughlan, E. (2020). *Strengthening social care analytics during the pandemic and beyond*. The Health Foundation. <https://www.health.org.uk/news-and-comment/blogs/strengthening-social-care-analytics-during-the-pandemic-and-beyond>

The King's Fund. (2019). NHS waiting times: Our position. <https://www.kingsfund.org.uk/projects/positions/nhs-waiting-times?gclid=EAIaIQobChMIsLvBi9O-7QIVGdN3Ch0KkwJbEAAYAiAAEgIrx_D_BwE; https://www>. At: <http://org.uk/projects/positions/nhs-waiting-times?gclid=EAIaIQobChMIsLvBi9O-7QIVGdN3Ch0KkwJbEAAYAiAAEgIrx_D_BwE>. King's Fund

Understanding Patient Data. (2020). *What do people think about third parties using NHS data?* <http://understandingpatientdata.org.uk/what-do-people-think-about-third-parties-using-nhs-data>.

## REFLECTIVE QUESTIONS

- From your own experience, where have you seen data and analysis used effectively to improve health and social care?
- In your area of practice, what data sources are available that could be used to understand how effectively your service is running? What are the gaps?
- How could you assess whether your service is delivering equitable care to patients? What questions do you need to ask, what data would you need, and what methods could be used to assess this?
- How can you develop analytical capacity to support your area of work?

# 10

# FINANCIAL MANAGEMENT FOR LEADERS AND MANAGERS IN HEALTH AND SOCIAL CARE

SIVA ANANDACIVA

## OBJECTIVES

*After reading this chapter, you should be able to:*

- Understand trends in health and social care expenditure and the current and future financial issues facing health and social care systems.

- Identify the different approaches countries use to fund health and social care systems and the impact this can have on equitable access to health care.

- Analyze efforts to reduce the growing costs of care by improving the efficiency of existing services and transforming how services are delivered.

- Discuss the role of leaders and managers in improving how resources are used to deliver health and social care services for patients and service users.

## INTRODUCTION

Leaders and managers in health and social care need to understand the financial context in which their organizations and staff operate. This chapter provides an overview of how much countries spend on their health and social care systems, the different ways these services are funded, and what the funds are spent on. With a special focus on the English National Health Service (NHS) and the broader United Kingdom (UK) NHS, the chapter then describes how countries are meeting the challenges posed by the rising costs of delivering health and social care services.

Since many countries finance their health and social care systems differently, health care will be considered before turning to social care. The final section considers how efforts to integrate the planning and delivery of health and social care services will impact the financial management of these sectors.

## TRENDS IN HEALTH CARE SPENDING

The level of spending on health and social care varies substantially across different countries. This is due to a wide range of macroeconomic, social, and demographic factors that affect both the demand for care and the cost of providing services.

For example, within the group of countries that make up the Organisation for Economic Co-operation and Development (OECD), the United States spent approximately 17 percent of its gross domestic product (GDP) on health care, while other countries, including Mexico and Turkey, spent less than 6 percent of their GDP on health care (OECD, 2019). The UK falls somewhere in between these extremes, spending 9.8 percent of its GPD on health care (OECD, 2019).

Although detailed patterns of spending will differ on a country-by-country basis, most OECD countries have seen health spending account for a growing share of GDP over the past half century. This trend of health spending outpacing wider economic growth was particularly pronounced during the 1990s and early 2000s. Health spending as a proportion of GDP fluctuated in the years that immediately followed the 2007–08 global financial crisis, but the share of spending on health care has remained relatively stable over much of the past decade (OECD, 2019).

The long-term trend of rising health care spending is driven by demographic factors (including the population size, changing age structure, and health status), income effects (including the increasing demand for health care as incomes rise), and other cost pressures (including technological advances that increase the range of available treatments that can be offered to patients) (Office for Budget Responsibility, 2017). These factors are expected to continue to affect health care spending, with health care's share of GDP in OECD countries expected to grow to 10.2 percent by 2030, compared to 8.8 percent in 2015 (Lorenzoni et al., 2019).

The NHS provides a useful microcosm of many of the broader changes resource-rich countries have seen over the past 50 years. Since 1949–50, annual public spending on health in the UK rose more than tenfold from £13 billion to £164 billion, with health spending's share of GDP more than doubling over this period from 3.6 percent to 7.4 percent (Warner & Zaranko, 2021). Despite some initial expectations that spending on services would fall after the NHS was formed and people's health improved (Alaszewski & Brown, 2011), over the long run, health spending has grown by 3.6 percent per year on average (adjusted for inflation).

There have also been particularly clear periods of faster or slower spending growth. For example, health spending rose by 6 percent per year during the Blair and Brown New Labour governments (1996–97 to 2009–10), but in real terms, growth in health spending fell to 1.1 percent during the coalition government (2009–10 to 2014–15) that followed the global financial crisis. More recent NHS funding settlements announced in 2018 and 2021 will see planned spending on the NHS rise by 3.9 percent a year (above inflation) until 2024–25. (Warner & Zaranko, 2021)

### SUMMARY POINTS

- There is substantial variation in how much countries spend on health care.
- Most resource-rich countries have seen health spending grow as a share of GDP over the past 50 years.
- Health spending is projected to increase in future years because of demographic changes, income effects, and other cost pressures, including technological change

## HOW ARE HEALTH SYSTEMS FINANCED?

We have seen that countries spend considerable sums on their health services and that spending on health care is rising. Where does this funding come from? The funding for health care comes from a variety of sources, although there is little evidence that one financing model or a particular mix of models is superior to another in delivering cost effective health care (OECD, 2010). Four common types of health care financing are explained in more detail to illustrate the different ways health care can be financed.

### Taxation

In countries like Australia, Canada, New Zealand, and the UK, tax revenues are collected to fund a large share of health care services. These taxes can include direct taxes on individuals, such as income tax, and more indirect taxes, such as those applied to goods and services. These taxes do not necessarily need to be specifically earmarked for spending on health and social care. Instead, government finance ministries can allocate spending limits to different public services—including health care—that are largely supported through tax revenues.

Taxation is generally an efficient way of raising money for health care services because many countries already have established systems for processing tax revenues, and the additional administration costs are low. Tax-based systems also pool financial and health risks, as the amount of funding contributed by individuals is not directly tied to their use of health care services. However, because health spending tends to rise over time, health services can consume an increasingly large share of public spending and may lead to tax increases or diverting funding from other public services (The King's Fund, 2017).

### Social Health Insurance

In countries such as Germany, a defined and comprehensive package of health care services is funded through financial contributions by employees and employers. Members of these schemes contribute a portion of their salary, such that an individual's financial contribution to the health care system is usually based on income rather than the need for health care. Participation in social insurance can be compulsory or voluntary (Robertson et al., 2014).

The package of health services can also vary across different social insurance schemes, but there is often a standard basic package of services that all funds must provide. Additional financing mechanisms can be put in place to cover populations that are unemployed or to cover health care services that are not included in the standard package of benefits (Doetinchem et al., 2010).

Social insurance systems can vary in how they operate, but they often share some common features. They pool financial risk by receiving contributions from a large population; that is, the system provides social health insurance rather than personal or private health insurance. Financial contributions are based largely on income rather than health care needs and generally include contributions from both employers and employees. The revenue raised is more explicitly earmarked for health and care services than would be the case under general taxation.

### Private Health Insurance

Individuals or employers offering corporate plans can take out health insurance policies offered by private organizations. People with private health insurance usually make regular contributions that are based on their probable use of health care services. This insurance will pay for private treatment should individuals fall ill (McKenna et al., 2017). Insurance packages can vary widely in the range of services that are offered to encourage people to choose according to their health needs and financial means.

Where individuals cannot afford private health insurance, countries will often provide access to publicly-funded health care—including for people on low incomes and older people. However, in some countries, such as the United States, there may be a significant proportion of the population (8.5 percent in 2018) whose health costs are not covered by insurance (Berchick et al., 2019).

Unlike general taxation or social health insurance, an individual's financial contributions are closely tied to their actual or potential use of health care services. Private health insurance also tends to require high administrative costs to assess the health and financial risks of the population, organize insurance premiums, and process insurance claims.

### Out-of-Pocket Spending

Individuals can also finance the health care services they need out of their own financial means—or pay "out of their own pocket." These payments can include "copayments," where individuals contribute toward the

cost of their health care (e.g., user charges for medical prescriptions or accessing primary care services) and hotel services (e.g., access to bedside entertainment systems in a hospital).

High out-of-pocket spending can have significant consequences for individuals and households. The financial costs of this spending can be a barrier to accessing treatment and have been linked to poorer adherence to medication regimes and delays in seeking care (Glied & Zhu, 2020).

## A FOCUS ON THE UNITED KINGDOM

The UK illustrates the mix of different systems that can be in use at any one time. Health care in the UK is predominantly funded through general taxation and national insurance contributions. Moreover, the majority of services offered by the NHS, including both planned and urgent care, are "free at the point of use."

However, patients in England, unless they are exempt (e.g., for pregnancy), are also required to contribute toward the cost of some services through charges for items such as prescription medicines. Private health insurance policies are held by a minority of the UK population and are mainly offered as part of corporate subscriptions offered to employees (NAO, 2003).

Qualitative research and public polling suggest there is support for future NHS funding to be provided in a way that is consistent with the current approach (Sussex et al., 2019). For example, the majority (54 percent) of respondents to the annual British Social Attitudes Survey 2019 say they would prefer additional NHS funding to come from higher taxes, with far lower proportions in favor of introducing further user charges for accessing primary care and Accident and Emergency services (Appleby et al., 2020).

### SUMMARY POINTS

- Countries use a range of different means to finance their health care systems, with few countries relying on only one scheme to raise revenue for health care services.
- Government schemes (including taxation) and compulsory health insurance are the principal

financing arrangements for funding health care systems in resource-rich countries.

- Different financing schemes seek to balance similar underlying goals, such as maximizing access to health care services, minimizing administrative costs, and pooling risks across populations.

## WHERE THE MONEY GOES— EXPENDITURE ON HEALTH AND SOCIAL CARE SERVICES

The high levels of expenditure on health care naturally leads to the question of what this funding is spent on. Although there are many ways to analyze what funds are spent on, three common ways are by where care is delivered, functional groupings of services, and the resources a health system has to deliver care.

### Where Care is Delivered

Health care spending can be analyzed based on the setting in which care is delivered. Hospital activity accounts for the largest share (38 percent) of health spending in most OECD countries (OECD, 2019). This includes care in acute hospitals that, for example, offer general surgery or deliver psychiatric services.

Ambulatory care providers account for the next largest share of spending (28 percent) and include GP and dental practices and providers of home health care services. A large share of the remaining spending is accounted for by retailers (largely pharmacies dispensing prescription and over-the-counter medicines) and residential long-term care facilities.

### Functional Groupings of Services

Alternatively, health care spending can be divided into broad categories depending on its purpose (OECD, 2019). The majority of health care spending is for "day-to-day" services. For example, delivering inpatient and outpatient services accounts for the largest share of health spending (around 60 percent) across the group of OECD countries.

Medical goods, including pharmaceuticals, account for a further 20 percent of spending, with long-term care accounting for an average of 14 percent of spending in 2017, although this share is growing (OECD, 2019). Delivering collective care services (e.g., prevention and

public health services) account for broadly 6 percent of spending.

Data on longer-term capital investment in buildings, equipment, and technology are often collected separately from data on day-to-day spending. Across the OECD countries, capital spending in health services accounts for approximately 0.5 percent of GDP (OECD, 2019).

Within these broad categories, there is a familiar story of variation in the costs of delivering different types of health care. For example, in the English NHS, the average cost for planned inpatient care was £4,078 in 2018–19 (NHS England and NHS Improvement, 2020); however, a complex procedure such as a bone marrow transplant could cost over £80,000, while a breast biopsy could cost approximately £500 (NHS England and NHS Improvement, 2020).

### Inputs—The Resources a Health System Has to Deliver Health Care

A third way of dividing health care spending is by looking at the "inputs" or resources it requires. These inputs include labor (the number of staff and their salaries); goods and services used to deliver health care (including a wider range of items from pharmaceuticals and stationery to cleaning and security services), and non-health care goods (including the energy and water costs of running health care facilities). In the NHS, staff costs make up the single largest share (40 percent) of overall spending (Charlesworth & Johnson, 2018).

### SUMMARY POINTS

- There can be substantial variation in the costs of health care based on the setting in which care is delivered and the type of care.
- A large share of health care funding is accounted for by care delivered in hospital settings and staff costs.

## CONTAINING THE GROWING COSTS OF HEALTH CARE

As discussed so far, many countries have seen sustained increases in how much they spend on health care. This section discusses four approaches that countries are taking to meet the challenge of rising health care costs.

## Reducing Costs or Spending

Some countries have attempted to reduce the costs of health care by paying or spending less on services. For example, in the UK, Portugal, and Spain, the remuneration of clinical staff was frozen or fell in real terms for several years after the global financial crisis (OECD, 2019). In recent years, the English NHS has reallocated funding that would otherwise be used for long-term capital investment in buildings and equipment to support the day-to-day running costs of the service (NAO, 2020).

Many of these schemes to reduce costs have yielded substantial savings in health care spending, but they are not a sustainable strategy. For example, wage freezes for clinical staff can impair recruitment and staff retention and periods of wage restraint are often followed by a rapid "catch up" in wages over subsequent years (Monitor, 2013). Underinvestment in the upkeep of hospital buildings, facilities, and equipment has led to a rising backlog of maintenance issues in the NHS estate in England. For this reason, countries rarely try to use these types of measures for sustained periods of time or as their only means of controlling the rising costs of health care.

## Reducing Waste

A report by the OECD (2017) suggests that up to one-fifth of health spending is at best ineffective and at worst wasted. Understandably, reducing avoidable spending on services has become a focus in many health systems. For example, the English NHS has developed a list of treatments that have limited clinical effectiveness, such as tonsillectomies and varicose vein surgery. National guidance has been developed to restrict the degree to which these procedures are performed by publicly funded health services (NHS England, 2018).

Countries around the world have tried to reduce avoidable harm and adverse events, which are distressing for patients and wasteful for the health care system. Hospitals have reduced medication errors by making greater use of electronic systems to manage and record prescription processes. Adopting safety checklists has reduced the incidence of wrong-site surgery and other harmful and costly errors in surgical care (OECD, 2017). These initiatives demonstrate that the pursuit of better quality health care can also result in lower health care costs.

## Reducing Variation

Another common area of focus is reducing the avoidable variation in how health care services are delivered. Several countries publish an "Atlas" of health care variation to highlight geographical or institutional differences in, for example, rates of elective caesarean procedures, the level at which cheaper generic medicines are used instead of more costly branded alternatives, and the cost of procuring clinical and non-clinical supplies.

In the English NHS, a national program—Getting it Right First Time—has been developed to collect data across a broad group of clinical specialties and highlight the unwarranted variation in the cost and quality of services. The program has helped save money in orthopedic services by, for example, reducing rates of revision surgery, reducing how long patients stay in the hospital before and after operations, reducing surgical infection rates, and reducing litigation costs (GIRFT, 2020).

## Changing How Services Are Delivered

Alongside efforts to improve how services are delivered, health care systems are also trying to change how services operate to improve quality and reduce costs. These changes include modifications to clinical practice; for example, the increased use of day-case surgery has reduced the amount of time that patients spend in the hospital. One-stop clinics for some services like urology bring together a range of professionals in one setting, which improves efficiency by reducing movement and referrals around different parts of the hospital and improves the patient experience with shorter waiting times and fewer visits (NHS England, 2016).

Adopting digital technology has also allowed primary care consultations and outpatient attendances to be completed without patients attending facilities for face-to-face appointments. In addition to improving convenience for some patients, this can improve productivity by allowing hospital outpatient areas to be repurposed for other services and by reducing the rate of missed hospital appointments.

The integrated care systems and population health management approaches emerging in the English NHS are a more fundamental example of how services can be transformed to better meet or even moderate the future demand for services. These systems bring together different parts of a regional health and social care system to deliver more coordinated care that meets the needs of their populations.

While providing cost-effective and accessible medical treatment, these systems also have a longer-term focus on moderating health care costs by tackling the wider determinants of care, for example by reducing obesity, excessive smoking, and alcohol consumption.

## SUMMARY POINTS

- Meeting the financial challenge of rising health care spending involves reducing costs, waste, and avoidable variation in how services are delivered.
- To contain the growing costs of health care in the longer term, more fundamental transformation is needed in how services are delivered, including the use of technology and focusing on the wider determinants of health status.

## FINANCIAL MANAGEMENT IN HEALTH CARE

Even if health and social care professionals are not directly managing budgets, it is useful to understand how these budgets are developed and managed and the impact this has on staff, patients, and service users. Some aspects of financial management are common to the different national and local organizations that make up a health and social care system. These include developing an annual and medium-term financial plan, monitoring delivery of the financial plan, and reporting financial performance both within the organization and publicly.

The English NHS is a good illustration of these processes. National regulators of health care require publicly funded providers of NHS services to develop long-term financial plans that set out expected income and expenditure over a three- to five-year period. Providers also develop detailed annual financial plans each year. Although the process of developing a plan can vary across organizations, it usually requires individual clinical divisions to develop their own income and spending projections. These plans then go through a process of internal scrutiny to test their assumptions and fit with projections made by central finance teams for the organization as a whole.

These financial plans often include planned efficiency savings, sometimes referred to as cost improvement plans (CIPs) in the NHS. These savings can be categorized as non-recurrent (e.g., by taking actions that are harder to sustain over a long period, such as not recruiting for a vacant post or holding down the growth in staff remuneration) or recurrent (e.g., sustainably changing clinical practice to deliver the same or better-quality clinical care at a lower cost).

Over the course of the year, the individual clinical departments and organization as a whole will report on their financial performance by, for example, assessing how their actual income, spending, and efficiency savings compare to the original plans. The final financial performance of the trust is audited and published in an annual report.

National bodies overseeing NHS finances also assess the financial performance of NHS organizations throughout the year. This includes measures of whether the organization is on track to achieve their planned financial position by the end of the year and whether they have sufficient cash to cover their operating costs (NHS England and NHS Improvement, 2019).

The description above may give the impression that financial management in health care is a relatively straightforward and technical process. In reality, it can be an incredibly complex and difficult task that requires both judgement and inter-relational skills. The process can be technically difficult—for example, individual services have to estimate the income they will receive from a complex range of sources, including government funding, income from private patients, charitable donations, and referrals for specialist care from other parts of the country or even overseas. These services also have to estimate the costs of delivering care, when many of the factors driving higher or lower costs, such as the availability of clinical staff, are not always directly within their control and may be affected by national decisions on staff pay, international recruitment, and immigration policy.

The process can also be complex because several layers of financial incentives and disincentives will be in use at any one time (Monitor, 2014). For example, NHS organizations can be fined for breaching national targets on infection rates or waiting times. In addition, they can receive additional funding through a different national incentive scheme by improving the quality of care they deliver.

The process of financial management itself can also place significant pressure on clinical and non-clinical staff, who are asked to deliver financial savings without compromising the quality of care or range of services that are delivered for patients (Anandaciva et al., 2018). Even though the task of financial management in health care is not an easy one, there are multiple examples of where it has worked effectively to reduce costs while maintaining or improving the quality of services (Jabbal & Lewis, 2018). These include the examples found in Box 10-1.

### SUMMARY POINTS

- Financial management concerns the effective stewardship of resources.
- Local leaders will continue to face the challenge of how to reduce costs while improving or maintaining the quality of services.
- Longer-term trends of involving clinical staff in financial decisions and focusing on value as well as efficiency may provide part of the answer to how this can be achieved.

## ADULT SOCIAL CARE FUNDING AND FINANCE

Adult social care services provide support to older people and working age adults to help them retain their independence and maximize their quality of life. These services can include help with daily living activities, such as washing and dressing, and more intensive care and support, including residential care in nursing and care homes.

The interdependency between health and adult social care services has received increasing recognition. However, there are often substantial differences in how health and social care services are funded and financially managed, which is highlighted by a more detailed look at how health and social care services are funded in England.

Unlike NHS services, adult social care services are not free at the point of use. Instead, people who need adult social care services are assessed by local authorities to identify the level of care they need and their eligibility for services. Only adults with high needs and limited means of paying for care will be assessed as eligible for publicly funded services (i.e., access to publicly funded adult social care is both needs- and means-tested). Adults who do not meet these criteria must self-fund the costs of their care, rely on informal care from relatives and friends, or forgo care.

Unlike the NHS, whose budgets are set and closely managed by the central government, there is no national social care budget. Spending on adult social care is instead individually determined by 152 local authorities in England (Social Care 360, Bottery et al., 2020) based on their local priorities, needs, and spending power. However, local spending can be indirectly affected by national policy decisions on how local government finances operate, that is, the degree to which local authorities can raise local council taxes on their resident populations.

In 2018–19, local authorities spent £22.2 billion on adult social care services. There are three main sources for local authority spending on adult social care services: the amount local authorities allocate from their central budgets, charges levied on the people who use social care services, and income from the NHS. Adult social care is the largest area of discretionary spending for local authorities in England, accounting for over 30 percent of spending on main services (Cromarty, 2019). There are no reliable estimates of how much private spending there is on adult social care in England, though the National Audit Office estimates that the size of this market was £10.9 billion in 2016–17 (Bottery et al., 2020).

Following the global financial crisis, local authority spending on adult social care services fell from £22.6 billion in 2010–11 to £20.6 billion by 2014–15 (all data in 2018–19 prices). Since then, spending has steadily increased, though the current spending of £22.2 billion in 2018–19 remains below spending levels in 2010–11 despite growth in the size and social care needs of the population (Bottery et al., 2020).

For over 20 years, there has been substantial national debate over how adult social care services should be funded and financed (Bottery et al., 2018). This has partly been driven by concerns over whether the current system of needs- and means-testing is contributing to unmet needs for care and catastrophically high care costs for some people. There have also been concerns over the fragility of the market for provider social care services, where a rising number of providers are going out of business or handing contracts back to local authorities.

Polling and qualitative research suggests the public has relatively little awareness of how social care operates and how services are funded. Polls have found that substantial proportions of the public think that social care is free at the point of use or provided by the NHS. Few people surveyed have started saving for the care and support they will need in the future (Bottery et al., 2018).

In more detailed focus group research and after people are given more information about how social care works, they recognize the issues with how social care is currently financed. Most people favored the idea of the state having greater responsibility for funding social care, with more risk-pooling so these services are available for whoever needs them (Bottery et al., 2018; Sussex et al., 2019).

In response to these growing concerns, in September 2021 the UK Government proposed reforms to how adult social care is funded. These changes include placing limits on the amount an individual financially contributes to their care and extending the eligibility for publicly funded care. These reforms will be supported through a new earmarked tax - the Health and Social Care Levy.

So far, the discussion has focused on the differences between the NHS and how adult social care in England is funded and financed. Adult social care for individuals is needs- and means-tested, rather than free at the point of use. Publicly funded social care budgets are largely set and managed by local governments rather than the national government. The growing acceptance of the need to reform how adult social care is funded has not translated into action.

Looking through a broader international lens at adult social care services, other countries face many of the same challenges but have chosen different ways of meeting them. Internationally available data often cover a broader definition of services than the one used to describe adult social care in England. For example, international data on "long-term care" includes palliative care as well as support with basic daily living activities, such as bathing, dressing, and walking (ONS, 2020). Accepting these caveats, spending on long-term care has seen the highest growth of any major area of health and social care spending in recent years. This increase is attributed to the aging of the population, leading to greater ongoing health and social care needs; rising incomes, increasing the expectations of the level of care provided to older people; and reducing the supply of informal care that could otherwise decrease the need for formal social care services (OECD, 2019).

There is substantial variation in how much countries spend on long-term care; the Netherlands spend 3.7 percent of GDP, which is more than double the average of 1.7 percent for all OECD countries, and higher than the 0.5 percent spent by countries at the other end of the scale, such as Estonia, Poland, and Latvia. The OECD notes this variation may be due to some differences in the population structures of these countries, but, for example, largely represents variation in how formally a country's long-term care system has been developed and the extent to which it relies on care provided by unpaid family members. Highlighting the issue of catastrophic costs, the cost of institutional care for people with severe long-term care needs can represent up to four times the median disposable income for people of retirement age (OECD, 2019).

In recent decades, some countries have put substantial effort into reforming the operation and funding of their social care systems. Two notable examples are Germany and Japan, where new national systems for funding and delivering social care have been developed. In Japan, the system is a mix of taxation, social insurance, and copayment, while Germany introduced a collective mandatory social insurance model (Curry et al., 2019).

Although they differ in the details of how they operate, these two systems share some common features, such as consistent criteria for eligibility, clarity over what level of benefit an individual is entitled to, increased stability and transparency within the care provider market, and greater pooling of risk (Curry et al., 2019). Countries around the world, including England, will similarly need to respond to the challenges facing social care services now and in the future.

## Integrating Health and Social Care

So far, this chapter has discussed health and social care services separately, but a key focus in many health care systems is to join up (or integrate) these services to deliver more coordinated and effective care for patients and service users (as alluded to by a number of authors within this book). In some cases, this move toward more integrated care has affected the financial management of health and social care services. The NHS in England offers a few examples of these joint working arrangements.

In 2014–15, the Government introduced Better Care Funds (BCF), a single pooled budget at the locality level. Funds from this budget were earmarked for schemes to encourage closer planning and working between commissioners and providers of both health and social care services. These included schemes to safely speed up discharges from hospitals to care homes and to provide more clinical support to social care and nursing homes to reduce hospitalization rates.

Alongside this national scheme, local areas have been exploring ways to integrate health and social care services. In Leeds, the health and social care commissioners developed the concept of a "Leeds pound (£)" to acknowledge that different organizations with individual budgets could work more closely and use their collective resources to improve the health of their citizens. Other parts of the country, such as Tameside and Glossop, have developed integrated commissioning funds, where the resources of the local health and social care commissioners are pooled as far as possible, with spending and investment decisions made as collaboratively as possible within the existing legal frameworks (Robertson & Ewbank, 2020).

None of these schemes fundamentally change how health and social care services raise their funds. However, once these funds have been raised, these schemes aim to use the separate budgets in a more collaborative and coordinated way to deliver more joined-up and effective services for patients and the public.

## SUMMARY POINTS

- Social care and health care often have very different funding arrangements.
- The costs of social care are growing substantially, in part due to demographic changes. Countries will need to ensure their social care systems have the resources they need to cope with rising demand. This may require substantial changes in how social care is funded and financed.
- Efforts to integrate health and social care services may have significant implications for how these sectors are funded and financially managed.

## CONCLUSION

Countries across the world dramatically differ in how much they spend on health and social care services and how they raise the money to fund these services. Yet many countries also face the common challenge of how to contain rising health and social care costs.

Countries are attempting to control costs by "doing things better" (e.g., reducing unwarranted variation in how services are delivered and minimizing error) and by "doing things differently" (e.g., moderating the demand for health care by supporting people in leading healthier lives and reducing fragmentation in how services are planned and delivered).

In the short term, these measures can help improve the productivity of health care systems—that is, the outputs a health care system produces from the resources it is given. However, in the longer term, these efforts—if sustained—aim to improve the *value* health care services deliver by improving the health outcomes and well-being of the population.

## REFERENCES

Alaszewski, A., & Brown, P. (2011). Making health policy: A critical introduction. Polity.

Anandaciva, S., Ward, D., Randhawa, M., & Edge, R. (2018). *Leadership in today's NHS: Delivering the impossible.* The King's Fund. <https://www.kingsfund.org.uk/publications/leadership-todays-nhs>

Appleby, J., Hemmings, N., Maguire, D., Morris, J., Schlepper, L., & Wellings, D. (2020). Public satisfaction with the NHS and social care in 2019: Results and trends from the British Social Attitudes survey. Research Report, Nuffield Trust and the King's Fund. <https://www.nuffieldtrust.org.uk/research/public-satisfaction-with-the-nhs-and-social-care-in-2019-results-and-trends-from-the-british-social-attitudes-survey#footnotes>

Berchick, E. R., Barnett, J. C., & Upton, R. D. (2019). Health insurance coverage in the United States: 2018. <https://www.census.gov/library/publications/2019/demo/p60-267.html>

Bottery, S., Varrow, M., Thorlby, R., & Wellings, D. (2018). *A fork in the road: Next steps for social care funding reform*. The Health Foundation and the King's Fund. <https://www.health.org.uk/publications/a-fork-in-the-road-next-steps-for-social-care-funding-reform>

Bottery, S., Ward, D., & Babalola, G. (2020). Social Care 360. The King's Fund. <https://www.kingsfund.org.uk/publications/social-care-360>

Cromarty, H. (2019). *Adult social care funding (England)*. House of Commons: Library. <https://researchbriefings.files.parliament.uk/documents/CBP-7903/CBP-7903.pdf>

Curry, N., Schlepper, L., & Hemmings, N. (2019). What can England learn from the long-term care system in Germany?: *Research Report*. Nuffield Trust. <https://www.nuffieldtrust.org.uk/research/what-can-england-learn-from-the-long-term-care-system-in-germany>

Doetinchem, O., Carrin, G., & Evans, D. (2010) Thinking of introducing social health insurance? Ten questions. World Health Report (2010) Background Paper, 26. <https://www.who.int/healthsystems/topics/financing/healthreport/26_10Q.pdf?ua=1>

Getting it Right First Time (GIRFT). (2020). A follow-up on the GIRFT national specialty report on orthopaedics. <https://gettingitrightfirsttime.co.uk/wp-content/uploads/2020/02/GIRFT-orthopaedics-follow-up-report-February-2020.pdf>

Glied, S. A., & Zhu, B. (2020). *Catastrophic out-of-pocket health care costs: A problem mainly for middle-income Americans with employer coverage*. The Commonwealth Fund. <https://www.commonwealthfund.org/publications/issue-briefs/2020/apr/catastrophic-out-of-pocket-costs-problem-middle-income>

Jabbal, J., & Lewis, M. (2018). Approaches to better value: Improving quality and cost. The King's Fund. <https://www.kingsfund.org.uk/publications/approaches-better-value>

Lorenzoni, L., Marino, D., Morgan, D., & James, C. (2019). Health spending projections to 2030: New results based on a revised OECD methodology: *OECD Health Working Papers, Number 110*. OECD Publishing. https://doi.org/10.1787/5667f23d-en.

McKenna, D., Dunn, P., Northern, E., & Buckley, T. (2017). How healthcare is funded. The Kings Fund. https://www.kingsfund.org.uk/publications/how-health-care-is-funded.

Monitor. (2013). Closing the NHS funding gap: How to get better value health care for patients. <https://assets.publishing.service.gov.uk/government/uploads/system/uploads/attachment_data/file/284044/ClosingTheGap091013.pdf>

Monitor. (2014). Research on financial and non-financial incentives. <https://assets.publishing.service.gov.uk/government/uploads/system/uploads/attachment_data/file/381930/FinanciaNonFinancialIncentives.pdf>

National Audit Office (NAO). (2003). International health comparisons: A compendium of published information on healthcare systems, the provision of healthcare and health achievement in 10 countries. <https://www.nao.org.uk/report/international-health-comparisons-a-compendium-of-published-information-on-healthcare-systems-the-provision-of-health-care-and-health-achievement-in-10-countries/>

National Audit Office (NAO). (2020). Review of capital expenditure in the NHS. <https://www.nao.org.uk/wp-content/uploads/2020/02/Review-of-capital-expenditure-in-the-NHS.pdf>

NHS England. (2016). Demand management good practice guide. <https://www.england.nhs.uk/wp-content/uploads/2016/12/demand-mgnt-good-practice-guide.pdf>

NHS England. (2018). Evidence-based interventions: Consultation document. <https://www.england.nhs.uk/wp-content/uploads/2018/06/04-b-pb-04-07-2018-ebi-consultation-document.pdf>

NHS England, & NHS Improvement. (2019). NHS oversight framework for 2019/20. <https://improvement.nhs.uk/resources/nhs-oversight-framework-201920/>

NHS England, & NHS Improvement. (2020). National Cost Collection 2019: For data relating to 2018/19: Commentary on headlines and introduction to the available data. <https://improvement.nhs.uk/resources/national-cost-collection/>

National Office for Budget Responsibility. (2017). Annuyal report and accounts 2016-2017. Crown copyright, Web ISBN; 9781474147125.

Office for National Statistics (ONS). (2020). Healthcare expenditure. UK Health Accounts: 2018. <https://www.ons.gov.uk/peoplepopulationandcommunity/healthandsocialcare/healthcaresystem/bulletins/ukhealthaccounts/2018#long-term-care-expenditure>

Organisation for Economic Co-operation and Development (OECD). (2010). *Health care systems: Getting more value for money* (pp. 2). OECD Economics Department Policy Notes. <http://www.oecd.org/eco/monetary/policy-notes.htm>

Organisation for Economic Co-operation and Development (OECD). (2017). *Tackling wasteful spending on health*. OECD Publishing. https://doi.org/10.1787/9789264266414-en.

Organisation for Economic Co-operation and Development (OECD). (2019). *Health at a glance 2019: OECD indicators*. OECD Publishing. https://doi.org/10.1787/4dd50c09-en.

Robertson, R., & Ewbank, L. (2020). *Thinking differently about commissioning: Learning from new approaches to local planning*. The King's Fund. <https://www.kingsfund.org.uk/publications/thinking-differently-commissioning>

Robertson, R., Gregrory, S., & Jabbal, J. (2014). *The social care and health systems of nine countries*. The King's Fund. <https://www.kingsfund.org.uk/sites/default/files/media/commission-background-paper-social-care-health-system-other-countries.pdf>

Sussex, J., Burge, P., Lu, H., Exley, J., King, , Cylus, J., ... Forder, J. (2019). *Options for funding the NHS and social care in the UK: How the UK general public would prefer extra funds to be raised*. Rand Corporation. <https://www.rand.org/pubs/research_briefs/RB10079.html>

Warner, M., & Zaranko, B. (2021). Pressures on the NHS. Institute for Fiscal Studies. <https://ifs.org.uk/uploads/Green-Budget-2021-Pressures-on-the-NHS.pdf>

## REFLECTIVE QUESTIONS

- From your own experience, how engaged have you been in discussions about how resources are used in your organization? To what extent do you feel that the "use of resources" is part of your role?
- From your own experience, when have you felt most engaged in the financial management of your organization? What factors led to this?

- How might you build a culture that allows you and colleagues to maximize value for money to improve services for patients?
- Do you think that sharing resources across local organizations is increasingly important, and if so, what role do you think you can play in making this process more effective?

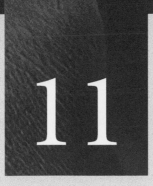

# 11

# LEADING AND MANAGING CHANGE

## LOIS FARQUHARSON

## OBJECTIVES

*After reading this chapter, you should be able to:*

- Critically analyze contemporary change management approaches and models in a health and social care context.
- Identify the key challenges that health and social care services face when implementing change programs, including resistance and readiness for change.
- Critically discuss leaders in their role as change agents in health and social care.
- Explore the role of social movements in aiding a cultural shift in a changing health and social care context.

## INTRODUCTION

Organizational change is a given in health and social care. Dynamic external factors, including governmental policies, financial cuts, and a need to improve quality, are often the key drivers of health care change (Anders & Cassidy, 2014). These forces together exert pressure on health and social care to maintain, improve, and in some cases, transform systems for the delivery of care. Research on various improvement projects across sectors show that 70–80 percent of all change initiatives fail (Burnes, 2009), and studies of organizational cultural change show that 90 percent never reach their targets (Burnes, 2011). There can be several different causes of failure, but the most common are connected with managing change, a lack of attention to corporate culture, employee resistance to change, and the leader's inability to drive change (Hughes, 2011). Countries cannot avoid the politicization of health and social care; it is a key priority of governments as they face ongoing economic and social pressures to improve the quality and efficiency of health and social care services (Gore & Parker, 2019). This in turn induces large-scale organizational change. Thus, global health and social care systems arguably fit within Morgan's (2006) view of organizations as political system metaphors as they remain pluralistic, large, highly complex, and operate in an interconnected way.

Jones et al. (2019) advise that health systems in high-income countries, such as the United Kingdom (UK) and the United States (US), often undergo large-scale changes despite limited evidence of clinical or financial benefits. Holton (2020) also suggests that improvements in health and social care systems in the UK have traditionally relied on top-down incremental approaches to changes for streamlining services and rationalizing spending. These approaches are challenged when leveraged against public pressure to sustain levels of service. The large-scale radical change needed in today's complex social and governmental environments requires a different approach to achieve the necessary outcomes.

Managing change is complex, as it involves not only the personal values of individuals but also how they operate within the culture of the organizations in which they work. In this context, this chapter explores the development of models and approaches that support organizational change management, the value of leaders as change agents, and the importance of addressing resistance and readiness for change.

# CHANGE MANAGEMENT APPROACHES

The language of change can be a challenge because many of the theories and concepts originate from a political, business, and societal context that has changed character over time. How change is described is often contradictory (Burnes, 2009), and the interpretation of approaches to managing change depends on the interpreter's ability to make sense of the change, background, and area of knowledge (Rosenbaum et al., 2018). Change approaches have been classified in three ways: scale and scope, rate of occurrence, and how change comes about (Senior et al., 2010). In the health and social care sector, the scale, scope, and rate of occurrence of change are highly relevant. As a roadmap for diagnosing and discussing it, Nadler (1998) describes four types of change (major transformation, adaptation, fine tuning, and new direction) (Box 11-1) in connection with chief executive officers' (CEOs) mastery of radical change in their companies.

---

**BOX 11-1**
## FOUR TYPES OF CHANGE

**Major transformation** indicates a change that comes with speed and has a dramatic effect on the core of an organization. For example, this change can be caused by new technology or be the result of a profound disruptive external event.

**Adaption** occurs when external factors put stress on an organization and apply pressure to reorganize. The organization still operates within the existing framework but may have to scale up or down with dramatic speed and consequences.

**Fine tuning** is change that is expected and allows the organization to stay within its current frame. Adjustments are small and stepwise within an existing framework. Most organizations are familiar with this type of change, which is characterized by continuous on-the-job improvements on a regular basis.

**New direction** represents change that is not sudden or unexpected but still forces the organization to handle a new situation outside the current framework. This change is often triggered by a major decision by key stakeholders, or by changed legislation or deregulation. When a change like this confronts an organization, it calls for transformation of the organization and culture.

---

Nadler, D. A. (1998). *Champions of change: How CEOs and their companies are mastering the skills of radical change*. Jossey-Bass.

---

**BOX 11-2**
## CHANGE AS THREE STAGES

1. **Unfreezing**—creating an understanding that change is required.
2. **Moving**—exploring ideas, issues, and approaches and initiating a change process.
3. **Refreezing**—identifying, utilizing, and integrating values, attitudes, and skills with those previously held and currently desired. A new status quo.

---

Lewin, K. (1951). *Field theory in social science*. Harper & Row.

---

Different approaches may be necessary to deal with these different change situations.

Building on the work of the early theorists, change has been consistently conceptualized in two ways: planned change and emergent change (Bamford & Forrester, 2003). Planned change has dominated the theory and practice of change management and is based principally on the work of Kurt Lewin; this approach views organizational change as a process of moving from one "fixed state" to another through a series of pre-planned steps. Lewin (1951) advises that change involves a three-stage process (Box 11-2).

This approach recognizes that, before any new behavior can be successfully adopted, the old has to be discarded. However, this model has limitations when the need for change may not be obvious. Lippitt et al. (1958) add three further stages to Lewin's (1951) original model: diagnosing the problem, examining the possible approaches to the problem, and selecting the best way to transform intentions into actions. Building on Lewin's work, many similar staged approaches have been developed. For example, Bullock and Batten (1985) develop a prescriptive four-phase model of planned change that draws on project management theory (Box 11-3).

Kotter (1996) observes that other initiatives such as total quality management, rightsizing, restructuring, and cultural change are also forms of change management. In this context, Kotter (1996) produces a model with eight steps, similar to those of Lippitt et al. (1958) (Box 11-4).

Planned change can be criticized. It can be argued that change from one stable state to another cannot occur in a turbulent environment; this supports the idea that change should be more cyclical than linear. Planned change can also be viewed as emphasizing isolated changes, with

**BOX 11-3**
**FOUR-PHASE MODEL OF PLANNED CHANGE**

1. **Exploration**—confirm the need for change and the supporting resources needed.
2. **Planning**—key decision-makers and technical experts build a change plan.
3. **Action**—actions are completed with feedback as necessary.
4. **Integration**—the changes are aligned with other areas of the organization and formalized via policies and communications.

Bullock, R. J., & Batten, D. (1985). It's just a phase we're going through: A review and synthesis of OD phase analysis. *Group and Organization Studies*, 10(4), 383–412.

**BOX 11-4**
**EIGHT-STEP CHANGE MODEL**

1. Establishing a sense of urgency
2. Creating a guiding coalition
3. Developing a vision and strategy
4. Communicating the change vision
5. Empowering employees for broad-based action
6. Generating short-term wins
7. Consolidating gains and producing more change
8. Anchoring new approaches in the culture

Kotter, J. P. (1996). Why transformation efforts fail. *Harvard Business Review, March/April*, 59–67.

**BOX 11-5**
**DIFFUSION OF INNOVATION THEORY OF CHANGE**

**Knowledge**—education and communication to expose staff to the change.
**Persuasion**—use of change champions to pique staff interest; peers persuading peers.
**Decision**—staff decide whether to accept or reject the change.
**Implementation**—putting new processes into practice.
**Confirmation**—the staff recognizes the value and benefits of the change and continues to use changed processes.

Rogers, E. M. (2003). *Diffusion of innovations*. Free Press.

an inability to incorporate radical change. The planned approach is also based on the assumption that everyone within the organization is willing to work in one direction, with there being no disagreement—this is clearly not realistic in any organizational cultural context. Thus, the emergent approach to change was born, focusing more on the external environment's role in shaping and driving change through people in organizations. Relevant to the health and social care context, Rogers's (2003) diffusion of innovation theory of change recognizes the core role of staff's perceptions and behaviors when moving forward with change. He suggests five change stages, each of which includes the core role of staff as key stakeholders in making change stick (Box 11-5). Firstly, knowledge is required and can be facilitated by offering education and communicating the details of the change to staff. Secondly, persuasion by using change champions assists in the change being supported and encouraged by peers. At stage three, staff decide whether to accept or reject the change. The final two stages involve the implementation of the change and confirmation when staff recognize the benefits and value of the change.

## TYPES OF CHANGE IN THE CONTEMPORARY ENVIRONMENT

### Incremental Change

Incremental change consists of frequent, purposeful adjustments that are small but ongoing and have a cumulative effect. Burnes (2004) refers to incremental change as happening when individual parts of an organization deal increasingly and separately with one problem and one objective at a time. Advocates of this view argue that change is best implemented through successive, limited, and negotiated shifts. Grundy (1993) suggests dividing incremental change into smooth and bumpy. Smooth incremental change evolves slowly in a systematic and predictable way at a constant rate. Bumpy incremental change, however, is characterized by periods of relative peacefulness punctuated by an accelerated pace of change (Grundy, 1993).

Dunphy and Stace (1988) suggest that a slower, progressive approach such as organizational development is preferable in environments like health and social care. Organizational development is "the organisation-wide application of behavioural science knowledge to the planned improvement, and reinforcement of the strategies, structures, and processes that lead to organisation effectiveness" (Cummings & Worley, 2014, p. 121). One of the major goals of organizational development is to create an environment where organizations will be more open and adaptive to learning as a means of becoming learning organizations.

## Transformational Change

Among the various types of changes an organization may have to handle, transformational change is the most challenging and can be protracted because it affects the whole organization (Balogun & Hailey, 2015). It is complicated because it embodies a fundamental change in an organization's culture, practices, and underlying assumptions. Successful transformation occurs through a series of iterative processes and is dialectic in approach, balancing discussions of the new and old to embed the change. It is recognized that leadership's role is extremely important in transformational change because it must engage and include all members of the organization to succeed. However, Pettigrew (2012) stresses that leadership is only one ingredient of transformational change, and the rationale, context, and content of change also play important roles. The pace, linearity, and process of transformational or radical change has been subjected to differing views, and empirical support is still needed. Transformational change can be achieved rapidly or through gradual steps. The sequence of change plays an important role in the outcome, starting with vital parts of the organization showing examples of change and providing strong symbolic meaning and signals. However, transformations are still difficult to effect, and outcomes are difficult to predict.

Evidence in health care supports the notion that changing institutional and market conditions creates a fertile ground for organizational transformation (Lee et al., 2012). Studies of organizational transformation in the US health care sector cite institutional change as an important factor for transformation, most particularly the shift from cost-based reimbursement to prospective payment (Lee & Alexander, 1999). In the UK, a pivotal institutional change that spurred organizational transformation efforts in the National Health Service (NHS) in the mid-1980s was the New Public Management (NPM), a range of policy reforms to stimulate competition; promote accountability; and produce efficiency, cost reduction, and service improvement (Kitchener, 1998). More recently, after an intensive consultation process, NHS England established a change model (NHS England, 2018) that was originally developed in 2012. It was designed to be an adaptable

---

**BOX 11-6**

**EIGHT COMPONENTS OF THE NHS MODEL OF CHANGE**

1. Our shared purpose—the starting point
2. Spread and adoption
3. Improvement tools
4. Project and performance management
5. Measurement
6. System drivers
7. Motivate and mobilize
8. Leadership by all

NHS England. (2018). Change model. https://www.england.nhs.uk/sustainableimprovement/change-model/

---

framework created for large or small projects with seven core principles and a focus around "*our shared purpose*." The change model (NHS England, 2018) has eight components, which set out the elements that should be considered when planning and implementing change (Box 11-6).

The change model is a framework, not a methodology, with components that provide an organized, systematic approach to help create an inclusive environment for successful sustainable change and is characterized by both soft and hard elements. The model provides leaders with ideas, prompts, tools, and resources to systematically use in their particular change situation and considering the critical dimensions that might affect change. As a relatively new model, there is limited feedback on the practicalities of its application in practice; however it has been noted that both clinicians and managers have implemented deviations from the model when implementing change projects (Lumbers, 2018).

## SUMMARY POINTS

- Change is inevitable in health and social care environments.
- Emergent changes are likely to be more common in the future due to changing external environments.
- Incremental change is associated with planned change over time.
- Transformational change requires engaging staff through leadership actions that provide meaning.

## THE ROLE OF LEADERS IN CONTEMPORARY CHANGE CONTEXTS

The leader's role is often emphasized as critical for successful change. Leaders are now expected to operate in a "new normal" environment that is characterized by constant change, both without and within organizations (Fleming & Millar, 2019). Thus, leaders and employees may experience organizational change as more disruptive (Bailey & Raelin, 2015) and sometimes emotionally disturbing. Jones et al. (2019) highlight that in health contexts, leaders must move beyond the managerialist, technical conception of health care as a system that can be managed and controlled using hierarchy.

Moran and Brightman (2000) suggest that, within organizational change, leadership capabilities must recognize the presence of emotional work and facilitate an emotional transition. De Klerk (2019) describes being fully present with compassion and acceptance during the moment change emotions evolve, connecting and serving authentically to be a catalytic instrument for individuals' healing and change transitions. De Klerk (2019) refers to the notion of "being-centeredness."

Fry and Kriger (2009) articulate a theory of leadership utilizing five levels of "being" as the context for effective leadership: the physical world, the world of images and imagination, the level of the soul, the level of the spirit, and the non-dual level. They explore how each level of being provides a means for advancing both the theory and practice of leadership. The leader becomes a facilitative instrument who assists the restoration of a healthy working environment, healed emotions, and change transitioning (Leybourne, 2016). Contemporary leadership approaches, including participative, authentic, empathetic, compassionate, and kind, have further developed the concept and practice of "being."

While leaders need to recognize the self and levels of being, it is also important that they are aware of how to lead in challenging and disruptive environments. These extreme contexts are described as

*one or more extreme events occurring or likely to occur that may exceed the organisation's capacity to prevent and result in an extensive and intolerable*

---

**BOX 11-7**
**FOUR CRISIS LEADERSHIP BEHAVIORS**

1. **Make decisions with speed over precision**—focus on business continuity as well as future success; priorities matter, be clear who the key decision-makers are, and encourage action including learning from mistakes.
2. **Get ahead of changing circumstances**—seek information from diverse sources, put on hold any initiatives that are not priorities, and strengthen connections with the front-line staff to gain on-the-ground feedback.
3. **Reliably deliver**—take personal ownership in a crisis, align team focus via metrics, and retain a fit mind and body.
4. **Take care of your team**—engage and motivate the team with clear communication, goals, and information. Remember the importance of positive messages.

Nichols, C., Hayden, S. C., & Trendler, C. (2020). 4 behaviors that help leaders manage a crisis. *Harvard Business Review*, April.

*magnitude of physical, psychological, or material consequences to—or in close physical or psychosocial proximity to—organization members.*
**Hannah et al. (2009, p. 898)**

Shared perspective, vision, trust, resilience, and a willingness to learn are especially important. Nichols et al. (2020) outline four key behaviors drawn from crisis leadership that can be used to lead organizational change (Box 11-7).

### SUMMARY POINTS

- Leaders must be prepared to facilitate the emotional transition of staff during change.
- Change leadership skills should include "levels of being" to enhance the meaningfulness of change.
- Crisis leadership offers significant insights for change leaders in current and future organizational environments.

## CHANGE READINESS: THE ANTIDOTE TO RESISTANCE

Resistance to change is common among employees and is defined by Peiperl (2005, p. 348) as "…. active or passive responses on the part of a person or group that militate against a particular change, a program of changes, or change in general." Since Coch and French's (1948) early work on overcoming resistance to change, various avenues have been taken to understand this phenomenon more fully (Nadim & Singh, 2019). Research suggests that psychological values are noteworthy (Hon et al., 2014), and studies of individuals and their interplay with complex organizational characteristics are useful (Ford & Ford, 2010). The existence of professional identities and boundaries in health care has been identified as a significant influencer of change processes through (re)negotiations of entrenched professional boundaries within organizational hierarchies (Huby et al., 2014). In the pervading complex organizational context, shedding more light on employees' attitudes and their readiness to change has become crucial (Bagrationi & Thurner, 2020). Change readiness is an individual concept, and every employee assesses the balance between the costs and benefits of maintaining or changing behavior (Vakola, 2014). Readiness factors such as individual beliefs, attitudes, and intentions help initiate change in organizations by creating employee support and involvement.

Kurt Lewin's (1951) studies of organizational and social settings led to his force field analysis theory, which includes individual and group behavior and describes the organizational background as a complex system surrounding individuals. Changes in behavior result either from a decrease in the power of restraining forces or an increase in the power of driving forces. Interestingly, one finding is that lack of workers' participation in discussions of the envisaged changes was directly linked to aggression and turnover rates. Hon et al. (2014) suggest two main aspects that remain important today. First, resistance is connected to shortcomings in the interactions between individuals and the organization—in the planning or execution of the process of change, through poor human resource management, or wrongly placed or missing incentives. Second, employees must actively participate in the change management process and the intersection between organizational factors and the focus on individual and group self-interests and/or psychological makeup. Choi and Ruona (2011) highlight that the relationship between change strategies and organizational culture can impact the perception of individual readiness for organizational change. Vakola (2014) develops this further by categorizing organizational readiness into three levels—micro-individual, meso-group, and

macro-organizational readiness—and by considering personality characteristics. Likewise, Wraikat et al. (2017) examine the readiness level, highlighting factors such as organizational structure, organizational climate, technology implementation strategy, and employee perceptions in psychological contracts on acceptance of change.

In a health and social care context, Packard et al. (2015) note that in 13 countries, change readiness, change capacity (management and organizational capability), and a participative leadership style are all important factors for sustaining change. Allied with this, Rogers's (2003) classical work on diffusion of innovation remains a useful model for its resonance within the health and social care sector, especially where the theory identifies the rates at which staff members are motivated to accept changes (Box 11-8). Five categories of acceptance of change are outlined within this model. Firstly, we have the innovators who are described as being passionate about the change and often suggest creative ideas to assist with it. The early adopters have leadership qualities, are respected by their peers and often take on the change first by acting as role models. Thirdly, are people with characteristics defined as the early majority who are willing to follow the early adopters. The fourth category of the late majority group are skeptical of the change but will eventually accept it and are often encouraged by social pressure from others. Finally, there is group categorized as laggards who are openly skeptical and resistant of the change.

During pre-change planning, leaders should assess their staff to establish which category they belong to.

---

**BOX 11-8**

### EIGHT CATEGORIES OF ACCEPTANCE OF CHANGE

- **Innovator:** passionate about change and technology; frequently suggests new ideas for departmental change.
- **Early adopter:** high levels of opinion leadership in the department; well-respected by peers.
- **Early majority:** prefers the status quo; willing to follow early adopters when notified of upcoming changes.
- **Late majority:** skeptical of change but will eventually accept the change once the majority has accepted it; susceptible to increased departmental social pressure.
- **Laggard:** high levels of skepticism; openly resists change.

Rogers, E. M. (2003). *Diffusion of innovations*. Free Press.

Most will likely belong to the early or late majority. Leaders should focus their initial education efforts on innovator and early adopter staff as they are often the most pivotal change champions and persuade the early and late majority staff to embrace change.

Building on this acceptance of change, Holt et al. (2010) form a conceptual framework to evaluate the readiness of caregivers for change. They focus on improving health care delivery, which they broadly divide into psychological factors, structural factors, and level of analysis. In an example of a wider view of perceived organizational readiness for change, Paré et al. (2011) explore introducing a clinical information system for home care, primary care, and integrated care networks. Ober et al. (2017) also apply organizational readiness to create a better implementation strategy to increase the quality of screening and evidence-based treatment of disease in primary care. Likewise, Nilsen et al. (2018) use organizational readiness to explore the implementation of palliative care-based evidence and guidelines for nursing homes.

## SUMMARY POINTS

- Staff reactions to organizational change can be challenging to manage.
- Understanding employee attitudes and their readiness to change has become crucial.
- Organizational culture and structure can significantly impact change readiness.
- There are five rates at which staff may accept changes (Rogers, 2003).

## THE VALUE OF STORYTELLING AND SOCIAL MOVEMENTS IN ACHIEVING CHANGE

Two less orthodox methods of managing change (storytelling and social movement) give additional insight into other models that may be useful when managing change within health and social care organizations. Storytelling is defined as "a recollection of events with collective associations that involve interactions of individuals to produce meaning that is applicable to future experiences" (Wilson, 2019, p. 18). The non-threatening character of storytelling can be seen as an asset in implementing change, particularly in the health and social care landscape, which is characterized by both a system of social relationships and a system of ideas, beliefs, and

ideologies (Jones et al., 2019). One of the benefits of storytelling is that in times of crisis, individuals search for understanding and thus sensemaking that is applicable to future experiences (Kopp et al., 2011). Dawson and Sykes (2019) advise that attention must be paid to the concerns, interpretation, and sense-making of those experiencing change and the ways these shared experiences enable or inhibit perceptions and behaviors that can affect the outcomes of change. Integrating storytelling into change management can therefore create an environment in which values and beliefs can be revised for the organization's survival (Wilson, 2019). Organizations can move from the uncertain to a clearer future by allowing employees to reflect on the organization's history, and sharing their stories with those experiencing similar situations allows a transition to a new future. Leaders must understand that commitment and loyalty to change efforts are built through shared communication of experiences (Gill, 2011). Organizations that engage in storytelling both proactively and reactively can greatly reduce many barriers to organizational learning and change (Kopp et al., 2011). Stories that resonate with deeply held values, beliefs, and emotions impact change by allowing for reevaluation through reflection. Thereby, the story can be key as a sense-making narrative when it comes to changing the mindsets, rules, objectives, and values of people and the system or organization they belong to.

We now move from the benefits of storytelling to another less orthodox method of supporting change, namely, the grass roots approaches of the social movement. The biggest difference between the traditional, planned approaches to change and the social movement approaches is that while prescriptive approaches focus on plans, social movement approaches focus on collective energy and take a bottom-up approach (Bate et al., 2004). Throughout history, social movements have played a key role in societal change, serving as moral movements that embody the emergence of a new ethos of what the good life should be (Crossley, 2002). The unique effectiveness of the social movement model of change is that it can enable large-scale systems such as health and social care to effectively mobilize often scarce community/system resources to implement and sustain complex change. Ganz (2010) proposes that shared values can serve as a means of attracting commitment for change by linking the need for change with personally held values at both the individual and community/system levels, thereby embracing inclusivity as the basis for creating strategic capacity and a sense of sustained collective commitment. Zald (2005) adds that social movement agendas can become part of a managerial strategy, but often present themselves outside the parameters of anticipated organizational policy.

Social movements have had an influential role in many US health reform agendas (Levitsky & Banaszak-Holl, 2010), including campaigns for universal health care (Hoffman, 2010), promoting services for marginalized groups (Kitchener, 2010), or introducing alternative therapies (Goldstein, 2010). However, movements can also oppose reform, such as the campaigns against "Obamacare" (Jacobs & Skocpol, 2015) in the US and contractual changes for junior doctors in the UK NHS (West, 2015). Bate et al. (2004, p. 64) suggest many "top-down" initiatives struggle to realize improvement because they fail to engage frontline clinicians, whereas a social movement approach enables service leaders to leverage the "latent potential" for change and secure "wider and deeper participation in a movement for improvement." However, relating to health care quality, social movements have shown the potential to engage and empower clinicians in "bottom-up" change (del Castillo et al., 2016).

## SUMMARY POINTS

- Storytelling is a key approach in supporting employees' understanding of change and making it meaningful for them.
- Commitment and loyalty to change efforts are built through the shared communication of experiences, often through storytelling.
- Social movements as an approach to change focus on collective energy and taking a grass roots or bottom-up approach.
- In health and social care, the power and engagement of social movements have been used to support as well as oppose health sector reforms.

## CONCLUSION

In the context of health and social care, change is inevitable due to ongoing pressures from governments and politicians to reform health care services and enhance quality and financial sustainability. For successful management, it is essential that organizations work hard to manage change. Some changes will be planned (new technologies, policy changes), whereas others will be more emergent based on shocks from the external environment. The change models discussed reflect the developing perspectives on managing change. This chapter has offered a traditional focus on prescriptive, often managerial, approaches to change, while also exploring the value of less orthodox approaches, which are proactive and malleable in changing contexts over time and have come to the fore more recently. The value of reflexivity and co-creation of meaning through storytelling has been suggested as crucial in health care organizations, where social relationships and ideas, beliefs, and ideologies are a core part of the organizational culture. Linked to this, the emergence of social movements as change agents in the US and UK health and social care sector has shown evidence of significant influence on major reforms. This approach emphasizes the need for various types and levels of staff to be involved and collaborate in change initiatives to embed the change. While the leader's role is critical in change programs in any sector, their role in the health and social care sector has been suggested as that of a facilitator, bringing together groups of staff who themselves act as change agents by using their skills to develop, support, and sustain change.

The culture and characteristics of the health and social care sector, such as embedded professional identities, entrenched boundaries, and hierarchies, have a significant impact on how change is managed and implemented and its relative success. This is further complicated by the proliferation of stakeholders across the public and private sector who now work in partnership to deliver services. Therefore, it is critical that within a health and care landscape, emphasis be placed on the human and emotional aspects of change to address potential resistance. Hence, it is vital that leaders understand the extent of change readiness so they can support a positive move toward successful change management.

## REFERENCES

Anders, C., & Cassidy, A. (2014). Effective organizational change in healthcare: Exploring the contribution of empowered users and workers. *International Journal of Healthcare Management, 7*(2), 132–151.

Bagrationi, K., & Thurner, T. (2020). Using the future time perspective to analyse resistance to, and readiness for, change. *Employee Relations, 42*(1), 262–279.

Bailey, J. R., & Raelin, J. D. (2015). Organizations don't resist change, people do: Modelling individual reactions to organizational change through loss and terror management. *Organization Management Journal, 12*(3), 125–138.

Balogun, J., & Hope Hailey, V. (2015). *Exploring strategic change* (4th ed). Prentice Hall.

Bamford, D. R., & Forrester, P. L. (2003). Managing planned and emergent change within an operations management environment. *International Journal of Operations and Production Management, 23*(5), 546–564. https://doi.org/10.1108/01443570310471857.

Bate, P., Robert, G., & Bevan, H. (2004). The next phase of Healthcare improvement: What can we learn from social movements? *Quality and Safety in Health Care, 13*(1), 62–66.

Bullock, R. J., & Batten, D. (1985). It's just a phase we're going through: A review and synthesis of OD phase analysis. *Group and Organization Studies, 10*(4), 383–412.

Burnes, B. (2004). *Managing change: A strategic approach to organisational dynamics.* Pearson Education.

Burnes. B. (2009). Reflections: Ethics and organizational change – Time for a return to Lewinian values. *Journal of Change Management, 9*(4), 359–381.

Burnes, B. (2011). Introduction: Why does change fail, and what can we do about it? *Journal of Change Management, 11*(4), 445–450.

Choi, M., & Ruona, W. E. A. (2011). Individual readiness for organizational change and its implications for human resource and organization development. *Human Resource Development Review, 10*(1), 46–73.

Coch, L., & French, J. R. P., Jr (1948). Overcoming resistance to change. *Human Relations, 1*(4), 512–532.

Crossley, N. (2002). Making sense of social movements. *McGraw-Hill Education*

Cummings, T. G., & Worley, C. G. (2014). *Organization development and change.* Cengage Learning.

Dawson, P., & Sykes, C. (2019). Concepts of time and temporality in the storytelling and sensemaking literatures: A review and critique. *International Journal of Management Reviews, 21*(1), 97–114.

De Klerk, J. J. (2019). Leading transitions in traumatically experienced change – A question of doing or being? *Journal of Organizational Change Management, 32*(3), 340–355.

del Castillo, J., Khan, H., Nicholas, L., & Finnis, A. (2016). *Health as a social movement: The power of people in movements.* Nesta.

Dunphy, D. C., & Stace, D. A. (1988). Transformational and coercive strategies for planned organizational change: Beyond the OD model. *Organization Studies, 9*(3), 317–334.

Fleming, K., & Millar, C. (2019). Leadership capacity in an era of change: The new-normal leader. *Journal of Organizational Change Management, 32*(3), 310–319.

Ford, J. D., & Ford, L. W. (2010). Stop blaming resistance to change and start using it. *Organizational Dynamics, 39*(1), 24–36.

Fry, L., & Kriger, M. (2009). Towards a theory of being-centred leadership: Multiple levels of being as context for effective leadership. *Human Relations, 62*(11), 1667–1696. https://doi.org/10.1177/0018726709346380.

Ganz, M. (2010). Leading change: Leadership, organization, and social movements. *Handbook of Leadership Theory and Practice, 19*, 1–10.

Gill, R. (2011). Corporate storytelling as an effective internal public relations strategy. *International Business Management, 3*(1), 17–25.

Goldstein, M. (2010). Complementary and integrative medicine in medical education. In J. C. Banaszak-Holl, S. Levitsky, & M. N. Zald (Eds.), *Social movements and the transformation of American health care.* Oxford University Press.

Gore, R., & Parker, R. (2019). Analysing power and politics in health policies and systems. *Global Public Health, 14*(4), 481–488.

Grundy, T. (1993). *Managing strategic change.* Kogan Page.

Hannah, S. T., Uhl-Bien, M., Avolio, B. J., & Cavarretta, F. L. (2009). A framework for examining leadership in extreme contexts. *The Leadership Quarterly, 20*(6), 897–919.

Hoffman, B. (2010). The challenge of universal health care: Social movements, presidential leadership, and private power. *Social Movements and the Transformation of American Health Care*, 39–49.

Holt, D. T., Helfrich, C. D., Hall, C. G., & Weiner, B. J. (2010). Are you ready? How health professionals can comprehensively conceptualize readiness for change. *Journal of General Internal Medicine, 25*(Supplement 1), 50–55.

Holton, J. A. (2020). Social movements thinking for managing change in large-scale systems. *Journal of Organizational Change Management, 33*(5), 697–714.

Hon, A. H. Y., Bloom, M., & Crant, J. M. (2014). Overcoming resistance to change and enhancing creative performance. *Journal of Management, 40*(3), 919–941.

Huby, G., Harris, F. M., Powell, A. E., Kielman, T., Sheikh, A., Williams, S., & Pinnock, H. (2014). Beyond professional boundaries: Relationships and resources in health services' modernisation in England and Wales. *Sociology of Health and Illness, 36*(3), 400–415.

Hughes, M. (2011). Do 70 percent of all organizational change initiatives really fail? *Journal of Change Management, 11*(4), 451–464.

Jacobs, L., & Skocpol, T. (2015). *Health care reform and American politics: What everyone needs to know.* Oxford University Press.

Jones, L., Fraser, A., & Stewart, E. (2019). Exploring the neglected and hidden dimensions of large-scale healthcare change. *Sociology of Health and Illness, 41*(7), 1221–1235.

Kitchener, M. (1998). Quasi-market transformation: An institutionalist approach to change in UK Hospitals. *Public Administration, 76*(1), 37–95.

Kitchener, M. (2010). *Social Movement Challenges to Structural Archetypes; Abortion Rights, AIDS and Long-Term Care. Social Movements and the Transformation of American Health Care* (pp. 128–143). Oxford University Press, Chapter 9.

Kopp, D. M., Nikolovska, I., Desiderio, K. P., & Guterman, J. T. (2011). "Relaaax, I remember the recession in the early 1980s…": Organizational storytelling as a crisis management tool. *Human Resource Development Quarterly, 22*(3), 373–385.

Kotter, J. P. (1996). Why transformation efforts fail. *Harvard Business Review, March/April*, 59–67.

Lee, S. Y., & Alexander, J. A. (1999). Consequences of organizational change in US hospitals. *Medical Care Research and Review, 56*(3), 227–276.

Lee, S. -Y. D., Weiner, B. J., Harrison, M. I., & Belden, C. M. (2012). Organizational transformation: A systematic review of empirical research in health care and other industries. *Medical Care Research and Review, 70*(2), 115–142.

Levitsky, S. R., & Banaszak-Holl, J. C. (2010). Social movements and the transformation of American health care: Introduction: *In Social movements and the transformation of American health care* (pp. 3–17). Oxford University Press.

Lewin, K. (1951). *Field theory in social science.* Harper & Row.

Leybourne. S. A. (2016). Emotionally sustainable change: Two frameworks to assist with transition. *International Journal of Strategic Change Management, 7*(1), 23–42.

Lippitt, R., Watson, J., & Westley, B. (1958). *The dynamics of planned change.* Harcourt: Brace & World.

Lumbers, M. (2018). Approaches to leadership and managing change in the NHS. *British Journal of Nursing, 27*(10), 554–558.

Moran, J. W., & Brightman, B. K. (2000). Leading organizational change. *Journal of Workplace Learning, 12*(2), 66–74.

Morgan, G. (2006). *Images of organization* (3rd ed.). SAGE.

Nadim, A., & Singh, P. (2019). Leading change for success: Embracing resistance. *European Business Review, 31*(4), 512–523.

Nadler, D. A. (1998). *Champions of change: How CEOs and their companies are mastering the skills of radical change.* Jossey-Bass.

N.H.S. England. (2018). Change model. https://www.england.nhs.uk/sustainableimprovement/change-model/

Nichols, C., Hayden, S. C., & Trendler, C. (2020). 4 behaviors that help leaders manage a crisis. *Harvard Business Review, April*

Nilsen, P., Wallerstedt, B., Behm, L., & Ahlström, G. (2018). Towards evidence-based palliative care in nursing homes in Sweden: A qualitative study informed by the organizational readiness to change theory. *Implementation. Science, 13*(1), 1.

Ober, A. J., Watkins, K. E., Hunter, S. B., Ewing, B., Lamp, K., Lind, M., ... Setodji, C. M. (2017). Assessing and improving organizational readiness to implement substance use disorder treatment in primary care: Findings from the SUMMIT study. *BMC Family Practice, 18*(1), 107.

Packard, T., McCrae, J., Phillips, J., & Scannapieco, M. (2015). Measuring organisational change tactics to improve child welfare programs: Experiences in 13 counties. *Human Service Organizations: Management. Leadership and Governance, 39,* 444–458.

Paré, G., Sicotte, C., Poba-Nzaou, P., & Balouzakis, G. (2011). Clinicians' perceptions of organizational readiness for change in the context of clinical information system projects: Insights from two cross-sectional surveys. *Implementation. Science, 6*(1), 15.

Peiperl, M. (2005). Resistance to change: *The Blackwell encyclopedia of management organizational behavior* (pp. 348–349) (2nd ed.). Blackwell.

Pettigrew, A. M. (2012). Context and action in the transformation of the firm: A reprise. *Journal of Management Studies, 49*(7), 1304–1328.

Rogers, E. M. (2003). *Diffusion of innovations.* Free Press.

Rosenbaum, D., More, E., & Steane, P. (2018). Planned organisational change management: Forward to the past? An exploratory literature review. *Journal of Organizational Change Management, 31*(2), 286–303.

Senior, B., Swailes, S., London, O. C., Times, P. H. F., Hardy, B., & Student, M. S. (2010). *Managing organisational change.* SOAS. University of London.

Vakola, M. (2014). What's in there for me? Individual readiness to change and the perceived impact of organizational change. *Leadership & Organization Development Journal, 35*(3), 195–209. https://doi.org/10.1108/LODJ-05-2012-0064.

West, N. (2015). Campaign against junior doctors contract must not lose momentum. *The Guardian.* https://www.theguardian.com/healthcare-network/views-from-the-nhs-frontline/2015/dec/21/junior-doctors-contracts-campaign-must-not-lose-momentum

Wilson, A. O. (2019). The role of storytelling in navigating through the storm of change. *Journal of Organizational Change Management, 32*(3), 385–395.

Wraikat, H., Bellamy, A., & Tang, H. (2017). Exploring organizational readiness factors for new technology implementation within non-profit organizations. *Open Journal of Social Sciences, 05*(12), 1–13.

Zald, M. N. (2005). The strange career of an idea and its resurrection: Social movements in organizations. *Journal of Management Inquiry, 14*(2), 157–166.

## REFLECTIVE QUESTIONS

- From your own experience or observations of a recent organizational change you have read about, why does organizational change fail?
- Explain which leadership capabilities will be needed to effectively manage change in the future.
- How might leaders deal with resistance to change?
- Which models of change do you think are appropriate for the changes faced in the future health and social care context?

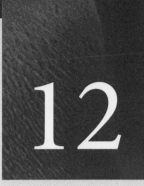

# 12

# RESPONSIBLE PROJECT MANAGEMENT IN HEALTH AND SOCIAL CARE

NIGEL L. WILLIAMS

## OBJECTIVES

*After reading this chapter, you should be able to:*

- Understand common project management terms and definitions.
- Identify the perspectives that have been applied to project management.
- Critically discuss the process of project management from the optimizing, adaptive, and responsible perspectives.

## INTRODUCTION

A project is defined as a temporary endeavor or enterprise that is created to deliver a unique output in the form of a product, service, or outcome (APM, 2019). Projects differ from operations because they are unique undertakings with defined start and end dates. For example, in the health and social care domain, these outputs can take the form of a new building (product), service (health advice), or outcome (increased screening rates). Project management therefore encompasses the application of knowledge, skills, relationships, and processes to deliver desired project outputs. Project management in the world of health and social care embraces these concepts, which are dynamic, complex, and interconnected. In addition, the specialist nature of health and social care provision requires the support and input of community stakeholders. Project managers working in these domains have a societal responsibility to health and social care beyond delivering defined outputs and should seek to apply inclusive approaches to project management, defined here as "responsible project management."

Projects form a significant part of many countries' economies and are the means by which health care organizations increase capacity, develop new capabilities, and respond to emerging scenarios (Shirley, 2020). For the National Health Service (NHS), projects enable realizing planned objectives and change responses (transformation, adaptation, and new direction) (NHS, 2019). They may be staged to implement a planned strategy such as increasing capacity or to take advantage of opportunities such as developing new treatment protocols. Projects can also be required to respond to new institutional demands, like meeting environmental laws and social value requirements. Finally, projects may be required to respond to public health crises such as the COVID-19 pandemic. On a macro scale, project management enables delivering large interventions such as building new hospitals and providing diverse types of health and social care. At the opposite end of the spectrum, on a micro scale, project management works on a day-to-day basis to support departments and practitioners in commissioning new equipment or services.

This chapter provides an overview of the origins and current perspectives of project management and discusses the key disciplines of project management. Finally, the reader is invited to examine the influence of their current organizational environment on project delivery.

## PROJECT MANAGEMENT FRAMEWORK AND TERMS

Health care projects are normally delivered for a host organization within a number of organizing frameworks or structures such as portfolios and programs. Within the host organization, projects may be delivered in a portfolio defined as a framework for achieving strategic organizational outcomes via coordinated management of programs and projects (APM, 2019). For example, portfolios used in health care could be utilized for expanding capacity to increase the number of patients served.

Programs and projects can also stand alone and exist outside of portfolios.

- A program is a structure designed to obtain complex benefits from a group of coordinated projects. From the previous example, a program within the capacity portfolio could focus on increasing primary care capacity.
- Projects are temporary initiatives created to deliver single or specific outcomes from a coordinated group of activities. In this case, a single project may be a new hospital building.

Project management uses a number of terms; they are summarized in Table 12-1 for greater understanding.

## PERSPECTIVES ON PROJECT MANAGEMENT

While there are many theoretical domains of project management, in practice, the current perspectives can be summarized as the optimizing perspective, adaptive perspective (Davies et al., 2018), and emerging responsible perspective (Thompson & Williams, 2019).

### The Optimizing Perspective

Also referred to as traditional project management and waterfall project management, in the optimizing perspective, project managers attempt to develop processes to manage and evaluate the project before activities are initiated. In health and social care, an example would be the redesign of a service, initiating a change in practice, or even building a new hospital. Project managers apply analytical approaches to predict future conditions and achieve planned outcomes. In this perspective, formal models are applied to identify possible options for the project's output, detailed planning of scope (outputs), time (scheduling), cost (budgeting), risk, and communication aspects.

**TABLE 12-1**

**Project Management Terms**

| Term | Description |
|---|---|
| Scope | The content and activities of a project |
| Requirements | The conditions or tasks that project outputs need to meet to achieve stakeholder aspirations |
| Schedule | A project time plan with start and end times for activities |
| Budget | A project cost plan with pricing methodology for items and activities |
| Stakeholder | Entities (persons, organizations, institutions) with an interest in the project activities and outcomes |
| Responsibility assignment matrix | A tool used to identify the delivery and evaluation roles of team members in a project |
| Risk | The uncertainty that can influence achievement of project outcomes |
| Milestone | Major decision point in a project schedule |

PMBOK. (2017). *Project management body of knowledge* (6th ed.). Project Management Institute.

For complex projects, programs, or portfolios, the planning process may also require associated planning on how project elements or components will be integrated in the final output. Since activities are predetermined, the cost of change can be high, as stakeholder commitments can occur long in advance of delivery. The optimizing approach does not work well in scenarios with rapid change or high uncertainty, such as in the COVID-19 pandemic response, in which activities needed to be developed and evaluated with little time for pre-planning.

### The Adaptive Perspective

In this perspective, the uncertainty of the external environment is recognized, and project processes are designed to respond to it. Instead of an extended period of planning, the project manager seeks to learn from experience as the project develops. Responding to the current pandemic by managing projects to quickly deal with situations is an example of this type of project management style. This learning process is enacted using shorter planning periods and performing experiments or developing prototypes and models that can be evaluated to support decision-making. Less formal processes are used, and there may be a greater use of consensus or trust-based agreements. Thus, the output may have a greater opportunity to meet stakeholder requirements in scenarios with high uncertainty.

### The Emerging Responsible Perspective

In the responsible practice management domain, the societal value and impact of projects are explicitly recognized from the outset. For instance, the NHS accounts for 25 percent of public sector carbon dioxide emissions in the United Kingdom (UK), with growing pressure to reduce its environmental impact (King's Fund, 2012). The emerging responsible perspective seeks to meet emerging demands for enterprises not only to reduce their impact on the natural and social environments but to also create positive effects (Geissdoerfer et al., 2017). Regarding the former, there is increasing recognition of the need to reduce the carbon emissions of organizational activities. This can include increasing the use of renewable energy, using low carbon materials, and reducing food and water waste. Organizations are now developing competencies in circular product and process design to ensure that outputs can be reused and recycled. Regarding social responsibility and workplace sustainability, activities are initiated to provide positive benefits for social ecosystems such as communities and employees. Specifically, in the domain of health and social care, the need to respond to evolving community and national needs requires sensitivity to the social environment. National regulatory frameworks such as Net Zero (Pencheon & Wight, 2020) for carbon emissions and social value (Banke-Thomas et al., 2015) are examples of national requirements that the NHS is required to meet. It is recognized that as the financial challenges for the health and social care sector increase, so too does the need for services to be delivered in ways that are environmentally sustainable (King's Fund, 2012).

### SUMMARY POINTS

- Projects may be viewed from multiple perspectives.
- The optimizing perspective may be best when the level of uncertainty is low, requirements are known, and appropriate solutions can be easily identified.

- The adaptive perspective can be appropriate when there is a high level of uncertainty.
- The emerging responsible perspective seeks to explicitly recognize complex, interconnected societal demands.

## SUCCESS OF PROJECTS

Projects are evaluated by outcomes, but a distinction can be made between project success, project management success, and societal success (Fig. 12-1). Project success is a project's beneficial output, while project management success is the appropriate management of delivery actions and processes (Ika, 2009). Societal success is somewhat more abstract but is concerned with the value communities derive from project processes and outcomes.

## PROJECT "FRONT END" (INITIAL CONCEPTION AND DECISION TO FORMALIZE A PROJECT)

Project success begins with the "front end," when the permanent organization (institution, organization, department, or team) requires a benefit from a particular change or outcome. The intended outcome of this stage of the process is to build consensus for a common understanding of the problem and gain support for the proposed solution, response to change, or planned activity. These benefits supporting the change can be identified by external trends such as national policy initiatives or internal analyses that identify a gap between organizational performance and patient experience requirements. It is at this stage that the initial need for the project, stakeholders, and source of the necessary resources are identified (Williams et al., 2019).

A formal stakeholder analysis process (NHS England and NHS Improvement 2020) is useful at this stage to identify the internal and external stakeholders and the extent of their involvement with the proposed project. Project managers are encouraged to engage with a wide variety of stakeholders drawn from the organization (staff, clinicians), community (patients and residents), and externally (suppliers and social organizations). This supports the planning processes and enables the project manager and team to make the

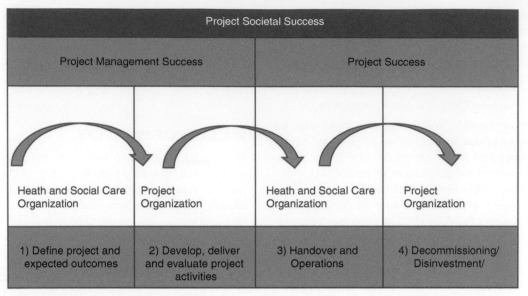

Fig. 12-1 ■ The extended project cycle and project success dimensions

time and effort to engage individuals, thereby reducing risks by minimizing any conflict among stakeholders. This decision is critical, as it influences project management success, project success, and societal success. The stakeholder analysis process as suggested by NHS England and NHS Improvement (2020), usually follows the steps outlined in (Box 12-1): The key project stakeholders (internal and external to the organization) are identified, and they are invited to offer their opinions on the emerging project initiative.

Stakeholders can then be classified by their degree of power and interest. This identifies those who should be prioritized for the appropriate engagement activities. In stakeholder discussions, it is important not only to examine formal or stated needs but also project stakeholders' latent biases, preferences, and interests, as they can influence the outcome.

The stakeholders involved at this stage need to find consensus on the types and characteristics of the project outputs. For example, what are the major desired outputs of the project? It can be useful to classify these outputs as mandatory (required by an external body such as a regulator or to meet a new legislated requirement for delivering care), project set up (required to enable the project activity), stakeholder engagement (required to obtain and maintain

stakeholders' support), and risk mitigation (required to reduce major risks identified at the front end stage). Despite the high level of uncertainty at this stage, early time and resource estimates are required for stakeholders to assess the value to be derived from the project and decide how best to meet the identified need. The formal justification for the project is captured in the form of a project brief, which at this stage documents initial thinking about costs, benefits, anticipated solutions, risks, and metrics for evaluating success. Project managers could also develop a more detailed document in the form of a project initiation document (PID). A PID extends the project brief to include background and rationale, project scope, constraints and assumptions, defined objectives, and project organizational structure. Approval for the PID is sought by the governing body at the host or commissioning organization. However, projects may not always follow this formal process as emergency responses (such as the COVID-19 scenario) require an urgent response with priority overriding formal business cases. Where a project can be planned, a high level of uncertainty still remains at this stage; however, defining the scope of the anticipated solution is important. A case study from Fife, Scotland, illuminates some key aspects of project management.

In addition to these general challenges, there were specific issues related to the Fife region. A review of the service identified that there were four "out of hours" GP centers with equal resources (staff and equipment) despite having varying demand for services at each center. The organization could not simply move resources to centers with higher demand; therefore, a new urgent care model needed to be designed to allow for responsiveness to the changing demand patterns of the people of Fife. The Fife Health and Social Care Out of Hours Urgent Care Review (2020) identified a need to respond to out of hours demand for services. To meet this need, a program was established with the overall aim to form a 24/7 community integrated health and social care model, ensuring individual partnerships of care that are sustainable and safe. The integrated program has three work domains (Box 12-3).

## CASE STUDY (FIFE, SCOTLAND): FRONT END (INITIAL CONCEPTION AND DECISION TO FORMALIZE THE PROJECT)

The front-end case history describes a new health and social care program in the region of Fife, Scotland, in the UK (www.fifehealthandsocialcare.org and adapted from https://www.fva.org/downloads/JUC_Summary_final_290618.pdf). This project has a number of policy and management differences compared to the NHS in England. In Scotland, organizations are funded to provide services, with no competition between providers. Additionally, Scotland offers free general medical prescriptions and personal social care for the whole population.

### Rationale for the Fife Project

Like many other NHS organizations, the Fife region faces the following general challenges (Box 12-2):

This program encompassed a number of projects; however, this case history focuses on the Urgent Care Dispatch, a resource hub for the region.

A multi-agent group examined the existing process and created a model based on a multidisciplinary team working from fewer centers, composed of an Urgent Care Dispatch (which coordinates service delivery) and two Urgent Care Centers (public care provision to Fife citizens).

### Project Initial Scope

The scope of the project is as follows:

1. Develop an information system that facilitates review and triage of requests. Visits can be booked via NHS 24 with support from a local clinical supervisor, where appropriate, at first contact. The information system will also have a dedicated direct phone line for palliative care patients who need rapid access to District Nursing. The information system will also track vehicles on home visits along with a shared diary and case status monitoring.
2. Reconfigure staffed centers from four to two Urgent Care Centers. Urgent Care Centers will deliver the range of urgent clinical care. They will be a safe venue that can be accessed by the public, located to make the best use of available workforce and facilities. These will be a venue to bring together all urgent care services, with each center delivering the same services. This would see a clinical model develop where urgent care is provided by a single team that provides a combination of GP services and handles minor injuries. Staff can undertake additional home visits as needed.
3. Increase diagnostic capacity after normal working hours. A range of diagnostics available after hours to minimize the need for additional appointments.
4. Develop and deliver a communications campaign. The team will work with communications colleagues to educate the public about when they should visit the Accident and Emergency Department instead of attending urgent care.
5. Develop and deliver the workforce model. Develop a workforce model that supports the new mode of health and social care delivery.

### The Fife Project Stakeholders

1. Patients who will use the new services.
2. Local support services (e.g., community pharmacy, Scottish Ambulance Service) who require direct access to the professionals in the Urgent Care Dispatch.
3. NHS Fife administration who will fund and evaluate the program.
4. Current frontline workforce who will be affected by the new working patterns.
5. Administrative staff who will have to use the new systems and deliver the communications campaign to educate the public.

### Fife Project Milestones

- April 2019: Establish an Urgent Care Dispatch and a new model of Urgent Care Centers.
- April 2020: Integrate urgent care resource hub and single point of access.

### Risks

The following risks were identified by the team at the front end:

1. **Clinical delivery**. The community does not accept the new clinical services, and they continue to be stretched with inequitable demand, inequitable access, and staffing challenges.
2. **Workforce**. New processes do not deliver the promised efficiencies and staff continue to experience cumbersome systems.
3. **Delay**. Delays in implementing program outputs will reduce the ability to meet identified demand and service capacity issues in Fife.
4. **Finance**. If the program is not delivered according to the scope and timeframe, efficiency benefits will not be realized, resulting in higher costs for health and social care.

## PROJECT DELIVERY

Moving away from the Fife case study and returning to a generic examination of projects, once a project has been initiated, it follows a path of development to conclusion. The rate at which this process occurs may be constrained by the organization's risk tolerance and the level of external uncertainty. The project pathway can be linear or iterative. A linear pathway model of project development is a sequential series of steps that align with the optimizing paradigm. However, iterative pathways may have non-sequential steps as project development follows the acquisition of insights from stakeholders. These are further explained as follows:

## Linear Mode

In the linear mode, the planning stage converts the concept and justification agreed upon in the front end into actionable activities that need to be completed for the project's success. Activities are delivered in a "push" mode, that is, following a predetermined time and resource schedule.

For the health and social care project identified in the Fife case study, the activities that need to be completed are numbered and described (see Table 12-2). It is also noted that each activity is mutually exclusive, with no overlap among elements.

The demarcation of activities to meet the project goals and objectives simplifies communication among the various stakeholders by providing an overview of the project and management elements. These activities can be further refined into work packages and assigned to team members for completion. Continual review of progress allows the project to respond to change.

### Resource Planning

Once an initial delineation of the activities has been completed and reviewed by stakeholders, it is possible to determine what resources may be required (e.g., IT support, office space, more personnel) and identify the source of these resources and the period in which the activities are to be completed. The team can draw upon the experiences of previous projects to estimate resource requirements, evaluate possible resource providers, and estimate the duration of activities.

### Sequencing and Scheduling

Once resources are confirmed, project teams can then determine the sequence of activities. While there are several patterns, most project activities can be staged in a series (one after the other) or in parallel (multiple activities at once). For example, in Table 12-3, activity 1.2 is in a series, while 1.2 and 1.3 are in parallel. Once the sequence is confirmed, project managers can then create a schedule. A simple version of a working schedule takes the form of a Gantt chart (developed by Clark in 1922), which displays activities using vertical and horizontal axes. On the horizontal axis, columns are used to display duration and person responsibilities. Work activities to be completed are listed from top to bottom on the vertical axis in the time order in which they will be executed. The durations of the work activities are displayed in graphical form as horizontal lines or columns, with the length showing the start and end dates for each line. This process can be done manually, using one of the many downloadable software Gantt chart templates or online tools. It is advisable to share any draft schedules with stakeholders for evaluation before the final schedule is published, as they may notice something that has been overlooked. This project information can also support the development of risk management activities where the initial risks identified in the front end can be elaborated on using the project planning data.

### Executing, Monitoring, and Controlling

In this phase, the project team, along with suppliers and community stakeholders, execute the actions described in the work activities needed to deliver the required outcomes. While these plans can guide the process, there is recognition that the project environment is dynamic, not static and linear, requiring the team to monitor and control activities to prevent unwanted outcomes. Throughout the project's implementation, the project team is required to continually evaluate performance against plans and communicate this progress to the stakeholders. If any variance occurs, it can negatively influence outcomes, making it important for the team to decide on the necessary corrective action.

### TABLE 12.2

**Activities for the Fife Case Study Project**

| Work activity number | Description of activities |
| --- | --- |
| 1 | Overall program |
| 1.1 | Information system |
| 1.2 | Reconfigured staff centers |
| 1.3 | After hours diagnostic capacity |
| 1.4 | Communications campaign |
| 1.5 | Workforce model |

**TABLE 12-3**

**Project Activity Sequence and Duration**

| WBS Element Number | Preceding Element | Element Description | Duration | Start Date | Finish Date |
|---|---|---|---|---|---|
| 1 | – | Overall program | 12 months | April 2018 | April 2019 |
| 1.1 | – | Information system | 2 months | April 2018 | June 2018 |
| 1.2 | 1.1 | Reconfigured staff centers | 3 months | June 2018 | September 2018 |
| 1.3 | 1.1 | After hours diagnostic capacity development | 6 months | June 2018 | December 2018 |
| 1.4 | 1.2, 1.3 | Workforce model development and implementation | 3 months | December 2018 | March 2019 |
| 1.5 | 1.4 | Communications campaign | 1 month | March 2019 | April 2019 |

## Iterative Mode

The iterative mode of delivery adapts ideas from lean and agile manufacturing systems such as those used in industrial production systems. Unlike the linear mode, while detailed project plans can be made in advance, they are reviewed closer to the time when the activity will be performed. This process is known as "pull planning," and it creates multiple levels of activities (Ballard et al., 2007). The highest level of this process is a master schedule that provides a roadmap of the overall project. Each successive level reduces the planning horizon, with evaluating weekly tasks being the lowest level of collaborative planning. Phased task scheduling ensures that the appropriate activities and resources are deployed to meet the overall project requirements; for example, this is particularly helpful to keep a project on track in situations where there is not enough time for planning. In addition, the schedules can be produced by working in reverse order from a target date in the master schedule. This process is aimed at only delivering work that is requested and needed by a subsequent phase. During this process, the team seeks to identify constraints that may hinder activities from being completed on time and remove these before tasks are assigned. At the lowest level, resources are assigned to responsible entities (team or individual), outcomes are evaluated, and corrective actions are taken. In this approach, work is planned closer to the time when it will be conducted, resulting in greater likelihood of completion within the agreed timeframe. In addition, the reduced timeframe can also make project risk management activities easier, as there is more detail available regarding the activities at the point of their delivery.

## SUMMARY POINTS

- Linear mode plans activities long before they are conducted but can be inflexible.
- Iterative mode only plans activities shortly before they are delivered.

## Reviving Stalled Projects

In both the linear and iterative modes of managing a project, there is always a chance that progress may not smoothly advance from initiation to conclusion. Frequently, projects may stall, that is, no progress is made beyond a certain point. There are multiple signs of stalling or stagnation, such as changing stakeholder priorities, making the project no longer seem important (NHS, 2013). Moreover, team members may no longer be participating in the project activities or supplying useful information.

To manage a stalled project scenario, the project manager should first determine the project status to confirm that the project is still required and that the outputs remain of value to the organization. If the project is no longer of value, then project teams can consult with the organization to consider cancelling the project. If the project is still of value, the project team can conduct an internal analysis of barriers and evaluate the project approach to identify avenues for reviving it. Some actions that can be taken by the project team include restructuring the project to ensure that the appropriate stakeholders are involved, obtaining executive support to signal to the organization that the project is still of value, and consulting with potential users to ensure that the aims of the project are understood and potential concerns are identified. After these discussions, the scope and business case of the project may need to be adjusted to meet the current realities, in addition to revising tools such as the Gantt chart and budget to ensure that resources are available to complete the project.

## Handover to Operational Use

The handover process at project completion can be overlooked by project managers, but it is critical for evaluating project management success, ensuring project success, and enabling societal success (Zwikael & Smyrk, 2019). As part of this process, project teams need to obtain end user or client acceptance of project outputs. In addition, as projects inevitably vary from the contractually agreed upon specifications, clients need to review and approve these changes. A process also needs to be established for resolving any outstanding project issues at the time of handover. For complex initiatives such as new technology, for example, when a new system of data entry is introduced into the health or social care environment, staff may need to be trained on the operation and maintenance of these outputs. The project team may also be required to establish or facilitate support arrangements for such projects after handover. The team will compile and hand over all project information along with the lessons learned during planning and delivery that can support the development of future projects and improve organizational project practice.

Handover and project closure need to consider not only the project outputs but also the organizational and societal outcomes; this is complex, as the period for utilization may not be fully known. Monitoring ambiguous future outcomes such as social value is also complex. To ensure that these outcomes are realized, the project team needs to identify resources and responsible stakeholders at handover. The team may also monitor the integration between the new project's outputs and existing services.

## Decommissioning

Decommissioning has been defined as a change in the provision of a service (National Audit Office, 2020), which can incorporate a range of outcomes from reducing the level of a service to replacing or terminating a specific health and social care service. A related action is disinvestment; this occurs when funding is removed from an enterprise, resulting in the cessation of a service. Since each service can be unique, this may require a project plan similar to front end planning (Topham et al., 2019). The organization will need to consider the national regulations existing at that point in time, as they may have changed since the project was delivered, along with the financial resources and environmental impact. This may be particularly complicated as financial demands may arise as part of decommissioning with no financial or service value to be obtained.

For health and social services, decommissioning is a critical activity necessary to meet changing health care requirements; activities therefore need to be aligned with overall delivery and development strategies. External stakeholders such as local communities also need to be engaged as part of planning decommissioning activities. Due to the sensitivities of removing or reducing services, public engagement can include the use of inclusive priority setting processes (Sabik & Lie, 2008).

The following stages can be used to assist with these activities:

1. Conceptualization of the issue to be addressed and specifying the project and program goals.
2. Decommissioning decision-making. Tools such as budgeting, local economic data, and modeling are used to inform the decommissioning process by identifying areas that may be of low benefit. The following areas are generally considered:
   - Impact on meeting health demands and the patient experience.
   - Impact on other organizations that may form part of service delivery.
3. Plan decommission program. This program can include activities such as relocating or replacing services or closure.
4. Implement decommission program.
5. Review and evaluate outcomes.

While decommissioning is proposed as a structured, dispassionate process, there needs to be recognition that stakeholders build personal bonds that will be disrupted when a service is removed. While there is no simple way to address the emotional loss that these stakeholders may feel, decommissioning planners must acknowledge the personal impacts and provide opportunities for discussing these along with approaches for minimizing harm during the process.

## SUMMARY POINTS

- Project team responsibilities do not end with the conclusion of scheduled activities.
- The handover process needs to be carefully managed if benefits are to be realized.

## CONCLUSION

As the demographics of regions change and technology creates new opportunities, health and social care organizations will develop projects to respond. Projects are required to meet the goals of organizations as well as emergent public health and social challenges. Before commencing a project, stakeholders engage in a consultation process to confirm the project's process and outcomes and identify how success will be evaluated. At a minimum, organizations may define the success of the project's output (project success and societal success) and the management processes for delivering the project (project management success). Once initiated, they may follow a prescriptive life cycle until handover or an iterative pattern of interim output delivery. In either scenario, changing priorities or waning interest can cause projects to stall. The project team may be required to re-engage stakeholders to ensure that the project is still necessary and the required inputs will be available to ensure that the initiative can be completed. The handover process needs to be carefully managed, as the project's benefits will only be realized if stakeholders (the organization and end users) can utilize the project's outputs. At the end of the project's life, it can be withdrawn or repositioned to serve evolving community demands.

Taking an extended life cycle view from initiation to decommissioning allows project organizations to seek maximization of stakeholders' long-term benefits. These benefits are not only linked to the operational or service value connected with the output, but also to social and environmental benefits linked to emerging societal values. As these trends continue to gain prominence, project managers need to ensure that their activities deliver the required outcomes for stakeholders in a manner that minimizes environmental impact and maximizes societal benefit.

## REFERENCES

Association for Project Management (APM). (2019). Body of knowledge. https://www.apm.org.uk/resources/what-is-project-management/#:~:text=A%20project%20is%20a%20unique,an%20agreed%20timescale%20and%20budget

Ballard, G., Hamzeh, F.R., & Tommelein, I.D. (2007). *The last planner production workbook-improving reliability in planning and workflow* (p.81). Lean Construction Institute.

Banke-Thomas, A. O., Madaj, B., Charles, A., & van den Broek, N. (2015). Social Return on Investment (SROI) methodology to account for value for money of public health interventions: A systematic review. *BMC Public Health, 15*(1), 582.

Clark, W. (1922). The Gantt chart: A working tool of management. https://ia902703.us.archive.org/16/items/cu31924004570853/cu31924004570853.pdf

Davies, A., Manning, S., & Söderlund, J. (2018). When neighboring disciplines fail to learn from each other: The case of innovation and project management research. *Research Policy, 47*(5), 965–979.

Geissdoerfer, M., Savaget, P., Bocken, N. M., & Hultink, E. J. (2017). The circular economy – A new sustainability paradigm? *Journal of Cleaner Production, 143*, 757–768.

Ika. L. A. (2009). Project success as a topic in project management journals. *Project Management Journal, 40*(4), 6–19.

King's Fund. (2012). Environmental sustainability in health and social care https://www.kingsfund.org.uk/publications/sustainable-health-and-social-care

National Audit Office. (2020). What we mean by decommissioning. https://www.nao.org.uk/decommissioning/before-you-start/what-we-mean-by-decommissioning/

NHS England, & NHS, Improvement. (2020). Online library of Quality, Service Improvement and Redesign tools: Stakeholder analysis. https://www.england.nhs.uk/wp-content/uploads/2021/03/qsir-stakeholder-analysis.pdf.

NHS. 2013. Reviving a stalled effort. https://improvement.nhs.uk/documents/2154/reviving-stalled-effort.pdf.

NHS. 2019. Project management: An overview. https://improvement.nhs.uk/resources/project-management-overview/

Pencheon, D., & Wight, J. (2020). Making healthcare and health systems net zero. *BMJ, 368*, m970.

PMBOK. (2017). *Project management body of knowledge* (6th ed.). Project Management Institute.

Sabik, L. M., & Lie, R. K. (2008). Priority setting in health care: Lessons from the experiences of eight countries. *International Journal for Equity in Health, 7*, 4.

Shirley. D. (2020). *Project management for healthcare.* CRC Press.

The Fife Health and Social Care Out of Hours Urgent Care Review. (2020). https://www.fifehealthandsocialcare.org/joiningupcare/out-of-hours-urgent-care-redesign/

Thompson, K.M., & Williams, N.L. (2019). *A guide to responsible project management.*

Topham, E., McMillan, D., Bradley, S., & Hart, E. (2019). Recycling offshore wind farms at decommissioning stage. *Energy Policy, 129,* 698–709.

Williams, T., Vo, H., Samset, K., & Edkins, A. (2019). The front-end of projects: A systematic literature review and structuring. *Production Planning & Control, 30*(14), 1137–1169. https://doi.org/10.1080/09537287.2019.1594429.

Zwikael, O., & Smyrk, J. R. (2019). Realising outcomes from projects: *Project management.* Springer.

## REFLECTIVE QUESTIONS

Thinking about a recently completed or current project, consider the following questions:

■ What has gone well and why?

■ What would you change about the project?

■ Will you use the same approach (linear, adaptive, etc.) in the future?

■ If you were involved in the front end of the project, to what extent did you consider the extended life cycle (from front end to decommissioning)?

■ How were community stakeholders represented in the project?

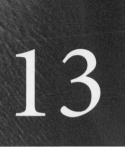

# 13

# COACHING AND MENTORSHIP FOR SUCCESSFUL LEADERSHIP

LIZ WESTCOTT AND ELIZABETH ANNE ROSSER

## OBJECTIVES

*After reading this chapter, you should be able to:*

- Demonstrate an understanding of the terms coaching, mentoring, and practice supervision and the value of each to leaders in contemporary health and social care.

- Analyze the effectiveness of coaches, mentors, and supervisors in today's health and social care practice.

- Identify the two main strategies used by coaches, mentors, and practice supervisors to support them in their roles.

- Critically discuss the impact of developing a successful coaching and mentoring culture.

- Critically analyze the value of creating an effective learning organization and the role of coaching, mentoring, and reflective practice in facilitating success.

## INTRODUCTION

Previous chapters have recognized the many unprecedented global challenges faced by contemporary health and social care leaders in both private and public organizations that operate in high-, low-, and middle-income countries. In particular, the United Kingdom has been experiencing ongoing issues in its efforts to integrate its health and social care workforce. Within this context, there is a movement toward interprofessional working, collaborative practices, new ways of working, and cultural changes; consequently, there is a need for a workforce that is flexible enough to adapt. Support structures are seen as key for facilitating leaders along their journey. In particular, mentoring and coaching have increased considerably in

recent years and, according to De Meuse et al. (2009), they are major components in leadership development practices in corporate organizations around the world. In health care, Hamer et al. (2019) acknowledge that effectively using such support roles can not only transform the trajectory of individual leaders' career pathways but can also shape the identity and success of institutions. When facilitated by experts in their roles, mentoring and coaching help leaders realize "their full potential, create and disseminate new knowledge, invoke positive institutional change, and build local capacity" (Hamer et al., 2019, p. 15). This chapter explores the principles of coaching, mentoring, and practice supervision and discusses the value of each for individuals, teams, and organizations. In addition, it examines the value of developing a coaching and mentoring leadership style and its impact on creating a "learning organization" (Berwick, 2013) that is able to respond to rapid change. Finally, the chapter considers strategies that mentors and coaches can use within the workplace, such as interprofessional teamworking, values-based practice, and reflective practice, to support leaders and managers in their roles and enable them to develop the teams and individuals with whom they work.

## COACHING, MENTORING, AND PRACTICE SUPERVISION

First, it is important to clarify certain terms as there has been some confusion over the terminology and concepts related to coaching, mentoring, and practice supervision. Moreover, there are recognized differences in generic understanding between Europe and the United States (Fielden et al., 2009).

## Coaching

There are a variety of definitions of the practice of coaching; the Chartered Institute of Personnel and Development (2020a, para. 1) suggests that coaching is about producing "optimal performance and improvement at work. It focuses on specific skills and goals, although it may also have an impact on an individual's personal attributes such as social interaction or confidence." Within UK health and social care services, coaching is often targeted at more senior organization leaders. However, an organization's investment in coaching leaders earlier rather than later in their careers can yield benefits as individuals develop.

The purposes of coaching can be diverse, but essentially focus on improving role performance and, as Fielden et al. (2009) acknowledge, involve developing human capital. The authors suggest that coaching can include helping a leader: (i) change from one role to another, (ii) cope with organizational change, (iii) address and resolve issues and problems, and (iv) advance their skills. According to Cox et al. (2017), coaching helps leaders develop greater understanding through discussion and reflective thought, enabling them to become more complete and authentic leaders.

The terms "executive coaching" and "leadership coaching" are both often used to describe the development of leaders' abilities and capabilities to help them more effectively undertake their roles. Coaching will enable leaders to understand themselves more fully and in turn, enable them to better understand their staff; moreover, coaching can be undertaken at any position in their career.

## Mentoring

Mentorship is used by organizations and individuals to develop staff and enhance learning (Garvey et al., 2018). It can be used to enhance both skills and knowledge (Godshalk & Sosik, 2003) and, similar to coaching, can involve a long-term relationship (Joo et al., 2012) that is focused on their career. In essence, a mentor relationship is built on mutual trust where the mentor is a more skilled and knowledgeable individual who is able and ready to share knowledge with

someone less experienced. Mentorship "entails informal communication, is usually face-to-face and sustained over a period of time, between a person who is perceived to have greater relevant knowledge, wisdom, or experience (the mentor) and a person who is perceived to have less (the protégé)" (Bozeman & Feeney, 2007, p. 720). Estimates indicate that in 2004, approximately 230,000 people undertook some mentoring activity within the UK Health Service (Healthcare Commission, 2004).

## Practice Supervision

Practice supervision offers staff the opportunity to reflect on and improve their practice and learn with a skilled and knowledgeable colleague. Practice supervision has also been found to provide peer support and guidance, which in turn reduces stress, increases professional accountability, and enhances skill and knowledge development (Brunero & Stein-Parbury, 2008).

More generally, beyond health care, supervision is accepted as a key role of first line managers, with "performance-oriented supervision" among their numerous other responsibilities (Hales, 2005, p. 501). In particular, first-line managers in social work recognize the importance of both individual and group supervision as part of their manager role (SCIE, 2012). As in health care, they acknowledge their role in leading the wider team, giving direction and support to team members, and making the best use of their resources in the informal supervisory process.

## Association of Concepts

As illustrated, the three roles have similarities but also differences. While they each offer support for the emerging manager and leader, it is important to consider the relationships among them. Fielden et al. (2009) suggest that professional coaching is defined as directly concerned with enhancing performance and skills; in the UK National Health Service (NHS), it is often seen as focused on supporting senior managers and executives. However, practice supervision, while also focusing on skills development, is usually provided to more junior staff. In coaching, the coachee is seen as the expert and the coach as a learning facilitator (Fielden et al., 2009), while mentors and practice supervisors are seen as the experts. Supervision

**TABLE 13.1**

**Differences Between Coaching, Mentoring, and Practice Supervision**

| Factor | Manager as coach/practice supervision | Mentoring | Coaching |
|---|---|---|---|
| Coach/mentor | Learning and development | Socialization | Self-awareness |
| | Performance improvement | Management development | Learning |
| | Retention | Understanding | Behavioral change |
| | | Organizational politics | Performance improvement |
| Coachee | Employees | Lower-level employees to those with high potential | Mostly executives and higher level managers |
| Process | Less structured | Revolves around developing the mentee professionally and giving advice, guidance, or support | Generally more structured in nature; meetings are scheduled on a regular basis |
| Focus | Partnership | Focus is on career and personal development | Focus is generally on development /issues at work |
| | Communication | | |
| | Development of skills in practice | | |
| Duration | Ongoing | Ongoing relationship that can last for a long period of time | Relationship generally has a set duration but can be long term |

Jarvis, J. (2004). Coaching and buying coaching services: A CIPD guide. CIPD. https://www.portfolio-info.co.uk/files/file/CIPD%20 coaching_buying_services.pdf

Joo, B.-K., Sushko, J., & McLean, G. N. (2012). Multiple faces of coaching: Manager-as-coach, executive coaching, and formal mentoring. *Organization Development Journal*, 30(1).

is normally a short-term relationship, while coaching and mentoring are longer term and are, for example, focused on projects, relationships, and career development. The Chartered Institute of Personnel and Development (2020a) suggests that the essential difference is that mentors give advice and teach, whereas coaches facilitate learning. Nevertheless, it is important that practitioners are clear as to the expectations of both parties at the outset of their relationship. This will ensure that the coach, mentor, and practice supervisor agree on any expected outcomes and the expected approach, as well as the time limitations.

Both Jarvis (2004, p. 20) and Joo et al. (2012, p. 30) have identified the connections between the manager as coach, executive coaching, and formal mentoring. Table 13.1 is a collation of concepts from Jarvis (2004) and Joo et al. (2012) related to practice supervision, coaching, and mentoring and may be helpful in distinguishing among the three roles.

## A Continuum of Coaching

While there are challenges to acting as a practice supervisor, mentor, or coach, there remains a clear relationship among them (Joo et al., 2012). E. J.

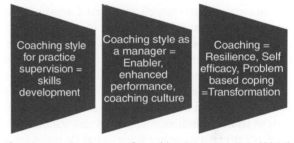

**Fig. 13-1** ▪ Continuum of coaching Westcott, E. J. (2014). *The role of coaching in the development of nurse managers* [DCM thesis, Oxford Brookes University]. https://radar.brookes.ac.uk/ radar/file/0dbe0087-8e59-4edf-9b51-59e279fe40df/1/west-cott2014role.pdf

Westcott (2014) developed the continuum of coaching identified by West and Milan (2001), and Hawkins and Smith (2010) translated this into a continuum with practice supervision at one end of skills development and coaching and transformation at the other end (see Figure 13-1). This concept of a practice supervision–mentoring–coaching continuum further helps illustrate the roles and value of these three areas of development.

## SUMMARY POINTS

- Given the current landscape of radical change, effective coaching, mentoring, and practice supervision are key for supporting leaders at all levels in health and social care, not only to develop themselves but also to help them motivate and maximize their workforce's performance.
- It is important to know the differences between coaching, mentoring, and clinical supervision and understand the value of each.
- Coaching and mentoring both facilitate the leader's role performance and can also focus on career development; however, they use different approaches to achieve this. Practice supervision tends to be used for skills development in the workplace and is normally short term.

## THE EFFECTIVENESS OF COACHING, MENTORING, AND PRACTICE SUPERVISION

The overall effectiveness of coaching, mentoring, and practice supervision is well recognized, especially the impact that these roles can have in supporting the development of emerging leaders. De Meuse et al. (2009) recognize that executive coaching is a multidisciplinary practice, and that there is no professional consensus as to what constitutes good coaching. Indeed, coaching skills are what make an effective coach, and the skills of facilitation and support help leaders (as experts) better understand their discipline and environment (Cox et al., 2017). Mentoring and practice supervision, however, are generally drawn from the professional group around the individual being supervised; the mentors and practice supervisors are the experts, supporting and nurturing the emerging leader. In education and with a focus on new head teachers, Hobson's (2003) review of the literature finds that both mentors and mentees, as well as their organizations, benefit from the relationship. Indeed, he finds considerable benefits for these new leaders, such as reduced feelings of isolation, stress, and frustration; increased confidence and self-esteem; enhanced rates of learning and professional growth; improved interprofessional and problem-solving skills; ability to surrender their previous professional identity; and finally,

friendship. Wahab et al. (2016) find similar benefits for mentees in interprofessional mentoring within medicine, nursing, and social work in Malaysia.

All three roles require expertise and experience to effectively support the individual, in addition to appropriate training and careful matching to ensure a successful "fit." Nevertheless, Straus et al. (2013) find that participants in North America identified a number of contributing factors that adversely affected their mentoring relationships and led to a lack of collegiality in their work. These factors included "poor communication, lack of commitment, personality differences, perceived (or real) competition, conflicts of interest, and the mentor's lack of experience" (Straus et al., 2013, p. 88). They offer a number of solutions to facilitate future success, such as being more cautious in approaching potential mentors, seeking an independent assessment from previous mentees, and having formal agreements in place. Indeed, the learning relationship between mentor or coach and the individual is what builds success and enables change (Connor & Pokora, 2012). It is the connection between them that encourages open dialogue on both sides: a willingness to share their ideas, listen, understand, and be open to new ideas. This is a relationship built on partnership working and not an unequal imposition of one's views on another's.

An evaluation of coaching in the NHS that was undertaken by the Institute for Employment Studies (IES) (Sinclair et al., 2008) and De Meuse et al.'s (2009) meta-analysis of empirical and retrospective studies that evaluate the effectiveness of executive coaching find many benefits of coaching. These include benefits at the behavioral level, such as increased confidence, self-awareness, and understanding, as well as better team management and improved leadership behaviors that lead to employee satisfaction and increased productivity, with beneficiaries taking a more strategic and objective approach to their role. Nevertheless, when managers act as coaches, rather than using a coaching style of leadership, it may adversely affect the team dynamics that the leader is charged with managing. Smith (2019) recognizes interpersonal conflict, which directly affects staff relationships, as one of the greatest challenges in teams in the United Kingdom. In particular, he notes that conflict in the workplace at the NHS is ever present and, across

Europe, hundreds of workdays are lost as a direct result of conflict (Chartered Institute of Personnel and Development, 2020b).

It is valuable to understand what is meant by the concept of manager-as-coach. Steelman and Wolfeld (2018, p. 42) clarify this term by stating it is "an ongoing method for improving problem work performance; recognizing and developing employee growth and potential; empowering employees and providing guidance, encouragement, and support." There is an especially important difference between this approach, which offers a coaching style of management, and a pure coach. L. Westcott (2016) illustrates the importance of not having a manager as a coach. She notes that one of many reasons managers seek coaching is to learn how to manage difficult situations with their own line managers; as such, the coach should not be the person's line manager.

Hobson (2003) reveals that head teachers highly valued mentors who provided practical advice and assisted with problem-solving. There was also an appreciation of mentors as an ongoing resource, in addition to their role in facilitating links to other individuals. Importantly, the mentors helped provide new leaders with emotional support and reassurance, the opportunity to "let off steam," and a sounding board for concerns and uncertainties. Nevertheless, as Wahab et al. (2016) acknowledge, in addition to providing funding, it is crucial that the coaches and mentors chosen have the desired characteristics and be trained to develop skills in giving support and feedback.

Coaching, mentoring, and practice supervision are gaining in popularity as part of organizational leadership development. These practices are undertaken by those committed to their role, who have been effectively prepared, and where relationships of trust and confidentiality have developed. They offer considerable benefits to organizations, those being supported, and those who accept these roles.

## SUMMARY POINTS

- Although there are some drawbacks, coaches, mentors, mentees, and their organizations experience many benefits from the outcomes of these relationships.
- Managers face a number of challenges when acting as either a coach or mentor to their staff.

- Mentors and coaches should have the appropriate training, expertise, and supervision; they must be committed to their role and develop a relationship of trust and confidentiality to be successful.

## STRATEGIES FOR SUPPORT

Organizations that survive and thrive depend on the success of their leadership and the quality and motivation of their workforce. The integration of health and social care services in the United Kingdom is used as an illustration. Until now, two services involving thousands of staff have always existed entirely separately and have been led and managed in silos, in spite of their close interface. Leaders and managers are now expected to introduce cultural change and educate themselves and their staff to better understand how they can work collaboratively, understand new information systems, and communicate using a common language. Two strategies will be considered regarding how coaching, mentoring, and practice supervision could assist leaders, managers, and their workforces adapt and embrace new ways of working and understand the nature of the new business. The two strategies considered are creating a coaching and mentoring culture and creating a learning organization using reflective practice.

### Creating a Coaching and Mentoring Culture

The benefits of successful coaching and mentoring have already been explored, but as Clutterbuck and Meggison (2005) suggest, it can only work when the organizational culture is supportive and there is trust between managers, coaches, and coachees, with all working together. They acknowledge that a coaching culture is one where coaching is the principal style of managing and working together and there is a commitment not only to grow the organization but also to grow the people within the organization.

Similarly, Garvey et al. (2018) emphasize the importance of a mentoring culture and summarize a mentoring organization as having:

- compatibility between individual and organizational aspirations,
- high employee commitment,

- a focus on collaboration and team development, and
- a complex web of practices and relationships that are supportive of and develop the individual and the organization.

When faced with this radical change of successfully integrating health and social care systems, a supportive culture is essential as successful change inevitably depends on the commitment of the people involved. It is the people who lead, manage, and commit to making change happen, combined with a workforce committed to change, that will ensure success. To enable the process, much depends on the leaders and managers helping their workforce understand the complexity of the changes and encouraging their motivation to succeed. Indeed, the idea of "superheroes" as leaders has long since passed (The King's Fund, 2011). The complexity of the NHS, in addition to that of amalgamating the health and social care services, demands an approach based on a shared and collaborative model of leadership. Integrating the two services requires that leaders and managers from diverse professions with competing viewpoints on priorities work collaboratively to meet the overall organizational aims. In this "post heroic" age of leadership, a collaborative style of leadership will enable and encourage these diverse talents to come together and successfully address the "wicked" issues that have no simple solution (The King's Fund, 2011). Collaborative leadership needs an environment that encourages asking questions, enables exploring new possibilities, and most importantly, offers a supportive climate.

Therefore, creating and developing a coaching leadership style and a coaching and mentoring culture within an organization will permit greater transparency and richer communication between health and social care organizations, conscious development of talent, and compassionate leaders committed to success (Horizons Unlimited, 2020). Organizations with a positive coaching culture encourage a high level of personal engagement and responsibility; there is a belief that to maximize the workforce's potential, it is important to engage with them rather than "tell" them. A coaching and mentoring culture is part of an overall culture of continuous learning and development to improve both workforce and organizational capacity

(Horizons Unlimited, 2020). Leaders and managers who adopt a coaching and mentoring style of leadership and management are better able to motivate and delegate to their staff, increasing team performance (Hawkins, 2012). However, cultural change is well recognized as difficult; therefore, sustaining and developing a coaching and mentoring culture across an organization requires commitment by all. Recognizing the value of a collaborative leadership that is shared, distributed, and adaptive, and where leaders need to focus on systems rather than organizations, is key to achieving high quality patient outcomes (The King's Fund, 2011).

Nevertheless, coaching and mentoring cultures cannot be viewed as the "cure-all" for the problems within organizations. They are most successful when fully embedded within an organization's psyche rather than separate from it. In particular, Clutterbuck and Meggison (2005) stress the importance of an organization embracing coaching and a coaching culture. Figure 13-2 depicts E. J. Westcott's (2014) Coaching Impact Circle Framework and illustrates the value of coaching to an organization. It demonstrates how coaching by an individual manager and leader can effect change in a team that leads to long-term improvements in care and outcomes; this in turn leads to enhanced organizational effectiveness. The circle can only be completed if the organization appreciates the value of coaching and has a coaching culture embedded within it.

In summary, an organization that values a mentoring and coaching culture will enjoy both enhanced outcomes and organizational success.

## Creating a Learning Organization

Given the importance of creating and developing a coaching and mentoring culture as part of an overall philosophy of continual learning, Law (2013) reinforces the need for any organization to continue learning if it is to survive in the current ever-changing world. Developing the right people with the right skills and values must be a key priority for health and social care services to meet their ongoing challenges and maximize learning; creating a "learning organization" is key to success. Law (2013) suggests that a learning organization is one that enables its workforce to learn from their mistakes, encourages adaptive behavior,

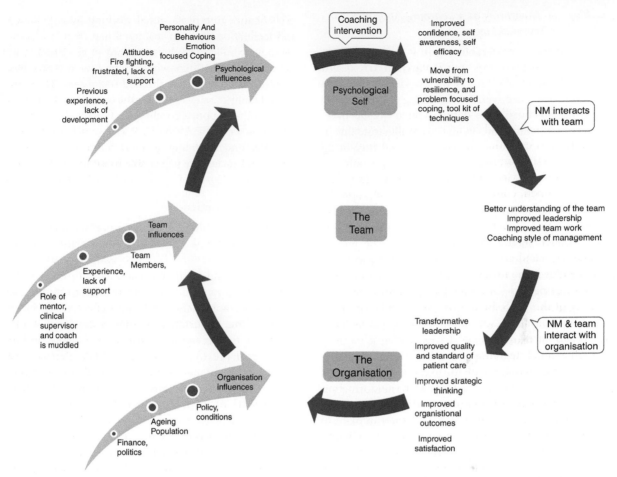

**Fig. 13-2 ■** Coaching impact circle framework. Westcott, E. J. (2014). *The role of coaching in the development of nurse managers* [DCM thesis, Oxford Brookes University]. https://radar.brookes.ac.uk/radar/file/0dbe0087-8e59-4edf-9b51-59e279fe40df/1/westcott2014role.pdf

detects and corrects errors, and collectively thinks in action. It is one committed to learning, and, as Berwick (2013) in his report on improving patient safety recommends, all health services should become learning organizations by embedding learning and quality improvement throughout the organization. He recommends that leaders at all levels mobilize the resources and commitment of others to achieve the goal of cultural change and lifelong education of all health care professionals, including managers and executives (Berwick, 2013, p. 15). He suggests that: "The capability to measure and continually improve the quality of patient care needs to be taught and learned or it will not exist" (Berwick, 2013, p. 9). To achieve such

an organization, Thurgate (2018) suggests that effective mentorship and a positive learning culture are key to success. Indeed, by encouraging organizations to embed practice supervision from the point of professional registration, encouraging all staff members to seek a professional mentor, and—from early leadership roles—promoting the use of coaching, leaders and managers can establish learning as an expectation. This supports staff in adapting to change, being open to new ways of thinking, and learning from their mistakes. Learning at work would become a state of being. However, such a vision is a theoretical concept unless and until there is a commitment by leaders and managers to make it a reality.

## Coaching and Mentoring as a Learning Approach for Effective Teamworking

In spite of the considerable funding devoted to formal leadership programs, particularly in UK health services, West et al.'s (2015) review of the literature questions their effectiveness. Coaching and mentoring programs, however, have demonstrated greater overall success. Stewart-Lord et al. (2017) illustrate this in their UK organization-wide coaching and mentoring program, which increased the skills of not only the coaches and mentors, but also individuals. They find that their program, which is open to all staff, supports a culture change toward greater transparency. It also makes staff feel valued and supports them in their new roles. Indeed, they seemed to recognize the importance of a coaching and mentoring culture, with the need for strong organization-wide program leadership and managerial support to enable staff participation.

In relation to the integrated care agenda, coaching and mentoring has a role in supporting and facilitating successful teamworking. In particular, it requires interprofessional working and collaborative leadership to build teams across the divide and provide a seamless service. From the 44 Sustainability and Transformation Partnerships set up in 2016 across England, 42 Integrated Care Systems have grown to replace them with plans to put them onto a statutory footing from 2022 (Charles 2021). The new leadership of these partnerships are drawn mainly from senior health managers, with very few leads from local authorities (The King's Fund, 2017). Therefore, health leaders and managers require considerable support to reach out and better understand and collaborate with their partners in social care to create new partnership working and truly integrated teams.

Smith et al. (2018) confirm that interprofessional rather than multi-professional working has been found to create greater teamworking and effectiveness in all of its aspects. However, teamworking is not a natural phenomenon, and Smith et al. (2018) advocate requiring the team leader to spend considerable time building the team and creating an environment of mutual respect. Interprofessional collaboration is not straightforward, especially as professionals have been tuned to work and communicate within their own professional teams. However, the recent emergence of values-based practice (VBP) is an opportunity to enhance interprofessional working and collaboration (Merriman et al., 2020). VBP can enhance interprofessional working by supporting and facilitating decision-making when there are complex and conflicting values (Fulford et al., 2012). This is particularly pertinent when attempting to merge two diverse teams, such as health and social care. There are indeed many parallels between the openness of an organization that supports coaching and mentoring and one that embraces VBP. Using VBP as a vehicle to develop a greater understanding of the different values within health and social care will enable more successful management of integration.

### Reflective Practice

Coaches and mentors who can support team leaders in creating time for and developing their teams' skills to achieve interprofessional collaboration, effective communication, and positive socialization through individual and group reflection can transform traditional supervisory approaches and more effectively achieve success. The importance of interprofessional working is key to successful integrated care teams, and as Wahab et al. (2016) confirm in their Malaysian study of interprofessional mentoring across medicine, nursing, and social work, it has considerable success. They find the benefits of mentoring include improved patient outcomes, shorter hospital stays, and reduced surgical morbidities. Connor & Pokora (2012) acknowledge that effective practice is reflective practice and involves the mentor and coach in a continuous cycle of preparation, engagement, and reflection on the mentoring and coaching interaction. Clark et al. (2019) recognize that reflection creates a relationship for learning, whether in a practice supervision, mentoring, or coaching relationship. They suggest that reflective supervision improves vision and nourishes the supervisory process, making communication purposeful. For leaders involved in driving radical change in the integrated care agenda, the opportunity to be supported in a secure and confidential partnership with a more senior practitioner contributes to positive outcomes by allowing them to continually review their vision and personal and organizational objectives (Clark et al., 2019). Reflection and reflective practice are also viewed as established parts of coaching, although caution is required to acknowledge that reflection is sometimes implemented to encourage acceptance of the existing culture rather than facilitate a change (Cushion, 2018).

## BOX 13-1

### REFLECTIVE PRACTICE MODEL (ROLFE ET AL 2001)

- "What?" Identifying and describing the problem: roles, responses, and actions
- "So what?" Analyzing and understanding the actions and consequences
- "Now what?" Learning how to improve future performance

Rolfe, G., Jasper, M., & Freshwater, D. (2001). Critical reflection for nursing and the helping professions: A user's guide. Palgrave.

While there are a number of frameworks recommended to assist in the reflective process (e.g., Kolb, 1984), it is more than just thinking about practice; it is a process of critical analysis, where learning from the issue or problem is the focus of the reflection. Essentially, reflective practice consists of three stages as identified by Rolfe et al. (2001) and is usually a cyclical process (Box 13-1).

With its roots in the seminal work of Schon (1987) and based on Dewey's (1933) earlier work, reflective practice has been particularly impactful in professions associated with health and social care; thus, it is pertinent to leaders in these professions and to the organizations in which they work. The contexts of health and social care practice are, as Kinsella (2010, p. 565) reinforces, "messy, complex and laden with value conflicts." Schon (1987, p. 3) refers to the realities of professional life as "swamps":

> In the varied topography of professional practice, there is a high hard ground overlooking a swamp. On the high ground, manageable problems lend themselves to solution through the application of research-based theory and technique. In the swampy lowland, messy, confusing problems defy technical solution.

In addition to the myriad considerations necessary to achieve the integration agenda, Chapter 1 illustrates a range of issues that challenge leaders in health and social care on a daily basis. They are required to navigate the "wicked" issues, such as the considerable workforce shortages and widespread developments toward digital transformation, and strive to lead where resources are diminishing. As Kinsella (2010, p. 565) confirms, "the swamps seem to be getting messier and messier." She suggests that leaders who are successful are those who are able to engage in reflective practice.

The roles of mentor, coach, and practice supervisor are situated more objectively outside the leader's immediate situation and are well placed to support those who find themselves in the "swampy lowlands," facing the challenges of leadership in complex, value-laden situations. It is difficult to reflect effectively and analytically alone. In addition, Horton-Deutsch and Sherwood (2017) observe that learning is not a destination but rather a continuous process of developing and enhancing the individual's understanding of "self" and their ability to gain meaningful insight into how they deal with real-life situations. Being supported in learning from experience helps the individual adapt to change and allows them to be creative, innovative, and essentially improve their practice. Not only is reflective practice valuable for supporting individuals at all organizational levels, but as Law (2013) reinforces, organizations that collectively think and reflect in action are successful learning organizations.

Creating an effective learning organization and using reflective practice creates an environment that supports the roles of supervision, mentoring, and coaching; these can transform an individual's leadership and relationship with their team, and enhance their resilience and self-efficacy. In essence, through analytical use of reflective practice, all three roles have the potential to enable a health and social care professional to take a problem-focused rather than emotion-focused approach to managing, while at the same time helping them shift their coping approach from being vulnerable to becoming resilient.

## SUMMARY POINTS

- Creating a coaching and mentoring culture is key to organizational success.
- Organizations need to value learning and reflective practice.
- Values-based practice can be an effective tool for enhancing interprofessional collaboration.

## CONCLUSION

Unpredictability and the rate of change continue to increase alongside economic uncertainty and local, national, and global influences. In this context, leaders need support to enable them to effectively manage their teams and ensure that their organizations flourish. The importance of effective support mechanisms for leaders cannot be underestimated. This chapter has illustrated how coaching, mentoring, and supervision all have the potential to effectively support individuals at each organizational level, and through a successful coaching and mentoring culture, positively impact outcomes. Strategies such as recognizing the value of creating a learning organization by using reflective practice can assist the coach, mentor, and supervisor in achieving success and leading their team as effectively as possible. Figure 13-3 brings together these concepts. It illustrates how the three pillars (individual leader, organization and support interaction) are intertwined in a continuous circle.

All individuals who work within health and social care have their own learning style, skills, behaviors, and values. These are developed over years of practice and are then reflected in their own management and leadership styles.

All individual leaders are in turn influenced by their contextual organization, which has a culture of its own and a context within which it functions. The context is influenced by global and financial pressures along with the tensions of working with a split health and social care market. An organization has its own culture which, as this chapter has illustrated, can be enhanced by having an open approach to learning, coaching, and mentoring, along with openness to reflecting in and on actions. The final pillar brings together the concepts from this chapter and demonstrates the support and development available to leaders. The use of coaching, mentoring, and supervision are all enhanced by reflection and reflective practice. The support of peers and managers and the demonstration of a values-based

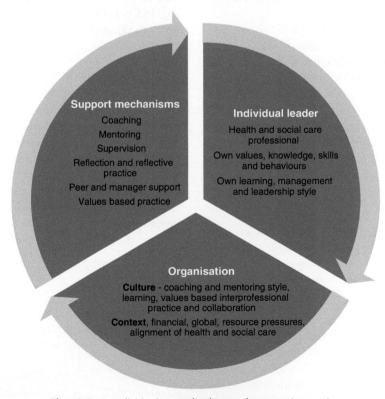

**Fig. 13-3** ■ Individual, organization, and support interaction

practice is essential for leaders and managers to flourish in their roles. There are so many opportunities available. However, as aspiring leaders, it is important to proactively seek out opportunities and identify your own support mechanisms to help you realize your potential in your role. The reflective questions at the end of this chapter will help in your journey.

## REFERENCES

Berwick, D. (2013). A promise to learn – A commitment to act. Improving the Safety of patients in England. National Advisory Group on the Safety of Patients in England. https://assets.publishing.service.gov.uk/government/uploads/system/uploads/attachment_data/file/226703/Berwick_Report.pdf

Bozeman, B., & Feeney, M. K. (2007). Toward a useful theory of mentoring: A conceptual analysis and critique. *Administration and Society*, 39(6), 719–739. https://www.researchgate.net/publication/249831334_Toward_a_Useful_Theory_of_MentoringA_Conceptual_Analysis_and_Critique.

Brunero, S., & Stein-Parbury, J. (2008). The effectiveness of clinical supervision in nursing: An evidenced-based literature review. *Australian Journal of Advanced Nursing*, 25(3), 86–94.

Charles, A. (2021). Integrated care systems explained: making sense of systems, places and neighbourhoods. https://www.kingsfund.org.uk/publications/integrated-care-systems-explained#what-are-ICSs

Chartered Institute of Personnel and Development. (2020a). What is coaching? https://www.cipd.co.uk/knowledge/fundamentals/people/development/coaching-mentoring-factsheet

Chartered Institute of Personnel and Development. (2020b). Stress in the workplace. https://www.cipd.co.uk/knowledge/culture/wellbeing/stress-factsheet

Clark, R., Gehl, M., Heffron, M. C., Kerr, M., Soliman, S., Shahmoon-Shanok, R., & Thomas, K. (2019). Mindful practices to enhance diversity-informed reflective supervision and leadership. *Zero to Three* https://www.zerotothree.org/resources/3010-mindful-practices-to-enhance-diversity-informed-reflective-supervision-and-leadership.

Clutterbuck, D., & Megginson, D. (2005). *Making coaching work*. CIPD.

Connor, M., & Pokora, J. (2012). *Coaching and mentoring in practice: Developing effective practice* (2nd ed.). McGraw-Hill: Open University Press.

Cox, E., Bachkirova, T., & Clutterbuck, D. (2017). *The complete handbook of coaching*. Sage Publications.

Cushion, C.J. (2018). Reflection and reflective practice discourses in coaching: A critical analysis. *Sport, Education and Society*, 23(1), 82–94. https://doi.org/10.1080/13573322.2016.1142961.

De Meuse, K. P., Dai, G., & Lee, R. J. (2009). Evaluating the effectiveness of executive coaching: Beyond ROI? *Coaching: an International Journal of Theory. Research and Practice*, 2(2), 117–134. https://psycnet.apa.org/record/2010-11441-003.

Dewey, J. (1933). How we think: A restatement of the relation of reflective thinking to the educative process. Heath.

Fielden, S. L., Davidson, M. J., & Sutherland, V. J. (2009). Innovations in coaching and mentoring: Implications for nurse leadership development. *Health Services Management Research*, 22(2), 92–99.

Fulford, K., Peile, E., & Carroll, H. (2012). *Essential values-based practice*. Cambridge University Press. ISBN: 9781139024488 https://doi.org/10.1017/CBO9781139024488

Garvey, B., Stokes, P., & Megginson, D. (2018). Coaching and mentoring: *Theory and practice* (2nd ed.). Sage Publications.

Godshalk, V. M., & Sosik, J. J. (2003). Aiming for career success: The role of learning goal orientation in mentoring relationships. *Journal of Vocational Behavior*, 63(3), 417–437.

Hales, C. (2005). Rooted in supervision, branching into management: Continuity and change in the role of first-line manager. *Journal of Management Studies*, 42(3), 471–506.

Hamer, D. H., Hansoti, B., Prabhakaran, D., Huffman, M. D., Nxumalo, N., Fox, M. P., … Rispel, L. C. (2019). Global health research mentoring competencies for individuals and institutions in low- and middle-income countries. *American Journal of Tropical Medicine and Hygiene*, 100(Suppl 1), 15–19. https://doi.org/10.4269/ajtmh.18-0558. http://www.ajtmh.org/content/journals/10.4269/ajtmh.18-0558.

Hawkins, P. (2012). *Creating a coaching culture*. Open University Press.

Hawkins, P., & Smith, N. (2010). Transformational coaching. In E. Cox, T. Bachkirova, & D. Clutterbuck (Eds.), *The complete handbook of coaching*. Sage Publications.

Healthcare Commission. (2004). NHS national staff survey 2004 – Summary of key findings. Healthcare Commission.

Hobson, A. (2003). Mentoring and coaching for new leaders. A review of literature carried out for National College of School Leadership. https://www.rtuni.org/uploads/docs/mentoring-and-coaching-for-new-leaders-summary.pdf

Horizons Unlimited. (2020). Create a coaching & mentoring culture. https://horizonsunlimited.com.au/pdf/Create_Mentoring_Culture.pdf. Online Publication

Horton-Deutsch, S., & Sherwood, G. D. (2017). *Reflective practice: Transforming education and improving outcomes* (2nd ed.). Sigma Theta Tau International.

Jarvis, J. (2004). *Coaching and buying coaching services: A CIPD guide*. CIPD. https://www.portfolio-info.co.uk/files/file/CIPD%20coaching_buying_services.pdf

Joo, B. -K., Sushko, J., & McLean, G. N. (2012). Multiple faces of coaching: Manager-as-coach, executive coaching, and formal mentoring. *Organization Development Journal*, 30(1).

Kinsella, E. A. (2010). The art of reflective practice in health and social care: Reflections on the legacy of Donald Schon. *Reflective Practice*, 11(4), 565–575. https://doi.org/10.1080/14623943.2010.506260.

Kolb, D. A. (1984). *Experiential learning*. Prentice Hall.

Law, H. (2013). The psychology of coaching, mentoring and learning. *John Wiley & Sons*

Merriman, C., Chalmers, C., Ewens, A., Fulford, B., Gray, R., Handa, A., & Westcott, L. (2020). Values-based interprofessional education: How interprofessional educational and values-based practice and are vehicles for the benefit of patients and health and social care professionals. *Journal of Interprofessional Care, 34*(4). http://www.tandfonline.com/10.1080/13561820.2020.1713065.

Rolfe, G., Jasper, M., & Freshwater, D. (2001). *Critical reflection for nursing and the helping professions: A user's guide.* Palgrave.

Schon, D. A. (1987). *Educating the reflective practitioner: Toward a new design for teaching and learning in the professions.* Jossey-Bass.

Sinclair, A., Fairhurst, P., Carter, A., & Miller, L. (2008). *Evaluation of coaching in the NHS: Report 445.* Institute of Employment Studies. https://www.employment-studies.co.uk/resource/evaluation-coaching-nhs

Smith, H. A. (2019). Manager as coach characteristics for dealing with team challenge. *Journal of Work-Applied Management, 11*(2), 165–173. Doi:10.1108/JWAM-06-2019-0022. https://www.emerald.com/insight/content/doi/10.1108/JWAM-06-2019-0022/full/html.

Smith, T., Fowler-Davis, S., Nancarrow, S., Ariss, S. M. B., & Enderby, P. (2018). Leadership in interprofessional health and social care teams: A literature review. *Leadership in Health Services, 31*(4), 452–467. https://doi.org/10.1108/LHS-06-2016-0026.

Social Care Institute for Excellence (SCIE). (2012). Managing practice: Supervision and team leadership. https://www.scie.org.uk/publications/guides/guide01/supervision/

Steelman, L. A., & Wolfeld, L. (2018). The manager as coach: The role of feedback orientation. *Journal of Business and Psychology, 33*(1), 41–53. https://doi.org/10.1007/s10869-016-9473-6.

Stewart-Lord, A., Baillie, L., & Woods, S. (2017). Health care staff perceptions of a coaching and mentoring programme: A qualitative case study evaluation. *International Journal of Evidence Based Coaching and Mentoring, 15*(2), 70–85. http://ijebcm.brookes.ac.uk/documents/vol15issue2-paper-05.pdf.

Straus, S. E., Johnson, M. O., Marquez, C., & Feldman, M. D. (2013). Characteristics of successful and failed mentoring relationships: A qualitative study across two academic health centers. *Academic Medicine, 88*(1), 82–89. https://doi.org/10.1097/ACM.0b013e318 27647a0.

The King's Fund. (2011). The future of leadership and management in the NHS. No more heroes. Report from the King's Fund Commission on Leadership and management in the NHS. https://www.kingsfund.org.uk/sites/default/files/future-of-leadership-and-management-nhs-may-2011-kings-fund.pdf

The King's Fund. (2017). Sustainability and transformation plans (STPs) explained. https://www.kingsfund.org.uk/topics/integrated-care/sustainability-transformation-plans-explained

Thurgate, C. (2018). Supporting those who work and learn: A phenomenological research study. *Nurse Education Today, 61*, 83–88. https://doi.org/10.1016/j.nedt.2017.11.010.

Wahab, M. T., Ikbal, M. F. M., Wu, J. T., Wesley, L. T. W., Kanesvaran, R., & Krishna, L. K. R. (2016). Creating effective interprofessional mentoring relationships in palliative care—Lessons from medicine, nursing, surgery and social work. *Journal of Palliative Care and Medicine, 6*, 290. https://doi.org/10.4172/2165-7386.1000290.

West, L., & Milan, M. (2001). *The reflecting glass – Professional coaching for leadership development.* Palgrave.

West, M., Armit, K., Loewenthal, L., Eckert, R., West, T., & Lee, A. (2015). Leadership and leadership development in health care: The evidence base. The King's Fund. https://www.kingsfund.org.uk/sites/default/files/field/field_publication_file/leadership-leadership-development-health-care-feb-2015.pdf

Westcott, E.J. (2014). *The role of coaching in the development of nurse managers* [DCM thesis, Oxford Brookes University]. https://radar.brookes.ac.uk/radar/file/0dbe0087-8e59-4edf-9b51-59e279fe40df/1/westcott2014role.pdf

Westcott, L. (2016). How coaching can play a key role in the development of nurse managers. *Journal of Clinical Nursing, 25*(17–18), 2669–2677. https://doi.org/10.1111/jocn.13315.

## REFLECTIVE QUESTIONS

### Individuals:

- From your own experience, would you value a coach or mentor or both to develop your leadership?
- Who would you choose to be your mentor?
- How would you start to find a coach?
- What are your health/life values? Do you consider and know what others value?
- How can you help your team members identify their own values?

### Organizations:

- What type of organization do you work in?
- What practical initiatives could you introduce to create a coaching and mentoring culture in your organization?

### Support Mechanisms:

- What steps could you take to help your organization move toward being a learning organization?
- What difference can you discern between thinking about your practice and reflective practice?
- How can you help your team introduce reflective practice as a way of being?

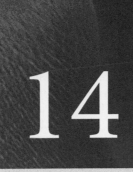

# 14

# GLOBAL CHALLENGES FACING HEALTH AND SOCIAL CARE LEADERS

ELIZABETH MADIGAN AND SARAH E. ABEL

## OBJECTIVES

*After reading this chapter, you should be able to:*

- Identify how migration impacts the delivery of health and social care.
- Critically reflect on your own cultural sensitivity and the importance of acting as a role model for your colleagues.
- Analyze the need for leaders and managers to provide resources to assist their workforce in developing cultural competence.
- Develop an understanding of the complex issues influencing health and social care workers as migrants.
- Discuss the importance of adhering to ethical recruitment codes.
- Critically analyze the importance of investing in and utilizing delegation.
- Discuss how effective communication can significantly enhance successful delegation.
- Critically analyze how global organizations can enhance the delivery of global health and social care.

## INTRODUCTION

All health and social care is global in nature, whether the provider recognizes it or not. Modern humans have been traveling and migrating at unprecedented levels, both voluntarily and involuntarily. Health and social care leaders have a responsibility to direct their organizations in ethical and responsible ways for the global world in which we all live. The intent of this chapter is to provide an overview of the challenges facing health and social care workers, with a focus on migration in general and the migration of health and social care

workers in particular. It also reflects on the importance of leaders and managers in addressing the issues relevant to diversity for an increasingly diverse workforce and its care recipients, including the challenges this brings to delegation. The globalization of society has in turn led to an increase in health and social care-related global organizations. The role of these organizations has evolved to become an essential part of the delivery and sustainability of healthy people.

## OVERVIEW OF MIGRATION

The United Nations (UN) estimates that 272 million people, or 3.5 percent of the world's population, live outside the country in which they were born (UN, 2019); this number includes both voluntary and involuntary moves. Europe hosts the largest number of migrants (82 million), followed by North America (59 million). By percentage of population, Oceania (Australia and New Zealand) lead with 21 percent of their population being migrants.

Involuntary migration includes asylum seekers and refugees and can be driven by natural disasters (tsunami, rising sea levels) or manmade disasters (war, criminality). There are also economic migrants who are driven to seek employment and remit their salaries back to family members in their home countries; there is a question as to whether these economic migrants are making voluntary or involuntary moves. From a health and social care perspective, it is also important to identify internally displaced persons: those who leave their homes but do not cross an international border. There are well-known involuntary migrations (the Syrian refugee crisis) but there are many others where the number of persons is smaller, and they therefore do not receive international attention.

The UN, through its member states, has issued a report on migration from 2016, "In Safety and Dignity: Addressing Large Movements of Refugees and Migrants" (UN, 2016, A/70/59), which provides some recommendations. The report presents a comprehensive background on past migration trends and how countries have responded. The key recommendations of the report are that migrants, regardless of the factors driving the migration, should be treated with safety and dignity in mind. In addition, the UN report calls for coordination between countries to address large-scale movements.

## CULTURAL COMPETENCE AND CULTURAL SAFETY

As a result of the increases in both voluntary and involuntary migration, all health and social care workers need a basic level of cultural competence to provide high-quality care to someone whose background and history are likely different than their own. While there have been a number of criticisms of cultural competence (Beagan, 2018, for example), the general intent of the approach was for the provider to consider the context and individual nature of the person seeking care, how cultural factors may influence the individual's care decisions, and the nature of the interaction with the care provider. Experienced providers all have stories that they can tell where they did not sufficiently understand the context and culture of a particular care seeker and were not able to provide the high-quality care that they wished to provide. In some cases, this can be as simple as a language barrier; in other cases, there are misunderstandings and miscommunications that are related to beliefs about health and illness by both parties involved. A common misstep is failing to ask about the care recipient's use of traditional medicine or herbal and nutritional supplements, which may be cultural in nature and interfere with prescribed medications or treatment plans (Bhamra et al., 2017). Leaders and managers need to build in education and structures to enhance culturally sensitive care.

Part of the critique of the cultural competence movement was the assignment of individuals to groups based on the assumption that the group members shared common characteristics and beliefs (Abe, 2020). This was often done based on race, ethnicity, or religion. It is now recognized as an over-simplification that did not recognize there may have been as much heterogeneity in beliefs within the "group" as between groups (Abe, 2020). A current example of this "group assignment error" is differences between generations, where evidence has found that there is as much heterogeneity within age groupings as between age groupings; beliefs like "Millennials are technology obsessed" are examples of this tendency (King et al., 2019), as discussed in preceding chapters. As a result of the critique of cultural competence, several professions have moved from knowledge acquisition to practice behaviors (e.g., social work) (Jani et al., 2016) or experiential immersion (e.g., nursing) (Harkess & Kaddoura, 2016). Leaders and managers can influence their workers' skills and abilities by building in practice and/or immersion in this area.

The other aspect to consider is intersectionality, where some aspects of an individual may be more important to them than others. For example, a black, gay, older person living in a white majority country may identify their age as having the most impact on how they interact with the health care system while the health care provider may identify their race or gender identity as most relevant. Loden and Rosener (1991), developed the Diversity Wheel, which identifies the various aspects one uses for identity (e.g., gender, ethnicity, age). The Diversity Wheel (Figure 14.1) was later expanded to include other aspects that may drive stereotyping, such as political beliefs and education. There have been additional iterations of the Diversity Wheel, and there are now many versions.

A more recent direction on how providers can best care for persons with different backgrounds and histories uses the term "cultural safety," where the provider works "to create a safe space for an encounter with patients that is sensitive and responsive to their social, political, linguistic, economic, and spiritual realities" (Kirmayer, 2012, p. 157–158). The other terms guiding work in this area are "cultural humility" and "cultural sensitivity." Regardless of the term used, the construct is that the provider recognizes there may be cultural

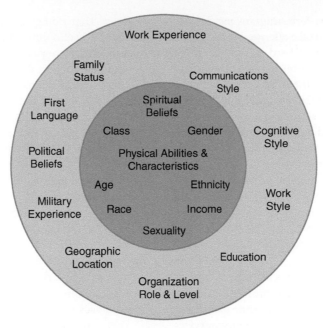

**Fig. 14-1** ■ Diversity wheel Loden, M., & Rosener, J. B. (1991). *Workforce America! Managing employee diversity as a vital resource.* Business One, Irwin.

and historical factors that will influence the provider–client interaction and trajectory of care.

Returning to culturally sensitive care for migrants, health and social care leaders need to provide their staff with access to resources on how to provide culturally sensitive care within their specific practice area. For example, the approaches used in the intensive care unit (ICU) for culturally sensitive care are not likely to be comprehensive enough or applicable for providers in psychiatry. For social and health care workers who provide care in the participant's home, even more sensitivity may be required because the care recipient's "turf" may need to be accommodated by the social care or health worker (Alvariza et al., 2020). A "one size fits all" approach does not work with true cultural sensitivity, and each unit or department may need different kinds of resources. Resources for culturally sensitive care may include knowledgeable members in the migrant community who can provide insight into experiences and beliefs, with the caveat that the generalizations are for better understanding and not to be used across the board. Other resources may be additional training in how to conduct sensitive conversations with care recipients and family members to elicit

their beliefs, regardless of the background. This is often uncomfortable for providers from the dominant group who fear being offensive or asking a question that may be misunderstood. These kinds of conversations can be even more fraught if there are language barriers or where English is not the first language of the care recipient or their family caregiver.

As one example, the Patient Centered Assessment Model (University of Minnesota, 2020) uses the social determinants of health as a framework to prompt health care providers to attend to patient-specific issues or concerns. The developers present a patient-focused questionnaire for the provider to use to identify the Social Determinants of Health (SDoH) and questions to ask patients to further elicit the impact of the SDoH.

Acculturation, the degree to which the migrant has adopted the norms, values, language, and beliefs of the destination country, will also drive provider decisions. Acculturation is not time dependent; some individuals never acculturate whereas others acculturate quickly. Even within families, there may be family members with varying levels of acculturation. Culturally sensitive providers do not assume a care recipient who is a longstanding resident has adopted the views of the destination country. Conversely, a short-term migrant may be very adept at the local culture and take offense at being treated as someone new to the system (Ward & Geeraert, 2016). Leaders and managers have the responsibility of making sure that their workers have the information they need on acculturation to avoid making assumptions based on time living in the new destination.

Beyond migration and cultural sensitivity, leaders also need to recognize that, even for populations within one region, there may be large cultural differences that have nothing to do with migration (persons who have always lived in the area) but reflect other SDoH, like socioeconomic status (Shick et al., 2019). Thus, the cultural sensitivity training and support for care of migrants will also benefit care for all recipients.

Finally, as the health and social care workforce becomes more diverse, leaders must consider the responsibility bestowed upon them to equip their teams with the resources to serve all persons seeking their services. Leaders must be aware of their own cultural sensitivity as they set the organizational tone and culture and drive change (Phillips et al., 2016).

## SUMMARY POINTS

- This is a global world with migration increasing worldwide.
- Cultural competence has been criticized and is increasingly being redefined as cultural sensitivity and cultural humility.
- It is important to recognize that one's cultural or geographic background does not indicate their personal preferences; one cannot use stereotypes to drive provider decision-making.
- Leaders and managers have a responsibility to ensure that their staff has access to information and education about culturally sensitive care that goes beyond the superficial.

## HEALTH CARE WORKERS AS MIGRANTS

In some migration crises, the first persons to leave may be professionals that are more educated and wealthier and who have the resources to relocate. In some cases, this professional class often includes health care workers. Depending on the timing and reason for migration, health care workers may not have all the documentation they need to start the process of becoming registered or permitted to practice in the destination country. Organizations such as CGFNS International (formerly known as the Commission on Graduates of Foreign Nursing Schools) can assist health care workers with restoring documents (CGFNS, 2019). Perhaps having more organizations to assist professionals in their transition would offer the individual and destination country additional resources for addressing health care shortages. Finally, in a classic work on nursing migration, Kingma (2006) notably identifies that, in many cases, nurses who left their home countries often return later in their careers. Thus, the term "brain drain" was reconceptualized as "brain circulation" or "circular migration," where the returning nurse brings the advantages and resources of having been in a higher resourced country back to the country of origin.

There are guidelines for the ethical recruitment of health care workers, including one from the World Health Organization (WHO, 2010). One criticism of the WHO code is that it discourages actively recruiting health care workers from lower resourced countries, which is seen as infringing on an individual health care worker's right to improve their status and personal situation. Other organizations have provided guidelines for ethical recruitment that recognize the certainty of health care worker migration. For example, the Alliance for Ethical Recruitment Practices (2017) certifies recruiters who meet ten principles for ethical recruitment (e.g., the right to move freely without economic coercion). Of note, health care worker migration is substantial and growing increasingly complicated. Traditionally, health care worker migration occurred from the global South to the global North, but it has lately been within regions in the global South as well as South to South and North to South (WHO, 2018). In recognition of the inevitability of health care worker migration, the WHO began work with the International Labour Organization (ILO) and the Organisation for Economic Co-operation and Development (OECD) to develop a framework for migration. This framework has not yet been approved by the World Health Assembly (WHA) of the WHO, but exists in draft form (WHO, 2020). The vision for the draft framework is "To maximize the benefits and mitigate adverse effects from health labour mobility through elevated dialogue, knowledge and cooperation" (WHO, 2020, p. 5).

The International Labour Organization (ILO) is a UN agency that focuses on standards for work and includes governments, employers, and workers. The OECD is an intergovernmental body that represents 37 mostly high-income countries that collaborate on a host of initiatives like health, development, and migration. Since WHO originated the development of the migration framework, its governing body, WHA, is responsible for approving the framework.

Even with the documentation in hand, the process of becoming recognized in a destination country for one's past training is often complex and time-consuming. In some cases, the initial training in the home country may not be sufficient for recognition in the destination country. Adding to the complexity is the different processes applied by the legal recognition body in the destination country. For example, in the United States, legal recognition and requirements for health care workers occur at the state level; therefore, each state may have slightly different requirements for foreign-educated health workers (FEHCs), with some states requiring a third-party verification of the educational and practice credentials through CGFNS (CGFNS, 2020). Leaders and managers may need to provide documentation of the need for a worker who is not from the host country, as well as provide support for the worker during the process—which may take years.

Assuming the FEHC accomplishes legal recognition for practice in the destination country, they then face the challenges of learning a new health care system. Going from even one well-resourced country to another well-resourced country is challenging, let alone going from a lower-resourced country to a higher-resourced country. Viken et al. (2018), in a systematic review of qualitative studies on the topic for foreign educated nurses (FENs), identify "being an outsider at work" (p. 458) as a main theme with two sub-themes: "loneliness and discrimination" (p. 458) and "communication barriers" (p. 463). Even FENs with previous nursing experience often reported shock and unfamiliarity with the health care work processes and equipment in the new setting. There were also unfamiliar cultural issues with patients and coworkers that were reported as stressful, particularly for FENs who came from countries with limited cultural diversity. Thus, organizational leaders need to keep these experiences in mind, particularly during the initial employment period, as this early period is often when the issues first arise. Viken et al. (2018) recommend strong mentoring for FENs along with efforts in reflective activity (see Chapter 13 for a further discussion on the value of mentoring and coaching).

Many health systems, organizations, or in some cases, countries have adopted a residency style orientation for those transitioning from student to professional nurse. Residency programs vary but generally include an extended onboarding or orientation process, designed to serve as a conduit in transitioning new graduates into the profession. They often include knowledge-focused activities (e.g., evidence-based practice) but may also include mentoring from more seasoned health care workers. These programs have proven effective at bridging transition-to-practice gaps, in addition to connecting new employees to the norms of the system or organization (Cochran, 2017). With increases in workforce mobility, it may be advantageous to incorporate a residency style program approach to assist in developing employee knowledge, skills, and abilities, including cultural norms for health care workers who are also immigrants.

## Social Care Workers as Migrants

There is significantly less information available on social care workers who are migrants, likely because many are not required to provide proof of education or registration/licensure, unlike the case with health care workers. This is despite the disproportionately large share of social care workers in many higher income countries, where migrants provide much of the workforce in the home and in domiciliary care. Social care workers who are migrants often provide care for the older population and for persons with disabilities (Doyle & Timonen, 2009). In the United Kingdom, for example, there are reports that approximately 20 percent of social care workers were born outside the United Kingdom (Franklin & Brancati, 2015) and half of these workers are not professionally educated (Hussein et al., 2011).

There are similar figures in other countries, like the United States, where social care services for care in the home and domiciliary care are often part of the health care system. One report from 2017 indicates that 27 percent of home care workers are migrants (Zallman et al., 2019). In Australia, there are reports that more than one-third of aged and disabled care workers were born overseas (Eastman et al., 2020), with increasing numbers from Southeast Asia and Africa. Of note, up to one quarter of the overseas-born care workers in Australia hold a bachelor's degree compared to 8.4 percent of the Australian-born care workers.

When it comes to recruitment of social care workers, although there are not the same sets of guidelines and codes for ethical recruitment, the same principles may apply. Hussein et al. (2010) note many of the same issues when recruiting health care workers. Managers will need to ascertain the guidelines and codes that may apply in their recruitment of social care workers.

Diversity, in the broadest sense of the word, within the workforce has its advantages. Significant research has shown diverse teams increase innovation (Lisak et al., 2016). The economy also benefits from workforce diversity, as it lessens the socioeconomic gaps within certain cultural groups (Furtado et al., 2018). Equipping an able workforce builds thriving, equitable communities (Strandberg, 2017). Leaders and managers should intentionally set goals to consider diversity within their workforce.

## SUMMARY POINTS

- Many health and social care workers are migrants, and the issues are complex.
- There are ethical recruitment codes that need to be incorporated.
- Additional training and support may be needed for these workers.

## THOUGHTFUL DELEGATION

As the demand and complexities of health and social care increase, leaders are challenged to design more efficient, high-functioning teams and systems (Porter-O'Grady & Malloch, 2018). Efficient teams rely on interprofessional and interdisciplinary delegation. It is essential that health and social care providers be knowledgeable of the scope, standards, and policies of their organization and regulatory bodies as they relate to delegating tasks. The health and social care provider who delegates tasks may be accountable for oversight and held liable for task completion or care delivered in the clinical environment.

Thoughtful delegation of tasks to subordinates allows a leader to focus on tasks that require a higher level of skill and vision. Ineffective leaders are often hesitant to invest in subordinates for fear they will leave the organization, wasting the leader's investment. The caveat to this way of thinking is that these leaders will have retained subordinates that are not equipped or empowered to assist in advancing the organization or leader's mission or vision. Subordinates and leaders are hired for their skills and knowledge; hindering their potential is counterintuitive. A leader's failure to see the big picture of empowerment will further cripple health care at every level (Asiri et al., 2016)

Subordinates often desire to be empowered through increased informal or formal power and opportunity for growth. This requires leaders to give them the authority, knowledge, or resources they need to be successful in completing their assigned tasks (Kanter, 1993; Kretzschmer et al., 2017). Leaders view the concept of power as either a scarcity that must be retained or an abundance that can be shared. Leaders that view power as a scarcity will struggle to delegate tasks, develop leadership succession plans, or retain creative thinkers. Those viewing power as an abundance may develop subordinates that supersede their own skill level (Covey, 2004). Rather than viewing subordinates as a threat, they will often consider this their legacy in the profession.

Health care providers are ethically, and in some cases legally, responsible for verifying the competency and understanding of the person that they are delegating to (Royal College of Nursing, 2017). Delegation for social care workers should follow the same principles, although the oversight will vary based on whether the workers are directly employed by the care recipient (e.g., the US situation) or the social care system (e.g., the UK situation). Closed loop communication, return demonstration, and asking open-ended questions can be beneficial in establishing expectations. Establishing initial clarity, albeit time consuming, can prevent errors, ethical dilemmas, and frustrations for all parties. Leaders are ultimately accountable for overseeing the delegation process.

The delegation process should include an appraisal of task, person, competency, message, time, and success. Leaders must identify and are responsible for delegating the right tasks to the right person. They should ask themselves: Is this a task I should/could delegate? Who is the right person for this task based on formal and informal power/authority? Is this person competent to complete the task or is more education required? If more education is required, can the person obtain the education? Is the message/instruction clear, concise, and complete? Is the person able to receive the task at this time? What is the timeline for completion? What does successful task completion look like? Evaluating delegation may be a quick mental checklist or require in-depth thoughtful planning depending on the complexities (National Council of State Boards of Nursing, 2005; The Nursing and Midwifery Board of Ireland [NMBI], 2015).

Communication may have additional complexities such as language and cultural nuances. As the world becomes more globally diverse, so does the workforce (see Chapter 15 for a further discussion). Evidence supports diversity in the workplace and the benefits it provides to an organization. However, there may be language barriers and cultural inflections that change the way a message is interpreted or delivered. Workplace diversity is beneficial but may require an investment of time and energy to be effective (Squires, 2018).

The art of delegation goes beyond passing tasks and authority to subordinates. Building a foundational rapport with interdisciplinary health care members can influence team dynamics and ultimately influence the care provided, outcomes, and efficiency. Health and social care providers and leaders need to establish mutual respect and trust, encouraging subordinates to have open communications and providing the opportunity to ask clarifying questions without judgement or repercussions. Being reluctant to communicate concerns increases patient risk and worsens other outcomes of poorly functioning teams (Wagner, 2018).

Over-delegating tasks without sufficiently balancing appreciation, feedback, and evaluation may also lead to poor team function and feelings of burnout. Providing positive reinforcement and affirming words can inspire confidence and lays a foundational culture of gratitude, a trait most organizations have the opportunity to improve upon. Leaders must role model this

behavior, as well as include positive reinforcement techniques as part of the delegation process in education and training (Porter-O'Grady & Malloch, 2018).

A lack of appropriate delegation can be detrimental to team efficiency and have financial implications for providing health care (Mayo & Woolly, 2016). An individual may be reluctant to delegate to or receive delegation from someone for a number of reasons, including but certainly not limited to a lack of understanding of scope of practice, a belief that it is faster to perform the task themselves, or a lack of trust in the other person. Delegation requires that a leader weigh the risks and benefits, often in high-pressure moments (Mayo & Woolly, 2016). The ability to identify tasks appropriately, communicate effectively, and build rapport sums up the art of delegation.

## SUMMARY POINTS

- Efficient, high-functioning leaders, teams, and systems invest and utilize delegation.
- Delegating requires leaders to artfully discern and appraise tasks and personnel.
- Effective communication is vital to successful delegation.

## THE ROLE OF GLOBAL ORGANIZATIONS

Global organizations are critical links in health and social care. These organizations can bring diverse innovators, visionaries, and researchers together to co-create, disseminate, advocate, and network (Sigma Theta Tau International, 2018). Improving global health and social care for all requires fewer silos and more action.

Examples of global organizations include those focused on specific professions (e.g., International Council of Nurses, Sigma Theta Tau International Honor Society of Nursing, World Medical Association, International Federation of Social Workers), interprofessional organizations (e.g., World Health Professions Alliance, International Network for Health Workforce Education), and clinically focused organizations (e.g., International Association of Gerontology and Geriatrics). Each organization has a focus area within health and social care. For example, some focus on workplace and workforce issues, while others concentrate on educational programming. Some are constructed from organizational membership (e.g., the national nurses associations in each country are members of the International Council of Nurses), whereas others are individual member organizations (e.g., Sigma Theta Tau International Honor Society of Nursing).

Leaders in organizations that are positioned to influence and impact global health and social care have an obligation to co-create tangible solutions for countries, organizations, or groups of people with no means or knowledge of how to achieve them, rather than devising mere theoretical concepts of a desired state of health (Cassagnol, 2017). Leaders in health and social care must become action-oriented organizations closing the implementation and knowledge gaps in best practices. During times of health crises, such as in a pandemic, the interconnectedness of health in communities and ecosystems and the chain reaction that local health practices can have on global health and economies need to be recognized. The requirement for timely evidence has come crashing into traditional modes of dissemination, such as the lengthy turn-around time for many peer-reviewed journal publications.

Scholarly dissemination of evidence is challenging for researchers, caregivers, and leaders. The research process itself can require a significant amount of time to design, implement, and evaluate results. Researchers have an inherent responsibility in the ethical conduct of research to disseminate (Derman & Jaeger, 2018). However, the process for disseminating evidence in a credible, timely manner to a wide audience has not been harnessed in an impactful way. The question must be asked: Whose ethical and moral responsibility is it to develop unbiased processes and infrastructures for global evidence dissemination?

Despite known best practices in routine health care, for example infant/prenatal health, the statistics for infant mortality remain significant (Edmonson et al., 2017). Leaders must leverage global organizations to harness the energies and assist in the dissemination and co-creation of evidence among health and social care professionals in a spirit of reciprocity. Ruchman et al. (2016, p. 738) challenge, "...that policies and innovations from settings abroad have the potential to transform health care..." Clinical and policy decisions

to improve health outcomes depend on the dissemination of research findings. Organizational leaders must recognize the opportunity to partner with stakeholders and become innovators in global evidence dissemination.

In this era of information and technology, sharing evidence-based practice would seemingly be easy (see Chapter 9 for further discussion). However, the public may be ill equipped to discern the enormous amount of health information and unsubstantiated evidence that is freely available and often widely disseminated. In both acute and chronic health challenges, transparency and dissemination of evidence can have a significant impact but often encounter political and educational barriers.

Beyond barriers to disseminating evidence, Premji and Hatfield (2016) suggest the concept of "global innovation flow," which fosters bidirectional sharing and co-creation of evidence-based solutions. They describe the current state as the colonial perspective, in which scholarship and training are unidirectional from high-income countries to low- and middle-income countries and recommend a transition to a more collaborative approach. Perhaps this approach would create a more equitable global health and social care network and foster further sharing.

Global organizations are well positioned to cultivate this type of networking (Kapucu et al., 2016). While some of these relationships may develop organically, organizational leaders should purposefully strategize ways to promote and support global co-creation and dissemination.

Leaders may often find it challenging to network and co-create between organizations. There may be conflicts in political or organizational values that deter partnerships, and it often requires more time to co-create. Moreover, forging new business models may require an investment of resources. However, organizational partnerships can be mutually beneficial for organizations and their constituents, exposing both to new opportunities and resources (Bell et al., 2013). One organization cannot be all things to all people, and therefore organizational leader collaboration is required to meet the needs of individuals (Karlsson et al., 2020).

There is no shortage of global health and social care organizations seeking to make an impact in the lives of others. However, there are many organizations working as independent entities to fulfill a narrow mission, resulting in wasted funds on administrative and infrastructure costs; in such cases, coordination could be advantageous (Bunger, 2013). For global organizations to cultivate innovation with limited resources, ongoing evaluation of the impact of programs and perhaps their subsequent retirement, organizational partnerships, and dedicated resources for innovation are necessary. As organizations struggle in times of economic downturn, the ability to properly balance and allocate investments in innovation could impact the organization's sustainability (Dutta et al., 2019).

Organizations must keep pace and be nimble in fulfilling their mission while maintaining trust with and value for influential stakeholders. Agile, influential leaders with skills in building trust, designing value-based organizations, promoting diversity, and advocacy should be highly valued within these organizations. It may be difficult to find and develop such leaders, as doing so requires time and resources some organizations may not be willing to invest (Vito, 2018). Global health and social care organizations have an opportunity to develop these types of leaders.

Advocacy is an essential skill for these leaders. Health and social care organizations are positioned to develop crucial advocacy skills in leaders. Health and social care leaders are often well versed in clinical and psychological human needs but may lack the skills to advocate for resources and policy changes within political or organizational networks (Ellenbecker et al., 2017).

Leadership development, although not linear in progression, can be fostered over time through such things as real or simulated experiences, educational opportunities, and mentorship. It is often difficult to measure the true impact of developing leaders (Crawford & Kelder, 2019). Organizations must create opportunities to propel the development of leaders. Funders must be open to innovative ideals and models to deliver this development; however, organizations need to cultivate innovative strategies to measure the impact.

Global organizations play a significant role in the current landscape of health and social care. To maintain relevance, effectiveness, and be good stewards of the resources entrusted to them, organizational leaders must examine endeavors through the lens of impact and innovation, asking themselves, "How can we do this better?" These questions are often propelled by outside forces that may include pandemics, disasters, or changes in political landscapes. Organizations may not get to decide when they are needed the most, but they can be nimble and equip the health and social care community to serve and advocate regardless of geographical, financial, or political barriers.

## SUMMARY POINTS

- Global organizations, through their diverse networks, can improve global health and social care by co-creating tangible solutions and agile ways to disseminate evidence.

## CONCLUSION

Health and social care leaders have ethical responsibilities and challenges in addressing the increasingly diverse patient population and workforce. As workforce diversity increases, additional support and training may be necessary. Leaders and managers should support educational opportunities, awareness, and practice implications regarding cultural sensitivity, communication, and delegation. Health and social care leaders of global organizations can enhance people's health through networking, co-creating, and evidence dissemination. Leaders will need to intentionally reflect on and strategize current practices and future opportunities to address the globalization of health and social care. However, strategy must be coupled with action.

## REFERENCES

Abe, J. (2020). Beyond cultural competence, toward social transformation: Liberation psychologies and the practice of cultural humility. *Journal of Social Work Education, 56*(4), 696–707. https://doi.org/10.1080/10437797.2019.1661911.

Alliance for Ethical Recruitment Practices. (2017). Health care code for ethical recruitment and employment practices. https://www.cgfnsalliance.org/wp-content/uploads/2019/03/Health-Care-Code-for-EIREP-Sept-2017_FINAL.pdf

Alvariza, A., Mjörnberg, M., & Goliath, I. (2020). Palliative care nurses' strategies when working in private homes—A photo-elicitation study. *Journal of Clinical Nursing, 29*(1-2), 139–151. https://doi.org/10.1111/jocn.15072.

Asiri, S. A., Rohrer, W. W., Al-Surimi, K., Da'ar, O. O., & Ahmed, A. (2016). The association of leadership styles and empowerment with nurses' organizational commitment in an acute health care setting: A cross-sectional study. *BMC Nursing, 15*(38), 38. https://doi.org/10.1186/s12912-016-0161-7.

Beagan, B. L. (2018). A critique of cultural competence: Assumptions, limitations, and alternatives. In C. Frisby & W. O'Donohue (Eds.), *Cultural competence in applied psychology*. Springer.

Bell, J., Kaats, E., & Opheij, W. (2013). Bridging disciplines in alliances and networks: In search for solutions for the managerial relevance gap. *International Journal of Strategic Business Alliances*, 3(1), 50–68. https://doi.org/10.1504/IJSBA.2013.058297.

Bhamra, S. K., Slater, A., Howard, C., Johnson, M., & Heinrich, M. (2017). The use of traditional herbal medicines amongst South Asian diasporic communities in the UK. *Phytotherapy Research: PTR*, 31(11), 1786–1794. https://doi.org/10.1002/ptr.5911.

Bunger, A. C. (2013). Administrative coordination in non-profit human service delivery networks: The role of competition and trust. *Nonprofit and Voluntary Sector Quarterly*, 42(6), 1155–1175. doi.org/10.1177/0899764012451369.

Cassagnol, J. (2017). *Partnerships among nonprofit organizations: Assessing the impact on global health*. Sigma Repository. https://sigma.nursingrepository.org/bitstream/handle/10755/621954/Cassagnol_83192_presentation.pdf?sequence=1&isAllowed=y.

CGFNS, (2019). *CGFNS presents refugee credential restoration project at Massachusetts Institute of Technology*. CGFNS International. https://www.cgfns.org/cgfns-restore-credentials-refugees-mit/#gs.vu88ix.

CGFNS, (2020). *Credentials evaluation service academic report*. CGFNS International. https://www.cgfns.org/services/credentials-evaluation/credentials-evaluation-service-academic-report/.

Cochran, C. (2017). Effectiveness and best practice of nurse residency programs: A literature review. *Medsurg Nursing*, 26(1), 53–57. 63.

Covey, S. R. (2004). *The 7 habits of highly effective people: Restoring the character ethic*. Free Press.

Crawford, J. A., & Kelder, J. -A. (2019). Do we measure leadership effectively? Articulating and evaluating scale development psychometrics for best practice. *The Leadership Quarterly*, 30(1), 133–144. https://doi.org/10.1016/j.leaqua.2018.07.001.

Derman, R. J., & Jaeger, F. J. (2018). Overcoming challenges to dissemination and implementation of research findings in under-resourced countries. *Reproductive Health*, 15(Suppl 1), 86. https://doi.org/10.1186/s12978-018-0538-z.

Doyle, M., & Timonen, V. (2009). The different faces of care work: Understanding the experiences of the multi-cultural care workforce. *Ageing and Society*, 29(3), 337–350.

Dutta, S., Lanvin, B., & Wunsch-Vincent, S. (2019). *The global innovation index (2019). Creating healthy lives—the future of medical innovation* ((12th ed)). Cornell. https://www.globalinnovationindex.org/gii-2019-report#.

Eastman, C., Charlesworth, S., & Hill, E. (2020). *Markets, migration & the work of care. Fact sheet 1: Migrant workers in frontline care*. UNSW. https://www.arts.unsw.edu.au/sites/default/files/documents/Migrant%20Workers%20in%20Frontline%20Care.pdf

Edmonson, C., McCarthy, C., Trent-Adams, S., McCain, C., & Marshall, J. (2017). Emerging global health issues: A nurse's role. *Online Journal of Issues in Nursing*, 22(1), 2. https://doi.org/10.3912/OJIN.Vol22No01Man02. manuscript.

Ellenbecker, C. H., Fawcett, J., Jones, E. J., Mahoney, D., Rowlands, B., & Waddell, A. (2017). A staged approach to educating nurses in health policy. *Policy, Politics and Nursing Practice*, 18(1), 44–56. https://doi.org/10.1177/1527154417709254.

Franklin, B., & Brancati, C. U. (2015). Moved to care: The impact of migration on the adult social care workforce. *Independent Age* https://independent-age-assets.s3.eu-west-1.amazonaws.com/s3fs-public/2016-05/IA%20Moved%20to%20care%20report_12%2011%2015.pdf.

Furtado, K. S., Brownson, C., Fershteyn, Z., Macchi, M., Eyler, A., Valko, C., & Brownson, R. C. (2018). Health departments with a commitment to health equity: A more skilled workforce and higher-quality collaborations. *Health Affairs (Project Hope)*, 37(1), 38–46. https://doi.org/10.1377/hlthaff.2017.1173.

Harkess, L., & Kaddoura, M. (2016). Culture and cultural competence in nursing education and practice: The state of the art. *Nursing Forum*, 51(3), 211–222. https://doi.org/10.1111/nuf.12140.

Hussein, S., Manthorpe, J., & Stevens, M. (2010). People in places: A qualitative exploration of recruitment agencies' perspectives on the employment of international social workers in the UK. *British Journal of Social Work*, 40(3), 1000–1016. https://doi.org/10.1093/bjsw/bcn131.

Hussein, S., Manthorpe, J., & Stevens, M. (2011). The experiences of migrant social work and social care practitioners in the UK: Findings from an online survey. *European Journal of Social Work*, 14(4), 479–496. https://doi.org/10.1080/13691457.2010.513962.

Jani, J. S., Osteen, P., & Shipe, S. (2016). Cultural competence and social work education: Moving toward assessment of practice behaviors. *Journal of Social Work Education*, 52(3), 311–324. https://doi.org/10.1080/10437797.2016.1174634.

Kanter, R. M. (1993). *Men and women of the corporation* (2nd ed.). Basic Books.

Kapucu, N., Yuldashev, F., & Feldheim, M. A. (2016). Nonprofit organizations in disaster response and management: A network analysis. *European Journal of Economic and Political Studies*, 4(1), 83–112. https://www.academia.edu/4164119/Nonprofit_Organizations_in_Disaster_Response_and_Management_A_Network_Analysis.

Karlsson, M., Garvare, R., Zingmark, K., & Nordström, B. (2020). Organizing for sustainable inter-organizational collaboration in health care processes. *Journal of Interprofessional Care*, 34(2), 241–250. https://doi.org/10.1080/13561820.2019.1638760.

King, E., Finkelstein, L., Thomas, C., & Corrington, A. (2019). Generational differences at work are small. Thinking they're big affects our behavior. *Harvard Business Review* https://hbr.org/2019/08/generational-differences-at-work-are-small-thinking-theyre-big-affects-our-behavior.

Kingma, M. (2006). *Nurses on the move: Migration and the global health economy*. Cornell University Press.

Kirmayer, L. J. (2012). Rethinking cultural competence. *Transcultural Psychiatry*, 49(2), 149–164. https://doi.org/10.1177/1363461512444673.

Kretzschmer, S., Walker, M., Myers, J., Vogt, K., Massouda, J., Gottbrath, D., ... Logsdon, M. C. (2017). Nursing empowerment, workplace environment, and job satisfaction in nurses employed in an academic health science center. *Journal for Nurses in Professional Development, 33*(4), 196–202. https://doi.org/10.1097/NND.0000000000000363.

Lisak, A., Erez, M., Sui, Y., & Lee, C. (2016). The positive role of global leaders in enhancing multicultural team innovation. *Journal of International Business Studies, 47*(6), 655–673. https://doi.org/10.1057/s41267-016-0002-7.

Loden, M., & Rosener, J. B. (1991). Workforce America! Managing employee diversity as a vital resource. *Business One Irwin, Homewood, IL.*

Mayo, A. T., & Woolley, A. W. (2016). Teamwork in health care: Maximizing collective intelligence via inclusive collaboration and open communication. *AMA Journal of Ethics, 18*(9), 933–940. https://doi.org/10.1001/journalofethics.2016.18.9.stas2-1609.

National Council of State Boards of Nursing. (2005). *Working with others: A position paper.* National Council of State Boards of Nursing. https://www.ncsbn.org/Working_with_Others.pdf.

Nursing and Midwifery Board of Ireland (NMBI). (2015). *Scope of nursing and midwifery practice framework.* Nursing and Midwifery Board of Ireland. https://www.nmbi.ie/Standards-Guidance/Scope-of-Practice/Considerations-in-Determining-Scope/Delegation-and-supervision.

Phillips, J. M., Stalter, A. M., Dolansky, M. A., & Lopez, G. M. (2016). Fostering future leadership in quality and safety in health care through systems thinking. *Journal of Professional Nursing, 32*(1), 15–24. https://doi.org/10.1016/j.profnurs.2015.06.003.

Porter-O'Grady, T., & Malloch, K. (2018). *Quantum leadership: Creating sustainable value in health care* (5th ed.). Jones and Bartlett Learning.

Premji, S. S., & Hatfield, J. (2016). Call to action for nurses/nursing. *BioMed Research International, 2016, article ID,* 3127543. https://doi.org/10.1155/2016/3127543.

Royal College of Nursing. (2017). *Accountability and delegation: A guide for the nursing team.* Royal College of Nursing. https://www.rcn.org.uk/professional-development/publications/pub-006465#detailTab.

Ruchman, S. G., Singh, P., & Stapleton, A. (2016). Why US health care should think globally. *AMA Journal of Ethics, 18*(7), 736–742. https://doi.org/10.1001/journalofethics.2016.18.7.msoc1-1607.

Shick, S., Adebambo, I., & Perzynski, A. (2019). Health disparities and social determinants of health. In A. Perzynski, S. Shick, & I. Adebambo I. (Eds.), *Health disparities.* Springer. ISBN 978-3-030-12771-8.

Sigma Theta Tau International. (2018). Global Advisory Panel on the Future of Nursing and Midwifery: Bridging the Gaps for Health. Report 22014-2017. Sigma Theta Tau International, Indianapolis. ISBN: 9781945157493.

Squires, A. (2018). Strategies for overcoming language barriers in healthcare. *Nursing Management, 49*(4), 20–27. https://doi.org/10.1097/01.NUMA.0000531166.24481.15.

Strandberg, C. (2017). *Maximizing the capacities of advanced education institutions to build social infrastructure for Canadian communities.* J. w McConnell Family Foundation. https://mcconnellfoundation.ca/wp-content/uploads/2017/08/Maximizing-Capacities-of-Advanced-Education-Institutions-to-Build-Social-Infrastructure.pdf.

The Global Advisory Panel on the Future of Nursing & Midwifery (GAPFON®) Report. (2017). Sigma Theta Tau International. https://sigma.nursingrepository.org/handle/10755/621599

United Nations. (2016). *In safety and dignity: Addressing large movements of refugees and migrants.* Report of the Secretary General. https://digitallibrary.un.org/record/828239?ln=en.

United Nations. (2019). *The number of international migrants reaches 272 million, continuing an upward trend in all world regions, says UN.* United Nations. https://www.un.org/development/desa/en/news/population/international-migrant-stock-2019.html.

University of Minnesota Department of Family Medicine and Community Health (University of Minnesota). (2020). *Patient centered assessment method.* University of Minnesota. https://med.umn.edu/familymedicine/research/faculty-research/pcam.

Viken, B., Solum, E. M., & Lyberg, A. (2018). Foreign educated nurses' work experiences and patient safety—A systematic review of qualitative studies. *Nursing Open, 5*(4), 455–468. https://doi.org/10.1002/nop2.146.

Vito, R. (2018). Leadership development in human services: Variations in agency training, organizational investment, participant satisfaction, and succession planning. *Human Service Organizations: Management, Leadership and Governance, 42*(3), 251–266. https://doi.org/10.1080/23303131.2017.1421284.

Wagner, E. A. (2018). Improving patient care outcomes through better delegation-communication between nurses and assistive personnel. *Journal of Nursing Care Quality, 33*(2), 187–193. https://doi.org/10.1097/NCQ.0000000000000282.

Ward, C., & Geeraert, N. (2016). Advancing acculturation theory and research: The acculturation process in its ecological context. *Current Opinion in Psychology, 8*, 98–104. https://doi.org/10.1016/j.copsyc.2015.09.021.

World Health Organization (WHO). (2010). *The WHO global code of practice on the international recruitment of health personnel.* World Health Organization. https://www.who.int/hrh/migration/code/code_en.pdf?ua=1.

World Health Organization (WHO). (2018). *The international platform on health worker mobility.* World Health Organization. https://www.who.int/hrh/migration/International-platform-HW-mobility.pdf?ua=1.

World Health Organization (WHO). (2020). *WHO global code of practice on the international recruitment of health personnel.* World Health Organization. https://apps.who.int/gb/ebwha/pdf_files/WHA73/A73_9-en.pdf.

Zallman, L., Finnegan, K. E., Himmelstein, D. U., Touw, S., & Woolhandler, S. (2019). Care for America's elderly and disabled people relies on immigrant labor. *Health Affairs, 38*(6), 919–926. https://doi.org/10.1377/hlthaff.2018.05514.

## REFLECTIVE QUESTIONS

- As a leader in a health or social care organization, what additional responsibilities does one have for determining and improving the team's cultural humility? How might this be achieved?
- For a leader in a health or social care organization that has a substantial immigrant workforce, what additional factors need to be considered? What strategies might you need to create a diverse workforce?
- When health or social care workers delegate tasks, what cultural aspects may come into play?

- In thinking about your work or future work site, are there specific global organizations you may want to consider joining or interacting with? If so, what do you hope to gain from these interactions?
- What gaps exist in your own leadership qualities or experiences? What ethical obligation do you have to continue your leadership development or the development of others?

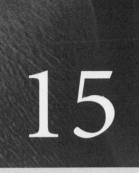

# 15

# FUTURE IMPLICATIONS FOR HEALTH AND SOCIAL CARE LEADERSHIP

CATE WOOD

## OBJECTIVES

*After reading this chapter, you should be able to:*

- Reinforce the current dynamic global context of health and social care leadership and management with a focus on integration.

- Understand why health and social care organizations need to invest in new types of leadership and management development.

- Explore the cultural values, characteristics, and skills required of future health and social care leaders.

- Discuss how interprofessional education can help prepare the next generation of integrated health and social care professionals.

- Revisit a selection of the attributes for leading and managing that were discussed in previous chapters.

- Reflect on the future global context of integration and leading in health and social care.

## INTRODUCTION

As witnessed in preceding chapters, in the dynamic world of health and social care—where epidemiological, demographic, and societal shifts are constantly evolving—successful organizations need both effective leadership and management. Economic, social, political and environmental changes combined with emerging technologies generate a complex global health agenda (Senkubuge et al., 2014). Definitions of leadership and management are surrounded by debate about their characteristics, style, and impact. John Kotter's often cited and now seminal interpretation presents the differences between leadership processes that involve setting a direction, aligning people, motivating, and inspiring and the processes of management that relate to organizational aspects such as planning, staffing, budgeting, controlling, and solving problems (Kotter, 1996). There is an anomaly in that not all managers are leaders, and some people lead without having management positions. Bass (2010) argues that despite the blurring of boundaries between management and leadership, the two activities are different. Leaders cope with new challenges and transform organizations, while managers maintain functional operations by using resources effectively. Current responses to change within health and social care organizations are a challenge for leaders and managers, requiring them to remain inspired, equipped, and supported in their roles. Their work must be dynamic to adapt and evolve to meet the needs of changing populations, embrace vital innovations, restructure for sustainability, and support increasingly integrated and personalized health and social care systems.

Global health and social care systems are moving toward a context of multiple professional group-working. Traditionally, groups are naturally located within different departments and specialties. Each group system has a unique set of complexities due to differing considerations imposed by disease specialties, multidisciplinary staff, and a variety of organizational directional goals. Inevitably, the interactions with each other and between groups in these complex environments are complicated. As an added intricacy, the variety of groups and their associated cultures and subcultures may be either supportive of or conflicting with each other. What type of leader will be needed to succeed in delivering this multi-professional integrated care? From a UK primary care perspective, Swanwick and Varnam (2019) describe a necessary shift from the traditional individualistic hierarchical leader who works within and for single teams to a collective leadership encouraging a compassionate and inclusive culture. De Meyer (2011) concurs with this view, advising that there is a need for responsible collaborative leadership that uses the skills of cooperation, listening, influencing, and flexible adaptation, a contrast to what he terms the traditional "command and control" top-down hierarchical approach. It is known that top-down approaches to leadership are the least effective ways of managing health and social care organizations, whereas inclusive and compassionate leadership helps create psychologically safe workplaces (Kline, 2019). Enabling staff to listen and support each other has been shown to result in fewer errors and staff injuries, less bullying and absenteeism, and reduced patient mortality (in hospitals) (Carter et al., 2008). However, "command and control" leadership is not extinct in all aspects of leading—for example, it can be necessary for surveillance, containment, treatment, and interventions for teams that manage infectious diseases, as well as for public health improvements, such as access to effective sanitation and clean water. In contrast, management of non-communicable diseases, which have increased globally, requires that multi-disciplinary professionals work collaboratively to provide an effective and seamless service (Calabretta, 2002). "Command and control" approaches would therefore not be appropriate in this environment. Similarly, prevention and control of accidents and injuries relies on collaborative work by even wider groups of people (beyond health and social care professionals) (Frenk et al., 2010). In broad terms, Britnell (2019) calls for transforming organizations from bureaucratic hierarchies to flat and agile learning organizations. In addition, he suggests that up to 36 percent of health care tasks will be automated by 2030, necessitating new teamworking and staff re-education that will be essential to face this digital upheaval.

Globally, health and social care providers are constantly tasked with many initiatives to keep pace with service demand, such as introducing new models of working and provision, designing new pathways of care, introducing a broader workforce, making greater use of technology, and encouraging peoples' ability for self-care while also working more closely with other teams and organizations (Ham et al., 2012). In this international high-pressure context, sustaining consistently high-quality organizational performance of health and social care services, irrespective of global differences, requires excellence in leadership and management. This chapter addresses how this may look, the leadership and managing skills required, and what educational underpinnings will support this, while reflecting on the content of previous chapters and looking toward the future.

## INTEGRATING AND RECONFIGURING THE WORKFORCE

Fragmentation, replication, and poor coordination encourage high-, middle-, and low-income countries to look to integrated care to tackle the universal financial and quality issues faced by health and social care providers (Goddard & Mason, 2017). Integrated care can be described as the combination of health and social care; acute and primary care; and mental health, learning disabilities, and intermediate care services. It is presented as a potential solution to some major challenges facing global health and social care systems (Kodner, 2009) and is promoted as the zeitgeist for future management. However, in the United Kingdom, a lack of success with these initiatives has been connected to gaps between policy and practice (Bussu & Marshall, 2018; Fulop et al., 2011; Lalani et al., 2019). Bussu and Marshall (2020) report that health and social care systems are often organized without aligning activities, resulting in disjointed care coordination and change that happens too fast. Goddard and Mason (2017) suggest that despite broad and shared understandings of the principles that underpin integrated care, there is wide variation in the implementation and details of the arrangements. Therefore, the reality of integrated systems often appears at odds with the philosophy.

Nevertheless, integrated care is known to offer several positive benefits, such as greater satisfaction and better experiences for professionals, patients, and their caregivers; more appropriate and enhanced preventive care; improved access; and fewer avoidable hospital and emergency admissions (Goddard & Mason, 2017). There is also evidence of wider benefits including prolonged independent living with delayed admission to institutional care, improved health status and quality of life, and enhanced cost effectiveness (Nolte & Pitchforth, 2014).

The literature suggests that when developing new partnerships, such as in integrated health and social care, individual relationship dynamics and control-based organizational forces are both essential (Valentijn et al., 2015). Creating an integrated workforce is complex and challenges the traditional and known ways of working while recognizing that the staff need to understand the benefits to embrace the change. When assisting with changes such as these, a manager's understanding of the organization's culture is said to be crucial (Carlström & Ekman, 2012). Busetto et al. (2016) summarize some workforce changes necessary for implementing integrated care, including new roles for leaders and managers; changes to professional roles; and different ways of working, such as using multi-disciplinary and team approaches to provide services. Multi-professional integration and collaboration necessitate new dimensions of leadership. Indeed, as professionals integrate across their traditional boundaries, leadership must also undergo a major shift and is viewed as part of a collective rather than an individual role (Folkman et al., 2019). Goddard and Mason (2017) report that the key elements for success and for integrated care to deliver its potential are alignment of vision, cultures across professional boundaries, and the degree of financial integration. Cameron et al. (2012) concur that shared financial arrangements facilitate and support integrated care.

## FUTURE LEADERSHIP FOR HEALTH AND SOCIAL CARE

A collaborative agenda will support international health and social care systems and delivery (Senkubuge et al., 2014), which are intended to improve quality, access equity, and service efficiency (Reich et al., 2016). Collaboration is not a new phenomenon, but leading change in systems, processes, and patterns of behavior for staff who are not normally used to working together is a new challenge. Building healthy communities across health and social care systems that incorporate integration and collaboration demands leadership that transitions from reactive approaches to those designed to improve lives in the longer term (Timmins, 2019).

Yammarino et al. (2012) describe collectivistic leadership as involving many individuals flexibly moving in and out of leadership roles over time, with both formal and informal relationships. This requires a new understanding of leadership and what it means to be a leader, encompassing being aware of collective identities, shared purpose, and altered attitudes toward power and change. Working in new environments across internal and external organizational boundaries with networks and teams collaborating and sharing resources to deliver innovative services for populations will progressively become the "new normal."

Collective leadership embodies and supports the collaborative agenda for the future design and delivery of health and social care. West (2014) advocates leadership as the responsibility of all instead of the few, with those having the necessary expertise taking leadership roles when appropriate, and everyone being accountable. Collective leadership is an emerging field, so there is no one definition. West and West (2015) posit it as shared leadership with a formal hierarchy, but where the power base shifts when needed to those with the required expertise. Leaders working together develop a shared culture of consistent leadership styles across the organization. There is an ethos of collaboration where leaders and staff unite through a common vision with associated improvements in team performance and staff engagement (Aime et al., 2014). The characteristics of collective leadership are based on collectives and are not individual, again diminishing the traditional top-down hierarchical models of leading and managing. The culture is one of cooperating and supporting each other across organizational boundaries with a common goal of delivering continually improving, high quality, inclusive, and compassionate care (West, 2014). The term compassionate care is explained as care that notices, feels, and responds to the suffering of others to endeavor to alleviate it (Dutton et al., 2006).

Within the context of the UK National Health Service (NHS), West and Bailey (2019) concur that all staff should consider themselves leaders. This reinforces the world view that regardless of the level of responsibility in an organization, all workers are encouraged at times to be collaborative leaders: everyone needs leadership skills. Indeed, there is capacity for all to be leaders in the new integrated and fluid world of health and social care, where teams develop through inter-team and cross-boundary working and are dispersed based upon need. The future health and social care leader characteristics comprise collaboration, flexible adaptation, listening, and influencing (Hardacre et al., 2011). Atchison and Bujak (2001) suggest that collaboration is a mutually beneficial relationship with clearly defined roles among many stakeholders to attain a common organizational goal. There is an ethos of individuals working together for mutual benefit, united by shared visions and values, to achieve outcomes that are bigger than individual efforts. Sharing knowledge and experiences and reducing organizational complexity through communication between various stakeholders assists these relationships (Lavis et al., 2005). In addition, Manion (2005) advises that understanding diverse cultures facilitates interdependency and integration among multiple parties. Evaluating collaborative leadership, Rouse (2013) reports that individuals are positively impacted by appreciating their interdependence and the opportunities offered for functional and organizational collaboration.

When reviewing the integration literature, Cameron et al. (2012) identify "teams" as a model of shared leadership that delivers a range of services within different organizational types and involves staff from health and social services. Second, they identify what they call "placement schemes," which offer an arrangement where staff from one agency are placed within another, for example, basing social care professionals within health settings and vice versa. Other examples of integration offered by Cameron et al. (2012) include structural integration, such as shared client assessments and other aspects of combined care management. However, they report that wide organizational, cultural, professional, and contextual issues can encourage or impede integration.

Drennan et al. (2005) describe the difficulties that occur when partnership organizations have a shared purpose but suggest that understanding each other's aims and objectives can assist with this. In addition, Regen et al. (2008) state that on a staff level, strong leadership contributes to people feeling more confident in new teams or roles. Integrity and trusting relationships are the foundations of strong leadership, which in turn facilitates everyone in an organization to reach their full potential. Strong leadership supports a responsive organization that communicates and cooperates well with all stakeholders to create solutions (Hardacre et al., 2011). As an example, in the United Kingdom, a flexible approach to organizing work in a specialist multi-agency team improved the responsiveness of the service, allowing the needs of older people with dementia to be met (Rothera et al., 2008). Communication is also highlighted as a factor in the success of shared initiatives. Not surprisingly, universal problems around information sharing, including lack of access to and incompatibility with information technology (IT) systems, hamper joint initiatives (Christiansen & Roberts, 2005; Regen et al., 2008).

## CULTURAL VALUES AND LEADERSHIP

As discussed, there is increasing acknowledgment that all professionals involved in health and social care provision can and will require leadership skills. How professionals lead is underpinned by cultural sensitivities; a style of leadership that may work in one culture (country or organizational) may fail in another. The behaviors and qualities of leaders are essential for enabling them to foster culturally sensitive and productive relationships with those they lead (West et al., 2017). Culture is multi-layered; some cultural codes are within countries while others can be integral within organizations and departments, adding extra levels of complexity to workplace integration and leading.

Global alliances and ventures, the economy, e-commerce, and technological innovation have the capacity to dissolve international boundaries, facilitating transformation of human relations and management of inter-cultural diversity. Despite globalization being thought of as universal with a common language, societal values, thoughts, and behaviors still have innate relevance in local, national, and international organizations. Global workforces, which often include people from diverse cultural backgrounds, enhance the need to recognize and manage diverse values, perceptions, worldviews, and behaviors of organizations, workforces, and the people they serve (Schneider & Barber, 2014). Intercultural communication and management can encompass and support cultural dimensions by influencing the interpretations, perceptions, and actions of those working in different departments within an organization (Saint-Jacques, 2011), facilitating management, communication, and effective interactions across borders.

Looking broadly to the cultures of countries, discrepancies can often originate due to different preferences, expectations, and culturally inherited values within a society. The Global Leadership and Organisational Behaviour Effectiveness (GLOBE) project founded by Robert House from the United States in 1991 is a longitudinal cross-cultural research study that examines leadership worldwide (GLOBE, 2020). Building on the findings of Hofstede (1980), Schwartz (1999), and Inglehart (1997), GLOBE has become a multi-phase, multi-method, multi-sample research project that was performed in 2004, 2007, and 2014; it examines the interrelationships between societal cultural values and practices, societal effectiveness, and organizational leadership. Measures of societal culture were initially identified and developed by researchers in 2004 during phase one of the GLOBE project, producing nine dimensions of societal culture. Several pilot studies measured cultural values and practices in different countries; 62 cultures (not necessarily country specific) were identified (House et al., 2004). They explored dimensions of cultural values and how cultures are similar or dissimilar in terms of their values. These "ways of being" or cultural values impact leadership and are important to recognize in a global arena. House et al. (2004) identify differences and similarities within norms, values, beliefs, and practices worldwide; understanding these are essential for managing and leading people and organizations. In the first dimension they outline performance orientation, referring to the amount of collective encouragement and reward given to group members for their performance and excellence. Secondly, is the extent to which individuals are assertive, confrontational, and aggressive in relationships with others. The third dimension assesses how much individuals participate in future-oriented behaviors such as planning, investing in the future, and delaying satisfaction. Fourthly, is the degree to which a collective encourages and rewards individuals, such as being fair, caring, and kind to others, they term this humane orientated leadership. The fifth dimension of institutional collectivism looks at the degree to which organizational and societal institutional practices support and reward the collective distribution of resources and actions. The degree to which individuals express pride, loyalty, and cohesiveness in their organizations is the sixth dimension of in-group collectivism. Gender egalitarianism is the seventh dimension, and is the attribute of the group minimizing gender differences. The extent to which the community accepts and endorses authority, power differences, and privileges of status is defined in the eighth dimension as a power distance. Finally, the ninth dimension expresses uncertainty avoidance, as how much a society, organization, or group relies on social norms, rules, and procedures to allay the unpredictability of future events. Uncertainty avoidance leads people to look for orderliness, consistency, structure, formal procedures, and laws as protection in their daily lives.

GLOBE's other major finding is that leader effectiveness is contextual and is embedded within the societal and organizational norms, values, and beliefs of the people being led. Put into cultural contexts, Lord and Maher's (1991) categorization theory suggests that through their socialization, everyone has an idea of what a leader looks like and how one behaves and acts. They advise that these ideas are built-in based on people's early experiences with leaders and are then shaped by both their culture and upbringing. These ideas form a baseline or barometer of what people gauge as good or poor leaders. GLOBE was the first study to investigate people's expectations of leaders on a broad scale and link them with cultural values and practices. They began with 112 leader characteristics, categorized them into 21 leadership scales, which were statistically and conceptually reduced to six global dimensions of leading.

The six global dimensions constitute the GLOBE notion of culturally endorsed leadership theory (CLT) and are defined in Box 15-1. These six global dimensions of leaders exemplify that cultural acceptance of styles is shown by specific behaviors. For example, leader characteristics such as being ambitious, enthusiastic, formal, logical, or a risk-taker are all valued differently around the world. A society's view of leadership risk-taking aligns with how much uncertainty a country tolerates (GLOBE 2020), but there are some leader characteristics that are universally accepted by all societies. People want leaders to be trustworthy, just, honest, and decisive, but how these characteristics are expressed and acted on may still vary across societies (GLOBE 2020).

**BOX 15-1**
## SIX GLOBAL DIMENSIONS OF CULTURALLY ENDORSED LEADERSHIP THEORY

1. **Charismatic/value-based leadership:** The ability to inspire, motivate, and expect high performance outcomes from others based on firmly held core values. It includes six primary leadership dimensions: (1) visionary, (2) inspirational, (3) self-sacrifice, (4) integrity, (5) decisive, and (6) performance oriented.

2. **Team-oriented leadership:** Team building and implementation of a common purpose or goal among team members. It includes five primary leadership dimensions: (1) collaborative team orientation, (2) team integrator, (3) diplomatic, (4) malevolent (reverse scored), and (5) administratively competent.

3. **Participative leadership:** The degree to which managers involve others in making and implementing decisions. It includes two primary leadership dimensions: (1) non-participative and (2) autocratic (both reverse scored).

4. **Humane-oriented leadership:** Supportive and considerate leadership includes compassion and generosity and it is patient, supportive, and concerned with the well-being of others. This dimension includes two primary leadership dimensions: (1) modesty and (2) humane orientation.

5. **Autonomous leadership:** Independent and individualistic leadership attributes, characterized by an independent, individualistic, and self-centric approach to leadership. It is measured by a single primary leadership dimension identified as autonomous leadership, consisting of individualism, independence, autonomy, and unique attributes.

6. **Self-protective leadership:** Ensuring the safety and security of the individual and the group through status enhancement; it includes five primary leadership elements: (1) self-centered, (2) status conscious, (3) conflict inducer, (4) face saver, and (5) procedural.

---

Global Leadership and Organisational Effectiveness (GLOBE). (2020). An overview of the 2004 study: Understanding the relationship between national culture, societal effectiveness and desirable leadership attributes.

Global health and social care organizations sit within their own societal backdrop of the six global dimensions of leadership GLOBE identified while also having unique organizational and professional cultures. Therefore, it is not surprising that integrating services is complex and difficult to achieve.

## ORGANIZATIONAL CULTURE AND COMPASSION

Looking to the cultures of organizations, Schneider and Barber (2014, p. 10) define them as "the values and beliefs that characterise organisations, as transmitted by socialisation processes that newcomers have, the decisions made by management, and the stories and myths people tell and retell about their organizations." The key to improving organizations is safeguarding cultures that work to implement, create, and support values that lead to a compassionate and inclusive leadership culture (King's Fund, 2020). The evidence for strong, shared vision and values as a foundation for high-quality care is clear; in the United Kingdom, Dixon-Woods et al. (2014) demonstrate that leaders at all levels in the highest-performing health care organizations championed high quality and compassionate care as a priority. They clearly articulated a vision of delivering high-quality care with explicit goals and a strategy to achieve them (value-based leadership of the GLOBE 6 dimensions). Returning to the need for collaborative and supportive cultures across organizational boundaries, common goals are paramount (West, 2014). Compassionate leadership is ensuring that everyone has a voice in the process of delivering and improving care, manifested in humility, which is stated as a key trait of many of the most effective leaders (participative leadership of the GLOBE 6 dimensions) (Ou et al., 2015).

de Zulueta (2016) offers a stark reminder that in many countries, there are concerns that modern health care has lost its ethical base and struggles to provide safe, timely, and compassionate care (humane-orientated leadership of the GLOBE 6 dimensions). Compassionate leadership creates conditions where the collective good is of greater importance than the need for status and individual agendas (West & Bailey, 2019). A compassionate culture can offer a new perception of what leadership is and what it means to be a leader. Decety and Fotopoulou (2015) support compassion and empathy as beneficial for patients' outcomes (including mortality) and satisfaction. The link between compassionate leadership and innovation is substantial (West et al., 2017). There is evidence that leaders' demonstrations of a commitment to high-quality compassionate care directly affect patient safety and experience; the health, well-being and engagement of staff; the extent of innovation; and clinical effectiveness. West and Bailey (2019) advise that compassionate leadership requires a large amount of courage and resilience, and a belief and commitment to be the best leader that you can be. They advocate self-compassion as the starting point for compassionate leadership, with a focus on yourself and an understanding of the challenges you face in your work and life, caring and helping yourself, and remaining close to core values that give meaning to life and work. The core values they suggest are compassion, wisdom, courage, and justice, which enable deeper, more authentic, and effective interactions between those who work together.

West et al. (2015) identify six key cultural elements for sustaining cultures of compassion: inspiring visions that are operationalized at all levels; clearly aligned objectives for individuals, teams, and departments; a high level of staff engagement; supportive and enabling people management; learning, innovation, and quality improvement all embedded in everyone's practice; and effective teamwork. Dixon-Woods et al. (2014) support this, articulating that leaders should focus on ensuring learning, innovation, quality improvement in the practice of all staff, and effective teamworking (team-oriented leadership of the GLOBE 6 dimensions). Indeed, how professionals work together effectively provides the foundation for quality care.

## TEAMWORK AND EDUCATING FOR COLLABORATION

The global demand for quality care necessitates that the corresponding professionals' development emphasize patient/client centered teamwork. However, in a UK health context, Dow et al.'s (2017, p. 677) research for evidence on interprofessional teams also found "networks of electronic collaboration among the healthcare professionals caring for each patient." They suggest a need to expand traditional ideas of interprofessional practice to include networking as an adjunct to traditional teamworking. Reeves et al. (2018) take interprofessional working a stage further by including collaboration and coordination (team-oriented leadership of the GLOBE 6 dimensions).

Reeves et al. (2010) review literature over a 30-year period and identify five common elements that define

the essence of teams: shared identity, clear roles/tasks/goals, interdependence of members, integration of work, and shared responsibility. They added team tasks (the predictability, urgency, and complexity of a team's actual work) as a sixth element. The six elements are placed on a continuum where a team can, for example, range from having a weak team identity to having a strong, shared team identity (Reeves et al., 2010). Kline (2019) indicates that teams are more effective and inclusive when they have a clear purpose, small numbers of agreed-upon team objectives, regular feedback, clear roles, good sharing of information, and a strong commitment to quality improvement and innovation. Taking a purely psychological perspective, Edmondson (1999) notes that creating an effective team is associated with the innate human need to belong in an environment where people feel safe.

The World Health Organization states that there is now enough evidence to support effective interprofessional learning (IPE) as a facilitator of collaborative practice (WHO, 2010). Teamwork can be supported, developed, and encouraged as a part of a professional's education. Internationally, IPE is recognized as vital for providing quality care and improving collaborative practice. Frenk et al. (2010) examine health professionals' education and conclude that attaining specific competencies must be defining attributes. For example, through education, students can acquire skills for collaboration such as teamworking, developing supportive relationships, role clarification, self-awareness, reflection, working across boundaries, interprofessional communication and teamwork, conflict resolution, and interpersonal skills. Dow et al. (2017) advise that "networking" as a distinct competency domain should be added to provide explicit opportunities for learners to engage with large ill-defined groups and equip them for reality. Staff can be brought together through education to teach the competency domains, enabling them to understand each other's worlds. Scragg (2006) advises that undertaking combined activities can help disciplines understand the potential of shared responsibility. In an educational sense, IPE reinforces collaborative competence; interactive learning methods encourage mutual understanding of each other's responsibilities and roles (Barr & Low, 2012). Placing the patient/service user at the center of care is also thought to encourage interprofessional working (Marshall & Gordon, 2005), allowing for experiential learning environments to promote collaboration across professions. Similarly, Santy et al. (2009) evaluate online case conferencing and note that working with different professional groups when providing care also facilitated interprofessional learning. A step further is to have interprofessional assessments, with individual professions setting outcomes for the achievement of competencies—assessed by professionals—other than their own. Integrated workforces can be supported through formal educational programs, and experiential learning also offers collaboration and leading skills that can be nurtured and embedded in future practice.

## ATTRIBUTES FOR LEADING AND MANAGING

Current thinking in the field of contemporary health and social care is presented by revisiting a selection of the attributes for leading and managing that were discussed in previous chapters. These thoughts are made accessible using the organization, team, and individual as themes, while recognizing that, in reality, each theme is interwoven, connected, and symbiotic.

### Organization

Organizations are not silos; all are impacted by global challenges within global societies, contributing to the need for dynamic health and social care systems and recognizing that despite differences, collectively, there are mutual challenges with potentially generalizable solutions. All countries have a political dimension behind their vision that impacts aspirations and influences leadership and management at all levels of health and social care provision. Whether rich or poorly resourced, health and social care systems must develop infrastructures (physical and digital) to enhance their services; successfully maintaining this requires investment, sustainable funding, ongoing education, and expertise. Integrating health and social care systems forms a part of this agenda. Many countries face the common challenge of how to control rising health and social care costs. Short-term measures can be used to improve the productivity of health care systems based on the resources allocated, and in the longer term, if sustained, the aim is to improve overall value

by increasing the health and well-being outcomes of populations.

### Groups and Teams

Teams, their leadership, and teamworking are complex, and yet are often cited as obvious solutions to configuring health and social care provision. Autonomous professionals are part of wider teams or groups of the same profession or those from allied disciplines, whether integrated or not. However, effective leadership is important for any team or group to function successfully. Effective team leaders enable members to understand the purpose and key roles of the team, clarify aims and values, and provide direction and vision. The days of "super heroes" as leaders are long past, with the move toward collective, collaborative approaches to leadership necessitated by the complexities of the evolving health and social care arena. With moves toward interdisciplinary working, both the leader and the team require multifaceted skills. Innovating and initiating new ways of working as well as of managing complex projects, and the changes they invoke, is demanding, in addition to the day-to-day provision of health and social care services to diverse populations.

### Individual

Globally, individual health and social care workers are the major cogs in the wheels of provision. With the shift away from the traditional individualistic hierarchical leader, all workers are encouraged to be leaders working with collective leadership responsibilities and encouraging a compassionate and inclusive culture. Individuals are now recognized as being part of a collective, and building resilient organizations is a prerequisite for ensuring stable health and social care workforces, as well as for the health and well-being of the individuals within them. There is a major need to develop resilience and manage self and risk. Supporting individuals by creating effective learning organizations and embedding the roles of coaching, mentoring, and reflective practice can facilitate success in this regard. If the common goals of health and social care systems can encourage nurturing the individual worker within an ethos of cooperation and support across organizational boundaries to enable delivery of continually improving, high-quality, inclusive, and compassionate care, the future is looking good.

## CONCLUSION

This chapter has raised culturally sensitive futures in integrating health and social care services within an ethos of compassion as a global approach to their leadership and management, while looking to the supportive practical knowledge of the authors of the preceding chapters. There is, however, an acknowledgment that the global playing field is not level; low- and middle-income countries have a completely different starting point than high-income countries. A major predicament for low- and middle-income countries in their human resources for health and social care is the availability of qualified workers (Nations General Assembly, 2015); their distribution, recruitment, and retention; performance/productivity; and quality of care (McPake et al., 2013). Chen et al. (2004) cite negative work environments, poor human resource regulatory and management systems, inadequate incentives (financial and non-financial), and insufficient capacity for education and training. There is an urgent call to address these global shortages and the poor distribution of the health and social care workforces (Kinfu et al., 2009). Effective health and social care delivery systems must have the right number and appropriate combination of workers, with the correct means and motivation to perform their roles (Anand & Bärnighausen, 2012).

The sustainable development goals (SDGs) for health and well-being outline large-scale global targets for disease reduction and health equity for 2030 (Nations General Assembly, 2015), including the provision of universal health coverage (UHC). Nevertheless, low- and middle-income countries continue to manage common infections, maternity-related health problems, and diseases of malnutrition that are no longer an issue in richer populations (Whitehead et al., 2001). Crisp (2010) reminds us of a shared responsibility, as health progress has not been distributed equitably across the globe. Health security is now challenged by new infections and behavioral and environmental threats compounded by demographic and epidemiological transitions (WHO, 2008).

The demand for and number and types of workers need to increase to meet global health and social goals and targets. Productivity in all countries can be enhanced by new configurations of skill mixes and integration across professional boundaries to enable fewer or more suitably qualified workers to provide the equivalent of the current level of services. Improved education, skill development, and institutional reform can also influence and reduce the shortage of workers predicted for 2030.

There is a global need for strong leadership and shared visions and values to underpin the provision of high-quality compassionate care. Leaders are a part of this vision with the suggestion that all health and social care workers need at times to be leaders. The six GLOBE culturally endorsed dimensions of leadership all have a place and need to be recognized as playing a part in the roles of future leaders in health and social care worldwide. Employing leader characteristics that are universally accepted in all societies in addition to nuanced culture-specific behaviors will assist in preparing culturally sensitive leaders and managers to sustain health and social care provision in the future.

## REFERENCES

Aime, F., Humphrey, S., DeRue, D. S., & Paul, J. B. (2014). The riddle of heterarchy: Power transitions in cross-functional teams. *Academy of Management Journal, 57*(2), 327–352.

Anand, S., & Bärnighausen, T. (2012). Health workers at the core of the health system: Framework and research issues. *Health Policy, 105*(2–3), 185–191.

Atchison, T. A., & Bujak, J. S. (2001). *Leading transformational change: The physician-executive partnership.* Health Administration Press.

Barr, H., & Low, H. (2012). Interprofessional education in pre-registration courses: A CAIPE guide for commissioners and regulators of education. *CAIPE.*

Bass, B. (2010). *The Bass handbook of leadership: Theory, research, and managerial applications.* Simon & Schuster.

Britnell, M. (2019). Human: Solving the global workforce crisis in health care. Nuffield Trust Guest Comment. https://www.nuffieldtrust.org.uk/news-item/human-solving-the-global-workforce-crisis-in-health-care

Busetto, L., Luijkx, K. G., Elissen, A. M. J., & Vrijhoef, H. J. M. (2016). Intervention types and outcomes of integrated care for diabetes mellitus type 2: A systematic review. *Journal of Evaluation in Clinical Practice, 22*(3), 299–310.

Bussu, S., & Marshall, M. (2018). *Organisational development towards integrated care: A comparative study of admission avoidance, discharge from hospital and end of life care pathways in Waltham Forest.* University College London. https://www.ucl.ac.uk/epidemiology-health-care/sites/iehc/files/newham_report.pdf

Bussu, S., & Marshall, M. (2020). Organisational development to support integrated care in East London: The perspective of clinicians and social workers on the ground. *Journal of Health Organization and Management, 34*(5), 603–619.

Calabretta, N. (2002). Consumer-driven, patient-centered health care in the age of electronic information. *Journal of the Medical Library Association, 90*(1), 32–37.

Cameron, A., Lart, R., Bostock, L., & Coomber, C. (2012). Factors that promote and hinder joint and integrated working between health and social care services. *Social Institute for Excellence*

Carlström, E. D., & Ekman, I. (2012). Organisational culture and change: Implementing person-centred care. *Journal of Health Organization and Management, 26*(2), 175–191.

Carter, M., West, M., & Dawson, J. (2008). Developing team-based working in NHS trusts. Report prepared for the Department of Health https://publications.aston.ac.uk/id/eprint/19330/1/Developing_team_based_working_in_NHS_trusts.pdf

Chen, L., Evans, T., Anand, S., Boufford, J. I., Brown, H., Chowdhury, M., … Fee, E. (2004). Human resources for health: Overcoming the crisis. *Lancet, 364*(9449), 1984–1990.

Christiansen, A., & Roberts, K. (2005). Integrating health and social care assessment and care management: Findings from a pilot project evaluation. *Primary Health Care Research and Development, 6*(3), 269–277.

Crisp, N. (2010). *Turning the world upside down: The search for global health in the 21st century*. Oxford University Press.

De Meyer, A. (2011). Collaborative leadership: New perspectives in leadership development. *European Business Review*, 35–40.

de Zulueta, P. C. (2016). Developing compassionate leadership in health care: An integrative review. *Journal of Healthcare Leadership, 8*, 1–10. https://www.ncbi.nlm.nih.gov/pmc/articles/PMC5741000/pdf/jhl-8-001.pdf.

Decety, J., & Fotopoulou, A. (2015). Why empathy has a beneficial impact on others in medicine: Unifying theories. *Frontiers in. Behavioral Neuroscience, 8*, 1–11.

Dixon-Woods, M., Baker, R., Charles, K., Dawson, J., Jerzembek, G., Martin, G., … West, M. (2014). Culture and behaviour in the English National Health Service: Overview of lessons from a large multimethod study. *BMJ Quality and Safety, 23*(2), 106–115.

Dow, A. W., Zhu, X., Sewell, D., Banas, C. A., Mishra, V., & Tu, S. P. (2017). Teamwork on the rocks: Rethinking interprofessional practice as networking. *Journal of Interprofessional Care, 31*(6), 677–678.

Drennan, V., Iliffe, S., Haworth, D., Tai, S. S., Lenihan, P., & Deave, T. (2005). The feasibility and acceptability of a specialist health and social care team for the promotion of health and independence in "at risk" older adults. *Health and Social Care in the Community, 13*(2), 136–144.

Dutton, J. E., Worline, M. C., Frost, P. J., & Lilius, J. (2006). Explaining compassion organizing. *Administrative Science Quarterly, 51*(1), 59–96.

Edmondson, A. (1999). Psychological safety and learning behavior in work teams. *Administrative Science Quarterly, 44*(2), 350–383.

Folkman, A. K., Tveit, B., & Sverdrup, S. (2019). Leadership in interprofessional collaboration in health care. *Journal of Multidisciplinary. Healthcare, 12*, 97–107.

Frenk, J., Chen, L., Bhutta, Z. A., Cohen, J., Crisp, N., Evans, T., … Zurayk, H. (2010). Health professionals for a new century: Transforming education to strengthen health systems in an interdependent world. *The Lancet, 376*(9756), 1923–1958.

Fulop, N., Walters, R., & Spurgeon, P. (2011). Implementing changes to hospital services: Factors influencing the process and 'results' of reconfiguration. *Health Policy, 104*(2), 128–135.

Global Leadership and Organisational Effectiveness (GLOBE). (2020). *An overview of the 2004 study: Understanding the Relationship between national culture, societal effectiveness and desirable leadership attributes*. https://globeproject.com/study_2004_2007

Goddard, M., & Mason, A. R. (2017). Integrated care: A pill for all ills? *International Journal of Health Policy and Management, 6*(1), 1–3.

Ham, C., Dixon, A., & Brooke, B. (2012). Transforming the delivery of health and social care. *The Kings Fund* https://www.kingsfund.org.uk/sites/default/files/field/field_publication_file/transforming-the-delivery-of-health-and-social-care-the-kings-fund-sep-2012.pdf.

Hardacre, J., Cragg, R., Shapiro, J., Spurgeon, P., & Flanagan, H. (2011). What's leadership got to do with it? Exploring links between quality improvement and leadership in the NHS. *The Health Foundation* https://www.health.org.uk/sites/default/files/WhatsLeadershipGotToDoWithIt.pdf.

Hofstede, G. H. (1980). *Culture's consequences: International differences in work-related values*. Sage.

House, R. J., Hanges, P. J., Javidan, M., Dorfman, P. W., & Gupta, V. (Eds.), (2004). *Culture, leadership, and organizations: The GLOBE study of 62 societies*. Sage Publications.

Inglehart, R. (1997). *Modernization and post-modernization: Cultural, economic, and political change in 43 societies*. Princeton University Press.

Kinfu, Y., Dal Poz, M. R. D., Mercer, H., & Evans, D. B. (2009). The health worker shortage in Africa: Are enough physicians and nurses being trained? *Bulletin of the World Health Organization, 87*(3), 225–230.

King's Fund. (2020). Improving NHS culture. https://www.kingsfund.org.uk/projects/culture

Kline, R. (2019). Leadership on the NHS. *BMJ Leader*, 1–4. https://bmjleader.bmj.com/content/leader/early/2019/12/05/leader-2019-000159.full.pdf.

Kodner, D. L. (2009). All together now: A conceptual exploration of integrated care. *Healthcare Quarterly, 13*, 6–15.

Kotter, J. P. (1996). *Leading change*. Harvard Business School Press.

Lalani, M., Fernandes, J., Fradgley, R., Ogunsola, C., & Marshall, M. (2019). Transforming community nursing services in the UK: Lessons from a participatory evaluation of the implementation of a new community nursing model in East London based on the principles of the Dutch Buurtzorg model. *BMC Health Services Research* https://bmchealthservres.biomedcentral.com/articles/10.1186/s12913-019-4804-8.

Lavis, J. N., Davies, H. T., Oxman, A., Denis, J. L., Golden-Biddle, K., & Ferlie, E. (2005). Towards systematic reviews that inform health care management and policymaking. *Journal of Health Services Research and Policy, 10*(Suppl 1), 35–48.

Lord, R. G., & Maher, K. J. (1991). *People and organizations, Vol. 1. Leadership and information processing: Linking perceptions and performance*. Unwin Hyman.

Manion, J. (2005). *From management to leadership: Practical strategies for healthcare leaders* (2nd ed.). Jossey-Bass.

Marshall, M., & Gordon, F. (2005). Interprofessional mentorship: taking on the challenge. *Journal of Integrated Care*, *13*(2), 38–43.

McPake, B., Maeda, A., Araújo, E. C., Lemiere, C., El Maghraby, A., & Cometto, G. (2013). Why do health labour market forces matter? *Bulletin of the World Health Organization*, *91*(11), 841–846.

Nolte, E., & Pitchforth, E. (2014). What is the evidence on the economic impacts of integrated care? WHO Regional Office for Europe on behalf of the European Observatory on Health Systems and Policies

Ou, A. Y., Waldman, D. A., & Peterson, S. J. (2015). Do humble CEOs matter? An examination of CEO humility and firm outcomes. *Journal of Management*, *44*(3), 1147–1173. https://create-value.org/wp-content/uploads/Do-Humble-CEOs-Matter.pdf.

Reeves, S., Lewin, S., Espin, S., & Zwarenstein, M. (2010). Interprofessional teamwork for health and social care. *Blackwell-Wiley*

Reeves, S., Xyrichis, A., & Zwarenstein, M. (2018). Teamwork, collaboration, coordination, and networking: Why we need to distinguish between different types of interprofessional practice. *Journal of Interprofessional Care*, *32*(1), 1–3.

Regen, E., Martin, G., Glasby, J., Hewitt, G., Nancarrow, S., & Parker, H. (2008). Challenges, benefits and weaknesses of intermediate care: Results from five UK case study sites. *Health and Social Care in the Community*, *16*(6), 629–637.

Reich, M. R., Harris, J., Ikegami, N., Maeda, A., Cashin, C., Araujo, E. C., ... Evans, T. G. (2016). Moving towards universal health coverage: Lessons from 11 country studies. *Lancet*, *387*(10020), 811–816.

Rothera, I., Jones, R., Harwood, R., Avery, A. J., Fisher, K., James, V., ... Waite, J. (2008). An evaluation of a specialist multiagency home support service for older people with dementia using qualitative methods. *International Journal of Geriatric Psychiatry*, *23*(1), 65–72.

Rouse, J. (2013). Nef consulting. Leadership for Empowered and Healthy Communities Programme Evaluation.

Saint-Jacques. B. (2011). Intercultural communication in a globalized world. In L. A. Samovar, R. E. Porter, & E. R. McDaniel (Eds.), *Intercultural communication: A reader* (13th ed., pp. 45–53). Cengage Learning.

Santy, J., Beadle, M., & Needham, Y. (2009). Using an online case conference to facilitate interprofessional learning. *Nurse Education in Practice*, *9*(6), 383–387.

Schneider, B., & Barber, K. M. (2014). Introduction: The oxford handbook of organisational climate and culture. In B. Schneider & K. M. Barber (Eds.), *The Oxford handbook of organisational climate and culture* (pp. 3–20). Oxford University Press.

Schwartz, S. H. (1999). A theory of cultural values and some implications for work. *Applied Psychology*, *48*(1), 23–47.

Scragg, T. (2006). An evaluation of integrated team management. *Journal of Integrated Care*, *14*(3), 39–48.

Senkubuge, F., Modisenyane, M., & Bishaw, T. (2014). Strengthening health systems by health sector reforms. *Global Health Action*, *7*(1), 23568.

Swanwick, T., & Varnam, R. (2019). Leadership development and primary care. *BMJ Leader*, *3*, 59–61.

Timmins, N. (2019). *Leading for integrated care: "If you think competition is hard, you should try collaboration"*. The King's Fund.

United Nations General Assembly. (2015). Transforming our world: The 2030 agenda for sustainable development. http://www.un.org/ga/search/view_doc.asp?symbol=A/70/L.1&Lang=E

Valentijn, P., Vrijhoef, H. J. M., Ruwaard, D., de Bont, A., Arends, R., & Bruijnzeels, M. A. (2015). Exploring the success of an integrated primary care partnership: A longitudinal study of collaboration processes. *BMC Health Services Research*, *15*, 32.

West, M. (2014). *Collective leadership: Fundamental to creating the cultures we need in the NHS*. King's Fund blog. https://www.kingsfund.org.uk/blog/2014/05/collective-leadership-fundamental-creating-cultures-we-need-nhs.

West, M., & Bailey, S. (2019). Five myths of compassionate leadership. King's Fund blog. https://www.kingsfund.org.uk/blog/2019/05/five-myths-compassionate-leadership

West, M., & West, T. (2015). Leadership in healthcare: A review of the evidence. *Health Management*, *15*, 123–125.

West, M., Armit, K., Loewenthal, L., West, T., & Lee, A. (2015). *Leadership and leadership development in health care: The evidence base*. The Faculty of Medical Leadership and Management, The King's Fund; The Center for Creative Leadership.

West, M., Eckert, R., & Collins, R. (2017). *Caring to change. How compassionate leadership can stimulate innovation in health care*. Kings Fund. https://www.kingsfund.org.uk/sites/default/files/field/field_publication_file/Caring_to_change_Kings_Fund_May_2017.pdf.

Whitehead, M., Dahlgren, G., & Evans, T. (2001). Equity and health sector reforms: Can low-income countries escape the medical poverty trap? *Lancet*, *358*(9284), 833–836.

WHO. (2008). Commission on social determinants of health. Closing the gap in a generation: Health equity through action on the social determinants of health. https://www.who.int/social_determinants/thecommission/finalreport/en/

WHO. (2010). Framework for action on interprofessional education and collaborative practice. https://www.who.int/hrh/resources/framework_action/en/

Yammarino, F. J., Salas, E., Serban, A., Shirreffs, K., & Shuffler, M. L. (2012). Collectivistic leadership approaches: Putting the 'we' in leadership science and practice. *Industrial and Organizational Psychology*, *5*(4), 382–402.

# INDEX

Page numbers followed by "*b*", "*f*" and "*t*" indicate boxes, figures and tables respectively.